Activate Your Super-Human Potential

"Offering one of the most powerful healing systems on the planet, Jerry is the real deal, a true and gifted healer and an amazing teacher. I have used Jerry's tools in my medical practice and the results are fast, lasting, and truly breathtaking."
— SHAWN K. CENTERS, M.D.(H), D.O., FACOP, professor of pediatrics and integrative medicine, director of medical education for AutismOne, and chief medical officer at Children's HOPE Center, Arizona

"I have witnessed cases like paralysis, where the brain cells are killed, resulting in loss of messages between muscles and nerves, damaging the nervous system and stopping it from coming back to life. The holographic healing available with the tools from *Activate Your Super-Human Potential* enables the revival of cells. Being a doctor, I can bring this work into the medical world."
— VANDANA RANNJJIT ASHAR, B.H.M.S. (Homeopathic Medical Science), Access Body Process facilitator and energy healer

"This new, surprising, and sophisticated healing system introduces us to powerful practical tools that support the full functioning of our DNA. It's a fast-paced and intriguing read, full of real human stories; advice on darkness, light, and love; details of sacred geometry, metaphysics, and mathematics; and transformational exercises of information, code, and frequency. Get ready, with love and discipline, to accelerate your personal evolution and contribute to planetary evolution."
— JULIA PAULETTE HOLLENBERY, therapist, speaker, teacher, and author of *The Healing Power of Pleasure*

T0265701

ACTIVATE YOUR
SUPER-HUMAN
POTENTIAL

The Ultimate 5D Toolkit

JERRY SARGEANT

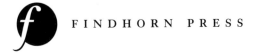

FINDHORN PRESS

Findhorn Press
One Park Street
Rochester, Vermont 05767
www.findhornpress.com

Findhorn Press is a division of Inner Traditions International

Disclaimer

The information in this book is given in good faith and is neither intended to diagnose any physical or mental condition nor to serve as a substitute for informed medical advice or care. Please contact your health professional for medical advice and treatment. Neither author nor publisher can be held liable by any person for any loss or damage whatsoever which may arise from the use of this book or any of the information therein.

Cataloging-in-Publication data for this title is available from the Library of Congress

ISBN 978-1-64411-529-9 (print)
ISBN 978-1-64411-530-5 (ebook)

Printed and bound in India by Nutech Print Services

10 9 8 7 6 5 4 3 2

Edited by Jacqui Lewis
Illustrations by Jerry Sargeant
Text design and layout by Damian Keenan
This book was typeset in Calluna Sans, Calluna with ITC Century Book Condensed
used as a display typeface.

To send correspondence to the author of this book, mail a first-class letter to the author
c/o Inner Traditions • Bear & Company, One Park Street, Rochester, VT 05767, USA, and we will
forward the communication, or contact the author directly at www.starmagichealing.com.

Contents

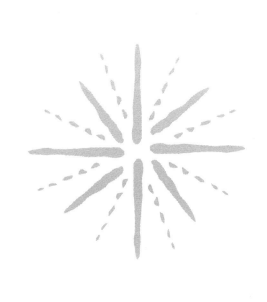

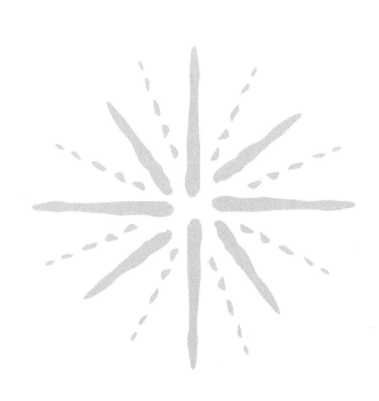

The Beginning:
How I Came into This World

It was the early hours of the morning on 8 March 1978. My birth mother was in a mother and baby home for women who were to give birth in secret, without their parents knowing. It was frowned upon back then to be pregnant out of wedlock, so she dared not tell anyone. At 2.50 a.m. my birth mother was taken into a room and left there in pain, with no medication for thirteen (an important number we will discuss later) hours. No one came to see her, no one came to comfort her or even check on her. She was left, in pain, wondering.

Just before 3.50 p.m., when I was born (the numerology of which adds up to eight, an extremely significant number in my life. And it's all about numbers), two men in black masks walked into the room, accompanied by a woman. They said nothing. They parted my mother's legs, got a huge pair of scissors, cut her vagina, reached in and ripped me out, cut the umbilical cord (something that should never be done because the child is still downloading cosmic code/information from the stars). I was taken into another room and left on a table. My mother was left bleeding, crying, and screaming in pain. They would not let her see me or touch me, and she never did until I found her twenty-six years later.

They left her for hours. She's not exactly sure how long as she was phasing in and out of consciousness with the pain and trauma and loss of blood. They came back in at some point and stitched her up. My mother was given no pain medication while she was in labour, before she was cut with the scissors or before she was stitched back up. I was left in the room on the table crying for some time. This was heavily traumatic for my mother, as it was for me. There was no bond, no love, just pure evil and massive predetermined trauma being created. A week later I was taken to my first foster-parents. I can even remember being in the arms of the woman, looking at the old burgundy/brown car pulling away from the drive after I was dropped off. I was a newborn baby, but the memory is so vivid. Soon after arriving I was raped. I only had the memory recall when I was much older.

At several months old I was adopted. My adopted mother used to bend me over the bed, pull down my pants and hit me with a wooden ruler three times, every time I did something that was bad in her eyes.

I remember going to school at five years of age. My first schoolteacher, Mrs Heskins, stood me on a chair in front of the whole class, pulled down my pants and smacked my arse.

I started life with a healthy dislike for the opposite sex. Women rejected, abandoned, raped, and beat me. I started life as an angry child who felt trapped. I am not sharing this story so you can feel sorry for me. I am sharing this because for me to succeed in this life, I have had to face my greatest trauma head-on: rejection. I was an insecure little boy, with big ears and darker skin, who got teased at school and was always in trouble for fighting. I felt like I didn't belong and for me to fulfil my life mission I had to face this fear and crush it, so I could come out into the public eye and share Star Magic with the world. The game of life is rigged. The game of life is designed in such a way that if you want to flourish and thrive you will have to crush and heal your biggest trauma to make it happen. No one can do this for you. This one is on you. The tools in this book will ensure that you crush and heal your biggest traumas and succeed.

If you have already done that, then these tools will take you to the next level and beyond. You will soon realize that the staircase of levels never ends, perfection is unattainable, and the envelope of your potential is greater than you could ever possibly imagine or dream of.

Introduction

So here we are at the start of another book. In this case we will start at the end, as consciousness floating in the ever-expansive darkness, the abyss of nature, the void, the womb of life, the empty space in which physical life forms were birthed from a shift in the vibratory rate of the universal field, when consciousness itself got curious and started the expansion process.

This spiritual journey is not an easy ride. It's a perilous journey for brave souls that know deep within that there is so much more. The most challenging encounters await the brave spiritual warrior who knows that love and light are mere signposts, guiding her or him towards their own divine and inherent natural power, an ancient wisdom that lies within the hearts of all women and men on Planet Earth.

I see so many people teetering on the edges of this infinite yet finite journey of the soul. Love and light is all that they preach and teach and in doing so they only ever make it to the edge of the cliff face. Hanging around staring at the views, soaking up the breathtaking beauty as they watch the sun rise and set; but little do they realize that the cliff face is the tip of the iceberg. Underneath the tip of this iceberg lies a gigantic mountain, riddled with mystery, and the only way to solve this mystery is through experience.

One must reach the edge of the cliff and jump into the void and trust that one's wings will grow on the way down. Beyond the masquerade of love and light, and all things fuzzy and warm, lies darkness, and beyond the darkness is sound, vibration, what we are at the core of our beings. It is so easy to pretend that love and light are all that there is and that the woman or man in question is good, caring, full of love and here to help the planet and its people move through the ascension process to bask in the so-called Golden Age of Enlightenment.

While this new dawn of enlightenment is certainly upon us, unfolding around us as I write, we must be aware of our spiritual ego, fighting tooth and nail as this last line of defence sets out its market stall to sell us all kinds of cheap and flattering gifts. Gifts such as "I must not shout or scream or be angry. I must always smile and be loving towards everyone. I must not think these thoughts towards another human being, they are not nice. She or he is bad because . . . And are not spiritual because . . . I'm spiritual so I must behave like this or not behave like that. I am supposed to be this or that. Judgement, blame, attack or defend . . ."

The list goes on . . .

The most treacherous space to enter is that of the loving, kind, considerate, planet-loving human who cares about everyone and everything else, pretending that this is who they are. Their spiritual ego goes into overdrive to keep them from looking in the most important place, within. Love, light, kindness is used as a heavy, powerless mask, worn to cover up the inner pain, that lies within the darkness of the woman or man in question. Their lack of self-worth torments them and to face such pain is tough. So, they stay in relationships, pretending all is OK, being directed by their spiritual ego, playing in the illusory light that hovers like gentle mist down country lanes in the morning. This powerless mask will not hold its own when the pain swells inside of the mind, body and spirit and these waters become icy-cold, forcing the human being to get out or freeze in their own misery and pain.

Sometimes the pain is where you must be. Often it is the foundation of your success, your brilliance, your truth. People often get out of the icy water and run. Those who stay start to understand something about themselves. Your sword of excellence strengthens as you dive into your trauma, face it, and heal. Much like a sword is beaten in extreme heat, the sword of excellence and success is forged in the inner cavern of your pain.

Within every human being there is the capacity to love, to hate, care, share, swear, steal, and even kill another human being. Somewhere deep in all of us lies the potential to make a decision to do something that we, as a human race, consider wrong. It's important at this stage that we accept there is no right or wrong, good or bad. They are forms of judgement and they only cause inner pain. We must, as a species, relinquish all forms of judgement, realize we are playing a spiritual game and see all things as experiences, releasing each experience in the moment, back into the eternal now.

Now is the greatest healer. Time itself is our greatest enemy. As we discuss the past, or try and plan, or worry about the future, we become disconnected from the present moment and lose our connection to the original information that is always streaming into our being.

This book is about you becoming all of you. You realizing that there is more to you than meets the eye. That beyond your physicalness, you are vibration or frequency, and that somewhere between the vibration or frequency at your empty but very rich core, and the physical being you see in the mirror every

morning, there are many layers that must be honoured, accepted, loved, and brought to the surface to be merged into the wholeness of who you are. I want you and every human being on Planet Earth to know themselves at the deepest possible level and in doing so, unleash their full Super-Human potential. Only by accepting all of you will you connect with this power.

I am going to share things with you in this book that you may well be hearing, seeing, feeling for the first time (in this reality anyway), so remain in your heart as you read on. The ego will not understand, the left brain will not compute, so you must feel this information and then embrace or disregard it. Your heart will guide you, so be still, pay attention, feel, and listen.

If you want to know the truth you must be prepared to live, experience, and embrace all facets of your inner world with open arms, a smile, and a grateful attitude towards every opportunity presented, for you to go deeper and deeper into your own heart to turn the key that will open the door of knowledge and wisdom and to be ready to face what guards this wisdom.

It will be worth fighting for. I know. I have opened the door, embraced the darkness, the demons that lurked there, fought the inner battle for my own soul, my consciousness, and lived to share the tale. So, too can you fight this battle and win. It won't be easy. Nothing ever worth fighting for is. What I do know is that this battle I speak of is a battle of will, fought on the spiritual planes of existence, down in the labyrinth of your powerful heart and the deep mines of your own fragmented soul, which you will, as you embark on this adventure with me, know how to piece seamlessly back together again.

You are the most extraordinary being on this planet and you have it all. There is nothing that you are not. You are it all. You are sound and light manifested into human form and within every cell of your being lies multiple universes.

Every star in the night's sky flows through your veins. Every tree, flower and plant is nourished by your thoughts and emotions. Every whale, dolphin, and shark swims in the ocean of bliss you call your heart.

I am going to guide you on an inner journey to "innerstand" you on a level of feeling, vibration, like an insect who communicates with another insect. No words are needed and yet everything is perfectly understood. The right brain and the heart will be your greatest allies. I will speak my truth; so many people find this difficult, but I know there is no other way to create freedom. I will share with you powerful healing ways (light technology I call Star Magic) that you will be able to use to accelerate the process and delve deeper into your own being, or use it to assist others, clients or friends, in their own spiritual awakening.

I am going to share ways of being that merge the mental, physical, emotional, and spiritual planes together, merging science and spirituality. I am a relentless savage who seeks out discomfort as discomfort is where the magic happens, the growth occurs, and the Super-Human is developed. I am not here on this planet to be average, mediocre, and neither should you be. You were blessed with gifts and the world is waiting to be inspired by them. Together we will embark on this process that will reactivate your soul code and activate and amplify the code of the heart.

Teamwork is mission critical on Planet Earth right now. An expanding of consciousness and an increase in frequency is naturally bringing aware people together, while those not seeing, locked in the illusion, continue to be manipulated and used as a food source by malevolent beings who know how to infiltrate the consciousness of those on a lower vibration. We will discuss this subject in more detail later on and I will share with you how to stop this happening to you. In turn you can share with those who are ready to to listen and thus support their raise of consciousness.

I spent years trying to sell sand to the Arabs, sharing my ideas, new-found philosophical ways, with everyone, whether it be ways to self-heal, my experiences with lower and higher vibrational beings, discoveries I had made about the corruption within the police force, the government, or the pharmaceutical industry. I soon realized that most people were not ready to hear the truth. It's easier for them to bury their head in the ground and pretend it's all OK. People want an easy life; let's face it, don't most of us? I don't, and neither should you, because there is no growth in easy. When the future of our planet and the potential chaos our children and our children's children may grow up living in bites at your ankles, it must be stamped out. It mustn't be eliminated through force, however. Love and compassion are the keys. With that said, your inner warrior must also be ignited, switched on, because we are in a spiritual war.

Love and compassion are only powerful once the individual has cracked the code and opened their own inner shell. Love and compassion can be façades, and dangerous ones to say the least if the human being in question has not done the inner work, glided through the light, opened themselves up, dived inside their own consciousness to bathe in the darker aspects of their consciousness, accepted all of who they are and then merged the dark and light aspects of their being together in perfect equilibrium. This is the only way to harness your power, to unleash your inner wisdom and be the mighty force of nature that you are. A master of dark and light. The ultimate spiritual warrior. A Super-Human.

I am going to offer you a way of being in this world and if you decide to adopt this all-encompassing approach to life, you will develop, grow, and expand aspects of your own inner world in such an incredible fashion that you will become an architect of your own physical reality. Once you remember these deep-rooted inner knowings, your life will breathe new information which will set you free to step fully into your power and be a Super-Human.

I am going to share some stories with you at the start of this book. Firstly, to give you some insight into my journey, and secondly to give you a glimpse into a life where magic and miracles have become second nature. You may need to keep an open heart and mind, because some of the stories I share are the kind you would see in a movie. I would like you to know that there was a time when I did not believe in anything spiritual. I had never heard of energy healing – and if I had, way back then, I would have dismissed it as nonsense. I thought that God and the universe, extra-terrestrials, angels or any other being or spirit or anything remotely associated, was complete garbage. I was, at one stage of my life, a criminal, smuggling drugs and other "interesting" commodities for business, as well as committing high-level bank fraud. An ego-driven maniac who only wanted material gains and to feed and support my false identity.

This book will open you up to a whole new world, furnish you with a way of being that will completely turbocharge your life, should you choose to adopt this new lifestyle. And let's be completely honest from the start: it is a lifestyle. You cannot dip in and out of discipline, achievement, success, love, motivation, unity, courage, action, determination, passion, enthusiasm. These ingredients are qualities that must become your spinal column. Let them be your medicine, until they flow from your soul as the elixir of life. You must harness them, encourage them, nurture them, and become them. You can read this book and go back to your old ways, habits, and beliefs; or maybe I will inspire you to take action, to think, feel, and act differently, to put these powerful ways of being (not ideas but ways) into practice and radically transform your life in a universally positive way.

If I can transform my life in the way I have, so can you. It doesn't matter what level in the game you are at (or think you are at), there is always another level. It's important to keep growing, diving deeper into your cosmic heart, and expanding, and what I share with you in the following pages will give you an infinite number of opportunities to accelerate and elevate your life on Earth in the most incredible, harmonious, and intelligent heart-centred way, where you step fully into your divine feminine and divine masculine balance and connect with that gateway of equilibrium, so courage, compassion, and authentic leadership of your own spirit flows from every cell and atom in your physical body and every bio-photon of light within your light body, as you exuberate a cascade of geometrical, spiralized code that fuels your life and gives you the tools to be the quantum architect of your own reality. A true Super-Human!

Do you want to be the big fish in the small pond or the small fish in the ocean, swimming with the sharks? This is an important question.

If it's the latter, carry on reading. If it's the former, put this book down and go read a book that's going to support your choices that take you down the easy road.

To truly grow and expand you must be willing to play in the ocean, getting small chunks torn out of you by the sharks. This is life. You must be willing to push through when it hurts, stay focused and undistracted among life's distractions, choose love not fear when your soul is under attack and stay on the path, swimming among the titans of the ocean, as you grow. Until one day you realize that every shark in the ocean is paying you respect; they are moving out of your way when you swim past, no longer taking bites out of the small fish because the small fish has not only become a shark but has grown even larger, understood the power of alchemy and become the entire ocean.

One thing you must accept before you go any further is death. I am going to take you on a journey, and you will die. This current version of you will, anyway. Also, the version after that and the one that comes after that one. You are going to die and be reborn, like a snake shedding its skin, over and over. It may be uncomfortable, but you will become the most extraordinary version of you. This I promise you. I have seen thousands of people change in our workshops and trainings and through our online events, simply by applying the positive protocols I share. You can start using the tools as you move through this book, or you can wait until the end, where I share with you a plan of how to best make use of these life-changing ways. Or you can work through the tools as you discover them (practising as you continue to read) and then apply the plan I share at the end, or create your own plan based on how you feel and what works best for you as a unique soul. You will discover your own way with these tools.

Many people of Earth talk about ascension. For one to truly ascend they must activate their DNA, their original twelve-strand blueprint, and be able to run enough frequency through the body so they can move through the planetary and universal Star Gate system and exit this matrix. (Star Gates are doorways for interdimensional and multidimensional travel.) This is real ascension. The tools in this book will enable you to activate your DNA and run the necessary light/frequency from the stars into your body and make it compatible to move through the Star Gates.

This is the start of something extraordinary. You're a part of the Super-Human Revolution unfolding on Planet Earth right now. Are you ready? Are you focused? I am going to show you the power that lies within your dormant DNA structure and share the precision tools that will ignite this formidable power, once and for all. It's time, beautiful soul. My sister, my brother, fellow warrior of both dark and light . . . let's do this!

PART 1

Preparing the Vessel

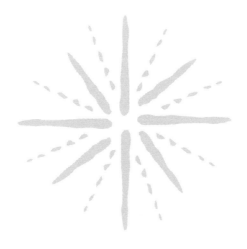

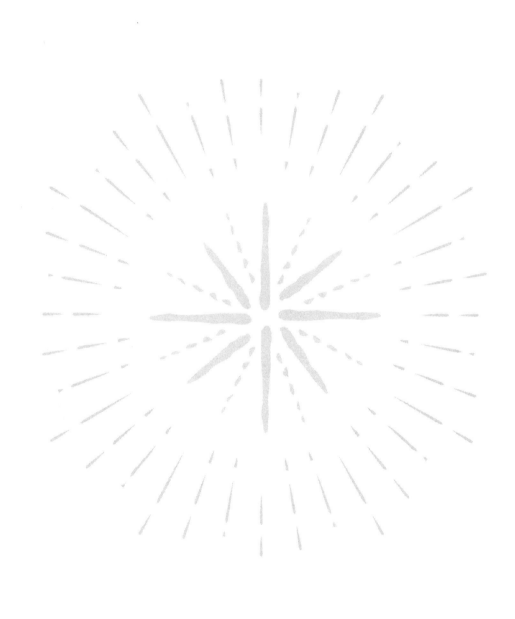

1

Mystical Experiences

El Cid – A Glimpse of the Truth

I want to share with you some interesting moments in my life that have been catalysts for me being exposed to life beyond the veil. I would call them mystical or magical experiences. Events that at the time of occurrence were unexplainable to me. Now I know more or have remembered more, I have clarity, but at the time they simply happened and I flowed with it. There was no other choice. These experiences will give you a glimpse into the Super-Human abilities that can be developed by each one of us, extraordinary beings on Earth.

It was 3.30 a.m. as I stirred in my bed, turned over and looked at my phone to see the time. I woke quickly, no time for blurry eyes. My mind was in full focus. I was switched on, ready! I was lying in a hard wooden bed in a stopgap apartment I had rented for two nights in the middle of Fuengirola, Spain. In the apartment below was Andrew, a man who would be flying a suitcase full of ecstasy tablets into Tenerife later that day. In the apartment above me was my driver, with the ecstasy tablets.

It was 2002. The Tenerife party scene was pumping. My driver had driven from Holland to Spain, with the ecstasy packaged into his dashboard. On arrival in Spain there were issues with the ferry, and he couldn't board the boat for three days. This would mean by the time the ship docked in Santa Cruz and we had driven the drugs down to Las Americas, we would have missed days of trade and a boatload of cash in sales. So, I called my friend. He let the driver leave the car in his underground garage. I flew to Fuengirola, took the dashboard out and removed the drugs. The driver took them to El Cid, a shabby block of apartments that you could rent for the equivalent of ten pounds per night; it really was a proper dive. Andrew had flown in later that day and was already holed up at El Cid, in a different apartment. I never let people in the chain meet each other. Degrees of separation were important for everyone's safety.

Flying with drugs in a suitcase is something you would never get away with with today's technology, but back then it was easier. Still a risk, but no one checked the bags on scanners like they do now. Also, Andrew would be flying business class, in a smart suit. Being a middle-aged man with glasses, he looked like a regular businessman. Back then I also felt no remorse if someone got caught. It was business and everyone knew the risks.

El Cid was a hole of a place but somewhere you could blend in easily and go unnoticed. Most single men staying in these apartments were bringing back prostitutes. As all three of us were staying alone, we fitted the bill perfectly. As I lay there in my apartment, listening to the creaks of beds in other rooms, people outside on the street still partying from the night before, the kettle turning itself on and off and the fridge humming me to death, I stared at the ceiling, contemplating my journey to the airport with Andrew, our flight back to Tenerife and the money we would make once the pills were back home.

My mind raced and my body was still. My heart felt like it was stopping, and then my mind slowed down, and I felt like I was falling asleep. My alarm clock was set, and I closed my eyes gently, feeling sleepy and expecting to drift off into dreamland. But something very different happened. With my eyes still closed, I "saw" the room I was in, and a sheet of glass appeared to my left-hand side. I saw colours and shapes that seemed to flow through the walls and surround me and I could feel myself sinking. As I sank I started to see my body from above, which seemed very strange. It was as though I was sinking and rising at the same time.

As I rose, I saw lots of people inside a building, all going places. I could see the people, but it was hard to make out where they were. It felt just like a dream, except unlike a dream I felt I was in control. I started looking around the crowds of people, from my slightly elevated position, and then I saw a sign that said ARRIVALS and I knew it was an airport. At this point I had no recollection of the bed, my physical body, or the apartment I was staying in. I was somewhere else completely. I then saw myself walking through customs and security checks and a horrible feeling came over my body. I felt nauseous, like something terrible was about to happen. The next thing this scene disappeared and I was above a red car. An old Fiesta that was parked outside a building. I tried to see the building, but it was out of focus. Then it became non-existent.

The next moment I saw policemen searching this car and again I felt very nauseous, as though I had been injected with the feeling of being on the Waltzers at a fairground, after being spun relentlessly for ten minutes, non-stop in the same direction. I could feel the nauseous feeling being pushed up as though my chest and throat were a tunnel and someone or something was trying to force a large boulder up inside the tunnel. It got more intense and then, once the boulder was forced through the tunnel, I saw a huge explosion of light.

The light vanished and I was up above my body, back in the apartment. I was looking down at my body asleep on the bed. How could I be looking at my body and be above it? With hindsight, I know I was having some kind of metaphysical experience, but at the time I didn't even know what the term metaphysical meant. I was just having this experience, going through it, being it.

As I looked at my body the sheet of glass that I saw at the start of this adventure started to bend. It bent over my body that was lying on the bed. It created an arch of what looked like glass, or maybe it was light, over my bed and over my body, from one side of the floor to the other. Then I started to free-fall. It was like one of those dreams where you are falling towards the ground, and you think you are going to die and then you wake up. The strange thing was I was only two metres above the bed, maybe less. and I was falling towards my body.

It was as though somehow the space between my body and where I was floating as consciousness, observing, was stretched, and I was falling really fast for what seemed like six or seven seconds; and then with a thud I opened my eyes. I felt so heavy, so stuck. What was even stranger was that when I was falling towards my body it was not my body. I was above my body but what looked like a giant red rose. The petals were so red and vibrant. When I hit the flower, I opened my eyes.

Then I just lay there. I knew inside me that something wasn't right and that today was not going to go to plan. I didn't know how or why but I just knew. I kept having hazy images appear in my mind of the red car and me walking through customs. Something was not right. I was meant to be with Andrew at the airport, but I could not see him in my vision.

I knew I had to change the flights, and that no one could know about it. When we set this deal up it was between my business partner and one other man. This other man we had not worked with before and he knew our flight schedule, but he didn't know who I had taken with me. He just knew we would be arriving back on this particular flight. Then I went down to Andrew's apartment and woke him up, saying: "We need to get you on an early flight out." I went to a phone box and booked him on to an early flight out that day. We flew him business class via Madrid. It was a long way round, but no one would be looking for anyone coming in from Madrid, especially business class passengers. I kept to the original flight.

Andrew arrived safely later that morning and I flew in the afternoon. When I arrived in Tenerife I walked through customs: no issues. My friend picked me up in a red car, exactly like the one I had seen in my lucid experience earlier that morning. As we drove down the motorway, he suggested we stop and have a drink. We stopped at a nightclub and went in. I had just ordered the second round of drinks when the music stopped, the lights went on and ten seconds later there were Spanish voices on the PA system. My Spanish isn't great, but I know what "Policia" meant. Everyone was asked to leave the club and as we walked out four police officers stopped us. They spoke in English and asked us if the red car was ours. They obviously knew who they were looking for. We said yes and they asked us to open it. They stripped the car as much as they could. Obviously there was nothing to find (as Andrew had rolled in safely earlier that day and the drugs were already being sold on street corners), so after 15–20 minutes of searching and radio calls, they let us go. It was obvious that the man who we had worked with for the first time had notified the authorities and tried to set us up, expecting me to have the ecstasy and that the police would find it in the car.

This whole experience was a blur but at the same time so precise and accurate. From my bed in the El Cid apartments I had been shown the entire scenario playing out, but I was shown it in a way that my brain didn't fully understand. There was a part of me, however, that knew the imagery and the information I was being shown and the feelings I felt, somehow, all translated into a decision. That decision was to put Andrew on a different flight.

At this time, I was a rogue, a criminal. A greedy, ego-induced nightmare with no love and compassion for humanity or respect for life itself. Why had I been helped by the universe? Or was it the universe? Maybe it was a spirit helping me, or an extra-terrestrial? I did not have these thoughts at the time. I just carried on, took it all in my stride and continued on my reckless path.

I have had many unusual experiences in my life and as I look back at them, I realize that some force was looking after me. I was destined to assist humanity in the long run, through my healing mission, Star Magic; there was a power, a mind greater than mine, an intelligence at work that kept me safe to do so. Living the life I have lived, I really should be dead or in prison, but neither have happened. As you journey with me through this book, I will share other mystical or magical experiences with you. You will know in your heart that my Earthly journey was predestined. The men in black masks who traumatized my mother when she gave birth knew it, as did many others. You see, we all have a mission on Earth. We knew it before we incarnated. We come down into this magical vessel we call our body and then have to figure it all out again, after our soul memory is blank-slated – wiped – on entry into this denser realm of the five senses.

You have a mission, and your heart will lead you into or onto it. You must listen to the inner wisdom, to the intelligence that is always communicating with us. I am going to give you the keys and codes and vital information to enable you to step into your power, your mission, your life and become a master alchemist, so you can fully "innerstand" what it means to be Super-Human. To be able to ignite mystical and magical experiences at will, just like the one I have shared, so you can connect with information streams beyond the veil of illusion, high-vibrational sources of light/energy that will open your heart and mind to a brand new and exciting world. A place that is available 24/7, 365, to every brave and fearless warrior who lives fiercely from the heart and is hungry for knowledge and truth.

The Indian Guru

I tell everyone I started my spiritual journey in 2005 after a few interesting experiences and a car crash in Romania, but writing this book now, and sharing with you, I know it started a lot earlier. I didn't have the awareness at the time to grasp what was happening, even though I did appreciate them on some level; I was too focused on making money and buying material things, trying to find happiness and complete myself, something I realized later on was futile as we are already complete, whole and at one with all things, living and playing in a magnetic and an electromagnetic universe, powered by a consciousness that thrives in harmony. Everything I did in my early years disconnected me from balance and harmony and this in itself was beautiful, because the depths of experience I had in darkness are now being mirrored on the opposite side of the spectrum, in high-vibrational light. I am merging the two.

One of my old business partners (I'll call him Vishal) introduced me to someone he called his guru. I didn't know what he meant at the time, but I went along with it. At the time I was still involved in crime. On this occasion I had to pick up a bag of money and drop off some forged invoices at a hotel. Vishal answered the door and told me his guru was inside. He did tell me his name, but I forgot it within seconds.

I walked into the room to be met by a man much taller than me, about fifty-five years old, dark hair, clean-shaven and wearing a cream suit that was far too big. He shook my hand and then told me to go outside, find a white flower and bring it back to him. What are you talking about? was the thought going through my head, but he looked at me with a deep penetrating glare and I knew I had to go. If anything, it was out of pure curiosity.

You expect me to find a white flower outside this hotel, which is in the middle of a gigantic roundabout, full of car fumes and smog, was the thought that continued to race through my head. I walked around the entire hotel area and then just as I was about to give up, there in a small patch of grass, in a corner, were two white flowers. So I picked them and went back into the hotel.

I handed the flowers to this guy. He opened his hand and looked at them, then told me to cup my hands and hold them out. He rubbed his own hands together and after about two seconds a white liquid started pouring from his hands and into my cupped hands underneath. I stared at this white liquid that looked like milk. He said, "Drink it." It *was* milk, the sweetest milk I had ever tasted. I couldn't believe it. I put my hands back under the gentle stream of white sweet liquid that was still trickling from his hands.

I stayed for a few minutes after drinking the milk and then I left (with a rucksack full of fresh fifty-pound notes). I walked down the stairs instead of taking the lift. I wanted to take my time and evaluate what had just happened. I had seen with my own eyes a man, made of flesh and blood, take two white flowers and turn them into milk in front of my very eyes. When he'd opened his hands the flowers, including the green stems, were gone. His hands were empty – and what was even stranger was that they were dry. What I also couldn't get my head around was the amount of milk that flowed from the two flowers. It was enough to fill a coffee cup.

It reminded me of the story of Jesus turning water to wine and bringing the fish from the bucket. After seeing this, tasting this and having this full-on undeniable experience, I fully knew and still know that turning water to wine is possible.

Is turning white flowers into milk a Super-Human feat? One hundred per cent yes. Do I feel it's possible for us all to develop this Super-Human gift? One hundred per cent yes. He was a normal human being, with arms and legs and blood that pumped through his veins. What is also interesting to note here is that this so-called guru, with spiritual superpowers, was mixing with hardened criminals. It goes to show that anyone can develop these gifts. I know that this guru took donations from my business partner to travel the world sharing his knowledge. If he could do this, it goes to show that you don't need to be a tree-hugging hippie, dressed in white, holding company with other spiritual people, all sharing rainbow streams of light from their heart, to embody these Super-Human powers. They really are accessible to anyone willing to do the work necessary to go beyond the five senses and connect with the quantum field, where all possibilities lie.

Since this day I have always been dazzled by women and men who have developed abilities in human form and can demonstrate them at will. I have met many more and each one of them has encouraged me to pursue my own journey, in search of my own Super-Human powers. After discovering Star Magic and being able to heal people at distance, from life-threatening diseases and injuries, I developed my own Super-Human ability. Performing psychic surgery that leaves physical scars and a body that has had its tumours removed, without a single touch, when I am in another country, town, or city from my clients, is a Super-Human power. Remember this and please keep this etched into your mind. If a man like me, a lad from the streets, who grew up as

a total sceptic regarding anything spiritual, who sold drugs and committed high-level fraud among other things, can start facilitating the healing of others and create rapid, massive change in their lives that lasts, so can you or any other man, woman, or child on this planet.

Each one of us is unique, gifted, and multidimensional and has the chemistry, biology, and metaphysical foundation (our soul) to bring these elements together, with practice, to perform what some call miracles. Remember the word miracle is just that: a word. It has been given a certain meaning, that of being something special, different, out of the ordinary. But we are all capable of creating miracles, by applying the right formula. By changing our energy and levels of consciousness and shifting our frequency to be able to connect to other, higher vibrational streams of information or light, each one of us can unleash Super-Human skills available to us all and have a profound impact on our reality and the lives of others, our human family.

An Angel with Wings

I have told this story in full in *Into the Light* and *Healing with Light Frequencies*, so I will keep it short and sweet here, but it's important to mention.

In 2006 I was involved in a car crash in Romania. The taxi I was in hit three ladies crossing the road early one morning. The first lady came through the windscreen, smashed me in the head and was sucked back out; the second lady had her feet cut off at the ankles, and the third lady was physically OK.

At the time I had no idea what had happened as I was asleep in the passenger seat, with my ex-wife and two kids in the back. When I got out of the car, I walked up the road, saw one lady with her feet cut off, the other lady crying and screaming, and I continued walking towards the lady who had come through the windscreen and died. As I walked towards her body (which I didn't know was a body until I got closer) I saw this energy source, hovering above. It was her soul. It stayed for several seconds and then fizzled off into the ether. This was another mystical experience that happened in my life.

It was six months after this that my healing abilities started to surface. My then-wife was lying on the bed with a migraine. I saw the headache in her head. It was green. I walked over, grabbed the green energy, and pulled it out. She got up off the bed without a headache. I used to think these things were strange at first but took them in my stride.

A little while after this, we moved to New Zealand, where I met a man who taught me to meditate. I had several mystical experiences, all of which I discuss in detail in the above-mentioned books, but the one that is important to highlight here is when I was picked up in a spacecraft and flown through a tunnel of light to Alpha Centauri, where I met many blue Lyran beings and received a huge download of light and geometric code. It was this experience, coupled with the car crash in Romania and then nine months in ancient mystery schools on my return to the UK, four years later, where I was shown how to use the geometric codes to heal, that kick-started my healing journey and from it Star Magic Healing was born.

It was in 2013, when I returned from New Zealand to England, that I was introduced to angels, fairies, and other beings. It was a strange time in my life, exciting but strange, transitioning from a life of crime to a life playing with fairies and healing people. A tough one to explain to my friends, colleagues, and business partners. They all thought I had gone completely nuts.

On arriving back in the UK I went to renew the passports for my two children, Aalayah and Josh, and myself at the passport office. I booked a same-day service where you go, hand in your paperwork, pay a fee, and then come back four hours later to collect them. When I returned, I was asked to go into another room where they presented me with two pieces of paper. On each piece was a picture of a passport. One with my name as it is now and the other with the name Daniel King. Daniel was one of the names I used through the years, and they wanted to know why I had two passports. Of course, this was illegal.

They told me they couldn't issue me my new passport and that I would have to come back later to collect it. They phoned me two days later, on a Friday, and asked if I could return the following Thursday to collect them. When I returned, I was asked to go into the same room I was questioned in before. They led me around to the right-hand side of the row of private offices inside the Newport Passport Office to two men and a woman standing there, along with a second woman from the passport agency: "Mr Sargeant, you are under arrest for conspiracy to defraud the Royal Bank of Scotland and holding a false travel document. You have the right to remain silent, anything you do or say can and will be used against you in a court of law. You have the right to a solicitor; one will be provided for you. Do you understand? Is there anything you wish to say?"

I kept my mouth shut, they cuffed me and led me out of the passport office and into an unmarked police car with blacked-out windows. I was taken to Newport Police Station for questioning. The events that followed this took me on an unexpected journey. One that led me to "innerstand" the corruption within our current system and one that would present me with a huge sign that I must fully embrace my life mission and start a healing business called Star Magic. And believe me, I needed that sign because I was tempted left, right, and centre to go back to my old ways of living, but the universe kept kicking my arse and steering me in the direction of Star Magic.

They released me from the police station after questioning and I spent the next two years on bail, up and down to London. Within these two years, I met some interesting people who gave me information that would help me get the conspiracy charge dropped. An old friend of mine introduced me to a different kind of lawyer. A lawyer who had trained in law school but then dropped out because of the corruption he witnessed. He decided on a different profession and decided importing cocaine was the way forward. This led him to an arrest and a court battle that would potentially earn him fifteen to twenty years in prison.

This man presented himself in court as a free sovereign being and used the words in the Bible to aid him along the way. Due to technicalities, they had no choice but to let him go. He was an extremely intelligent human being who knew the system inside and out and knew exactly how to behave in a court. I came to know and "innerstand" the corruption of our corporate legal system after speaking to him and he told me he could get me a document that would prove my innocence in the bank conspiracy charge.

Just so you know, I was being charged for stealing mortgage money. They alleged that I had raised mortgages for several million pounds and instead of buying the properties I had worked with a corrupt solicitor, drew the money down to pay for the properties and instead of paying the builders/vendors/sellers, sent the money to other accounts, drew it out in cash and kept it for myself. The police had bank statements and an informer that they had picked up through their investigations. This coupled with my false passport meant the odds were stacked against me. I took advice from Robin, the cocaine-smuggling lawyer.

If you know anything about mortgages, you will know that the banks that lend the money pull so many stunts that are completely corrupt, yet they

get away with it because we as humans trust them and never look into what is happening behind the scenes. This is not an education on mortgages, so I am not going into this in detail.

What Robin provided me with was a huge document with 62,000 properties in it, that included all those mortgages that were loaned against properties throughout the UK, in the time period that the properties I was being accused of loaning money against, were in. This document totalled 2.7 billion pounds. It showed that all of these properties had mortgages against them. It also showed that the mortgages were then sold to a company in America (called Aran Property Group), by the Royal Bank of Scotland, where they were traded on the New York Stock Exchange and turned into billions. Something that is highly illegal. What this document would enable me to do was prove that the Royal Bank of Scotland did not lose any money and so why were they chasing me for it?

Firstly, it's not easy to get your hands on a document like this and secondly, to do so leaves an electronic trail. This document arrived in my inbox and later that day it vanished. The next morning, I left the gym and was driving home. I was pulled over by an unmarked BMW X5 with armed police inside. They harassed me at gunpoint for a worn-down tyre. A little excessive, don't you think? Within an hour of this happening, two police officers turned up at my mum and dad's house, saying they were looking for Daniel King. They were rude to my parents and applied a lot of pressure. Again, a little excessive, particularly because they knew who Daniel King was – me – and that I didn't live at the house of my mum and dad. They also knew my parents were stressed because my dad had cancer, but they still treated them in an inhumane way. This is the game we are playing.

It was clear to me that they were upset, to put it mildly, that I had access to this document.

I phoned Robin who printed the document out for me. On my next bail visit to the Metropolitan Police station in London I presented the document. They dropped the charges within forty-eight hours. I still had the false passport document charge hanging over me.

All throughout this two-year game/battle, I was being exposed to different spiritual experiences, I had written my book *Into the Light* and was really starting to take this healing journey seriously. I had also travelled to the Philippines with my daughter Aalayah to rebuild homes and schools and put permaculture projects in place after the typhoon Haiyan had hit. I was really starting to enjoy this "giving back" experience even more.

There was something still holding me back, however. I was still being offered opportunities to make money illegally, some of which I took. Slowly, though, my willpower increased and I stepped away. I went to a couple of local spiritual fairs and gave away some free healings to test my abilities; the results were amazing. The issue for me was that I still had this court case hanging over my head. If I went to prison, it was all over. So, I made a pact with the universe. I said in no uncertain terms, if you want me to start a healing business, bring Star Magic into the world, and go full steam ahead with this Earthly mission, you are going to have to make sure I stay out of prison.

The police continued with their course of action and I was given a court date to appear in London. I made some plans for my family as I knew there was a possibility of me not coming home that night. I arrived at court, met my solicitor and went into the court room where they locked me in a transparent, bullet-proof dock. (*As a sovereign being you should never stand in the dock, have a legal representative and do certain things in court, but due to certain things wrapped around my personal situation, I did.*) The judge and his two assistants walked out into the court room. The judge was male and his two assistants

were female. The lady to his right looked at me and smiled and, as crazy as this sounds, I could see she had wings on her back. I thought I was going crazy. I was shaking my head. She looked over at me again and winked. It was as though she could read my mind, like she was listening to my thoughts. Something inside me said this is going to be OK. My whole body relaxed. It was as though it was over already and a huge sense of peace came over me.

The prosecution gave their side of the story and presented me to the court in the ugliest manner possible. They brought up the smallest of things, all the way back to arrests when I was fourteen and fifteen years old. They painted the worst picture of me they could. Next up my solicitor gave our side of the story. The judges were also given letters from the people involved in the humanitarian work we were doing. The judges went out to deliberate and the arresting police officer was looking happy at the back of the room. She thought I was in the bag, signed, sealed, and delivered and off to serve time under Her Majesty at HMP (Her Majesty's Prison).

Within twenty minutes the judges were back and the angel with wings winked at me again. "Everybody please rise", was the order in the court room. The judge looked at me and said, "Mr Sargeant, we can see that you are a changed man. We are giving you a one-year conditional discharge (which means if you get in trouble within the next twelve months you will be sent to prison without any questions) and an eighty-pound court fee." I was elated, grinning like a Cheshire cat. The first thought that came into my head was Star Magic. I had already decided on the name. Once they let me out of the dock, I walked over to my solicitor to say thank you. As I was walking, I looked over at the angel with wings and there was this feeling, this knowing on a deep level, that from this point forward I would remain on the right path. It was as though an unknown force had orchestrated my freedom from above. I don't know how but something mystical and magical happened that day. Was this lady even human? Did a spirit take over her body? How did this happen? These questions were racing through my head, and I felt huge gratitude in my heart.

I had decided to start Star Magic the following February. It was now September. I wanted to spend a few months practising my healing, so organized stands at other mind body spirit fairs to give myself an opportunity to connect with people, talk about healing and practise.

These next few months were amazing. I absorbed as much knowledge as I could through meditation and my communications with other beings. I met some awesome Star Sisters and Brothers and they guided me. I was facilitating some incredible healings and collecting video testimonials ready for the launch of our Star Magic Healing website in 2016.

I was being fast-tracked. It was as though I was on a mystical roller coaster, following the signs. There were so many coincidences and unexplainable happenings in my life, just as if I was an instrument and the universe was playing me. I surrendered to it all, let go, and flowed with it. Whoever or whatever the angel with wings in the court room that day was or is, I will be forever grateful. I feel much work was done behind the scenes to orchestrate the unfolding of events that day and this keeps me focused. I was chosen for this mission. Or maybe I chose myself? All I know is that nothing will stop me sharing this frequency and being a catalyst for transformation in the lives of my Super-Human family.

The Cross of Clouds

Many extraordinary events have unfolded in my life surrounding the people that I have facilitated the healing of. I always say facilitated and not healed as I am simply a vessel carrying information, a portal between the physical and non-physical worlds. Even though I am instrumental in the healing, it's an energy, a frequency, a quantum exchange of information that is taking place so the healing can happen. I simply set up the environment for the energetic exchange.

It's all mathematics, patterns, rhythms, and numbers. It's all spiralized geometry and numerical code. It's about seeing and "innerstanding" the code, knowing how to move it and change it. There is always a presence too. Other beings at work, assisting and guiding. These other beings I feel are other aspects of me, in higher-dimensional spaces, creating on other frequency bands within the quantum field; and the key to being a Super-Human partly rests on your ability to hold the frequency of all of your multidimensional selves in this now space.

Imagine, if you could take all the energy and information, all the knowledge from all these other versions of you, just for a moment, and bring it all into the same space when facilitating a healing, miracles and magic can take place.

A few years back I got a phone call from a lady who told me her boyfriend needed healing. He was riding his pushbike and was involved in a collision with a speeding car. His head had gone through the quarter light window, his neck and back were broken and his nose had been pushed into the back of his head. The man, Steffan, was in intensive care and in a bad way. He had what looked like a million tubes hanging out of him, his face was black and blue with rows of stitches. He was fighting for his life, on all sorts of heavy medication and not responsive. As I walked into the room, I could see, at the end of Steffan's bed, something very strange. It was a man but not any ordinary man. It was the Devil.

I didn't mention this to anyone. I simply went in, cleared the energy of the room (as best I could with that fella sitting there) and then went to work. I spent about three hours with Steffan.

I first worked on the geometrical coding, flowing through the universal fabric, that was linked into his skeletal system. I then worked on his lungs and then looked into any other parallel realities, where Steffan's soul was having experiences, and seeing if there was anything that needed working on.

There were several unhealthy incarnations that had created patterns of unworthiness that required healing. As I went through the process of collapsing the timelines and bringing his soul fragments into healing, the Devil was talking to Steffan, asking his soul to come with him. On a super-conscious level, communicating through telepathy, Steffan refused. All I could do was observe and do my job. We all have free will. There were some very powerful beings/spirits in the room with me, assisting and guiding. I always have a super-powerful spirit squadron with me but on this particular day, they all brought their halos out of the closet and came to play.

After I finished my work, I walked over to the window and looked up into the blue sky. It was a sunny day and there were no clouds in the sky – apart from this one. It was in the shape of a perfect cross. When I turned away from the window and looked back towards the bed, the Devil was gone. I touched Steffan's leg for a moment, thanked him and then left.

The next day I got a phone call and was told Steffan had woken up, pulled all of the tubes out of his mouth and was breathing on his own. Two days after that they X-rayed his back and neck and what had showed as broken bones just days earlier had completely healed. The doctors were flabbergasted.

Steffan's partner was told at the start that he would be in intensive care for at least three months, possibly much longer. But he was back at work in five weeks and his face, which had been cut to ribbons and smashed to pieces, looked really well.

When I spoke to Steffan later, he told me that he had seen the Devil at the edge of the bed and that he was telling him that all the bad things he had done in his life could be made up for, trying to persuade Steffan to go with him.

Is this a Super-Human feat? Yes, it is. Does it make me special? No. I am simply showing you what's possible for every single human being on this planet. Healing broken bones, saving lives and holding space, so rapid, lasting transformation can take place, is something every human is capable of. You too can create miracles like this if you are on the right frequency. Should you believe me that the Devil was there? No. Should it make you scared if you do believe that this being was there? No. In any given moment you get to choose: love or fear, opposites on the emotional spectrum. I always choose love and continue to do so. I have experienced many different aspects of reality: low and high vibration; and I know that unconditional love in all situations is a necessity.

When it comes to believing, none of us should. All thoughts, when you trace them back to their origin, are based on one of three things: time, distance, or measurement. And none of them really exist in the quantum field, which is where real change is initiated; belief systems are therefore false. There is only ever now. Once we transcend belief systems and come into a space of internal knowing, living from the frequency of the heart, following our life compass, the best satellite navigation on the planet, we will step fully into our power and recondition our consciousness to that of a Super-Human.

2

A New Aeon

A Platinum World

Our world is changing so quickly, however, it often seems that it's taking for ever while we are down here on Earth. Our lifespan is small. Other life forms live for hundreds, sometimes thousands of years and these beings (which are us also, as we have experienced and are experiencing lives with much longer lifespans right now, in other quantum galactic realities) have a completely different perspective on time, and how long things take and if it's happening quickly or slowly. We, as a human species (maybe because on a deep level we know we are here on Earth for a short period, in the vast ocean of time) on the whole are rather impatient and want things done now. When you know you have hundreds, even thousands, of years, you can kick back and allow a little more. Be in a surrendered state of consciousness.

Extremely high-frequency beings (certain extra-terrestrials for example), who are pure energy in some realities, have no concept of time because they are eternal. We humans were also originally eternal, but we lost the essence of our true gene code and our original twelve-strand DNA blueprint (in some cases twenty-four and forty-eight strands), that which we had when we first came to our 5D Earth (known as Tara) as angelic humans. We carry the potential for eternal life in our DNA once it is fully activated.

A lot of people talk about the golden age of Atlantis coming back and while this is true, we must look at what it really means. When Atlantis went under it was because the power

and energy being generated there was used in the end to manipulate and control and the beings in control misused their power. An entire species was genetically raped, and the crystalline grids of the planet were misused. Atlantis was a thriving, beautiful space (I've travelled into many incarnations I have had there) and the golden age of Atlantis that people refer to was a state of consciousness. Telepathy, telekinesis, healing, astral travel, bi-location, were all everyday abilities that every being had. They were as common as running, jumping, skipping, talking, laughing, and dancing.

But I say we should create something new, not try to relive or rebirth something old. Let's use our creativity and carve a compassionate, sovereign new world, exactly the way we want it!

We are expanding our consciousness here on Earth rapidly and are developing spiritually as a species. Light, information, codes, frequency, are the keys to our development as a species here on this planet. Higher vibrational light streams/information streams, coming from outside of our local cosmic environment (from planets and stars deep in space, in our galaxy and other galaxies and universes) are carrying codes. These codes are little crystalline keys that are triggering a deep remembering within our human system. On a DNA level, knowledge is stored, and once certain light streams (containing codes and keys) connect with our DNA, an activation of sorts occurs. Ancient cosmic wisdom is released, and we remember truths, we know/remember who we are at the core.

Our DNA is beyond comprehension. So much can be stored there. If you stuck the DNA in one cell together it would be six feet long. If you stuck the DNA from every cell together and uncoiled it, it would be at least 10 billion miles long. Let me put this into perspective. The Earth is 93 million miles from the sun. So, at its minimum your DNA could stretch from the Earth to the sun and back again sixty-one times.

We can store 35,000 terabytes of information in our DNA, the equivalent of 35 million hours of high-definition video. Our DNA is like computer code and can be written and rewritten. We can literally upgrade ourselves from the inside out. Just in case you have any doubts that you have the capacity to be a Super-Human, now you know. You are one of the most advanced computer systems in the universe. It's not inside of you. You *are* it. Each cell emits 100,000 photons per second. That means it must also be receiving vast amounts of data per second.

Did you know that per cubic centimetre, the human body produces 10,000 times more light than the surface of the sun? We are stars in human form. The protons in our cells, which are black holes are turning this light into a particle state and that is why you are not blinding every human being around you with your light.

So we have to take your light body into consideration and then there is your soul. Both of these, again, store huge amounts of data. Scientists say that one bio-photon can store ten megabytes of data. Our light body is vast and expansive, made up of trillions upon trillions of bio-photons. Mind-blowing. We have five densities and within each density there are three dimensions. This fifteen-dimensional time matrix is what we operate inside of right now. Operating effectively in 5D means being able to access all fifteen dimensions and move around freely, and ultimately move out from this time-based matrix and into the primary light and

sound fields, and then God Worlds beyond.

What I see each day, when I am working/creating/healing, is the patterns of light and spiralized geometrical code that is entering our space, shifting. I see this reality for what it truly is, nothing more than a game. We are living in a holographic reality, literally. On one level we are human, and, on another level we are like robots, controlled and programmed by information streams. Look at it like this: you are like a laptop, plugged into a hard drive. The only information you can access is that on the hard drive you are plugged into. If you want to access new information, you must unplug from it and plug into another, or plug in a second drive and have access to both sets of data, on both hard drives at the same time.

As a species we are plugged into geometrical data, which is allowing us to perceive reality in a certain way. When your third eyesight is developed (something we will be discussing), you can see the empty space is actually rich and bountiful and not empty at all. You realize that there is so much energy and so much information streaming through you and the space at all times, and actually you are a continuation of the space and the space is a continuation of you. The issue is, this information is on a different frequency and so you cannot see it, access it, utilize it and so in a way it's useless. Until you know how to tap into this vast, cosmic ocean of knowledge, your life will stay pretty much the same. With the right tools and a little discipline, though, you can have full access to a wealth of knowledge, and I am going to show you exactly what to do.

The new age of information is a platinum, diamond, and chromium world. We are going to delve deeply into these later. Our light body, our newly activated, high-vibrational light body, which will come online once you do the work or may have come online already, if you have done or are doing the work, is platinum. How do I know this? Because I see it. I see its colour and see and feel its frequency. We all have a light body, which is a metaphysical element of who we are as beings. We have a physical and a non-physical part of us. There are many colours/frequencies travelling through the invisible world, so vibrant and magical. We just can't see them with our physical eyes. All we see is what we are tuned into, the spectrum between infrared and ultraviolet.

Ancient Frequencies

The highest vibrational and most powerful light source in the universe (that I have encountered) is kaleidoscopic chromium. Again, we are going to go into this in detail later on but it's this particular frequency and all of the other subsets of information/frequency streams/light codes contained within kaleidoscopic chromium that give it so much power. It's the cosmic coding, contained within kaleidoscopic chromium, that activates and brings online our 5th-density platinum light body. I will show you an extraordinary way to activate any human being's 5th-density light body later in the book. You will be able to have a huge impact on people's lives, very quickly.

The Earth herself is switching her own frequency. She has, embedded within her cosmic body, an ancient architecture (ley lines/grids/networks to carry high-vibrational energy/light to and from Star Gates and around the planet) that was created along with the Earth, ready for the species that inhabited it to activate this architecture once the collective frequency was high enough. That time is now. Humans were and still are the original Guardians of the Star Gates on Earth. High-frequency Krystalline currents have been available on our planet since 2012, consciousness has been evolving faster on Earth. There are two primary sets of mathematics running on our planet. The activation of our sacred diamond hearts is making it possible, for us as a species, to take the cosmic information from the stars and ground it down into the planet, to feed and activate this ancient diamond architecture. Another timeline is in motion, a new/old set of spiralized geometries and mathematics, known as the Krystal Spiral. The Krystal Spiral runs alongside the Fibonacci Spiral, both of which are potentials we can tap into. The Fibonacci Spiral is the lower-density, corrupted mathematical version of the world we live in. The Krystal Spiral is the original/new and elevated, incorruptible mathematical version of the world we live in. Both sets of geometries and mathematics are playing out. One will keep you locked into a 3D/4D reality field and the other will see you spiral up/inwards, as you enter the multidimensional spectrum on your ascension path, being able to access all dimensional fields. The mathematics of the Krystal Spiral are what we must utilize for ascension.

We will discuss these two sets of mathematics later.

What is important to know at this stage is that your frequency can only change when you are able to access new information/light/energy. Once you do, the data lying in your DNA, activated by light, like a laser scanning CD technology and accessing the information on it, comes online. Once you tap the new frequency streams available, this will enable you to activate elements of your invisible/quantum self and expand your consciousness massively. Your 5th-density platinum light body is integral in controlling the ebb and flow of light codes from the stars so that your human system can handle it. What you must do as a human being is prepare your physical body as much as possible through high-vibrational nutrition, exercise, meditation, breathwork, qigong, yoga and a good, solid connection to Mother Earth. The Mag in Magic and the Mag in magnetic and the Mag in Magdalene, is the essence of our life force. Mag means motion and it's this ever-flowing motion/mag, that fuels the feminine energy and gives us eternal life. When you bring Earth's magnetic frequency up through your physical body, it draws the electromagnetic frequency from the stars back down into the Earth's grids and all life flows. It flows in a never-ending loop. We call this Infinity.

It is important to understand that Mother Earth is magnetic. You are taking high-vibrational (kaleidoscopic chromium) light from the stars, which is electromagnetic, passing it through 45 miles of electrical wiring (your human nervous system) and grounding it into the planet, which is magnetic. The source of light (electromagnetic and male/positive) is information, and the source of energy (magnetic and feminine/negative) is our power. The knowledge comes from up above and the energy comes from below, hence it's mission critical to have a good connection to the Earth. That means being in nature. Get your shoes and socks off and connect with the Earth. Not the grass but the Earth. Be with her, vibrate with her, talk, and connect with her. We also receive magnetic frequencies from our celestial sisters and brothers and also there are electromagnetic frequencies flying around the Earth's grids. But it's the Earth herself and the stars themselves that are feeding us. They are like batteries that send and receive, and we as humans are the connection point.

The 3 Ms. M in numerology is 13. Thirteen is the number of the Divine Goddess. 3 x 13 = 39. 9 + 3 = 12. The number that represents creation. The feminine is the sacred giver of life and as a species we must be connected to the sacred giver of life, energetically, at all times. To lose the connection with the magnetic is to stop our flow of life force.

You are an electromagnetic being streaming high-vibrational light codes from the stars, through your body/nervous system and into the planet. If your body is not able to accommodate this source of light (because it's unfit or unhealthy), firstly your journey of activating your 5th-density light body will be harder; it will certainly take longer and may not even happen in this lifetime, and you will not get to experience the magic that is available right now when your vibration elevates.

Look at your body as a vehicle. Let's say a Volkswagen Golf, with a 1.6 litre standard engine. It comes with a certain chassis. If you were to take the engine out and fit a Lamborghini Gallardo engine and drive it full throttle, the chassis would probably break apart because it wouldn't be able to handle the force and power of its upgraded engine. It's simple: if you want to upgrade the engine, you must upgrade the vehicle. If you want to bring in the kind of light that can expand you into a Super-Human, you must prepare your physical body, as mentioned, hence I am mentioning high-vibrational nutrition, exercise, meditation, breathwork, chi gong, yoga. The good, solid connection to our Magnetic Mother Earth is particularly vital because Earth is your outlet-point for this high-vibrational energy/light.

Star Consciousness

We are not entering a golden age, it's a platinum and diamond age. Our platinum light body will activate our diamond heart centre and our consciousness will expand exponentially. The state of consciousness that we will be unlocking will surpass that which the Egyptians, Sumerians, Atlanteans, Lemurians all knew. We are activating our star consciousness. Our extra-terrestrial (5th-density platinum light body) consciousness. We are unlocking a platinum and diamond world and it's going to be a breathtaking journey.

This will require effort and a disciplined and dedicated approach. You can sit by and watch or get off the bench, put on your space helmet and get involved. The choice is yours, beautiful soul. All I know is there is a whole universe of potential, waiting for us to tap into it, so we can be Super-Women and Super-Men.

3

Master of Dark and Light

To be able to access the information that is held in the geometry of your 5th-density platinum light body, you must do the work; and because we live in a world of polar opposites, there is dark and light and so you are most likely going to experience some opposing forces trying to derail your cosmic train.

Like Luke Skywalker, you must overcome the temptation of the darker side of the force, harness it and bring it into balance, knowing all the while it's a part of you that you must accept, embrace, and tame, like a wild beast fighting for survival. It takes strength, willpower, wisdom, and discipline to become your own master. And let's face it, if you don't become your own master, something or someone else will . . . and for a brave spiritual warrior like you, that is not an option.

There are many others who would like to be your master and control you. Some are your masters right now. When the police sound their sirens, and flash their blue lights, you pull over and move out of their way. When your government sends a council tax bill through your letter box, you pay it or they will threaten you with a fine or jail time. Your parents may expect you to go and see them every week and even though their lower vibratory rate takes its toll on your frequency (because you allow it), you still go, out of duty.

Duty is a terrible word. We must never do anything out of duty. We must make our own decisions and make every move because it is the best move in the moment and it's what we, as unique individuals/beings, want to do. Whatever that reason for doing or being is, it's OK. You must do what you must do, in the moment (with zero future or past consideration), and others' opinions must not enter your decision-making process. Unless of course you ask. And then you must question this information and ultimately make your own decision.

Walking the road I have throughout my life, being a drug addict and an alcoholic at a young age, working for a high-profile criminal organization, smuggling drugs and other commodities and engaging in high-level bank fraud, before moving into a space where I facilitate the healing of others and know only love and compassion as a way of life, having tamed my inner darkness and brought the dark and light aspects of who I am into equilibrium, I know I am in the perfect space to share this message. If I can do it, so can you; anyone can.

I am a role model for transformation. There are many like me who have taken a 180-degree U-turn in their lives, and now it's your turn. Maybe you already have, and this book is simply confirmation for you. Maybe you are on this path and struggling with your inner battle and are reading this to accelerate the process and take you across the finish line, which really is just the start. Either way is perfect. You are perfect. The perfection is in the imperfection. Know this. Zero judgement. Love all of you right now. Any woman or man who achieves in life knows that perfection is a myth. Once you get to where you are going, you acclimatize for a short period and then simply set your sights on the next mountaintop or the next goal to reach.

Every decision you make alters timelines. Every choice and every action determines which path you take and on that path you will have an impact on the lives of those you meet; and in turn they will make choices, often off the back of the choices you have made and the path and flow of natural evolution that took place in the space you entered, after the choices you made and the direction you travelled. You must choose wisely.

The stories I share in this book are not shared to create fear but simply to enlighten, to open your heart and mind so you can know the truth. I know some of it may be hard to swallow but please, for your sake, feel it. Don't analyze any of this information, simply feel it. Internalize it, place it inside of your heart and feel it as your truth, or not. You cannot fake vibration. The heart never lies. It's your life compass and will always lead you in the direction of bliss, when you allow it. I am not saying it's an easy journey, as love makes us do crazy things, but it will be the perfect journey once you let go and trust. Remember this. In every situation you get to choose love or fear and there is gold to mine from every encounter.

I want you to be happy, free, full of joy and bliss, living in a world where everyone cares and shares. This beautiful, peaceful world I know, exists. Everything exists if we see and feel it. Our imagination is actually reality. We can create anything. The observer affects the observed and also creates the observed within the space of the heart and mind. Remember, your heart is just like a brain too. It's intelligent. When you combine what you see inside of your mind with what you feel inside of your heart, these two powerful forces of nature, through magnetic and electromagnetic streams of light, go to work and create this.

But the funny thing is, it's already created. We simply create and observe and then align with the observed reality through our frequency.

All is now. All is one. All is available. All is frequency. If all is now, one and frequency then surely you, me or anyone else must simply align with the frequency of what they are seeing and boom, it manifests. No more waiting. Yes, we live in a world where certain things appear through events and circumstances, delivered on timelines, but these events and circumstances are speeding up and life is moving faster and manifesting rapidly. Timelines are becoming obscured; they are collapsing, and the eternal now is becoming ever more prevalent. The veil between the material and non-physical worlds are thinning. Light/information/colours/fractals are merging into kaleidoscopes of spiralized geometrical beauty.

To truly know your power, you must accept life, you and everything and everyone in this world in its totality. All the good and not so good. All the light and darker aspects of reality must be embraced, accepted, and that includes all of who you are as a multidimensional, extra-terrestrial being, having an earthly experience. We, as humans, carry in our DNA genetic encodements from a vast array of species from many planets, stars, and star systems. It's no wonder that many of us are lost, easy for external forces to infiltrate, or feel strange living on this planet and often dream of "going home". The geometry of our planet is wrong. The geometry of our species is wrong. The geometry of nature is wrong. Imagine: someone gets a mould and pours a liquid into that mould. The liquid will take the shape of the mould and then solidify. Our entire system has been fitted into a mathematical mould that stops our Super-Humanness rising to the surface. Everything you see around you in nature looks beautiful. From seashells to leaves, to spirals in tornados. They all follow a pattern, a code. But this code is not pure. It's been manipulated. I know this sounds crazy and it's tough to accept, that everything you have ever known and is, is created from a corrupted mathematical blueprint that doesn't have your best interest at heart.

We will be diving into the mathematics of the universe later. For now, just keep an open heart and know this. You are a quantum architect, and everything can be changed and transformed. It must be created in the quantum first and then the physical will change its geometry, structure, and appearance. It's not huge shifts that need to take place. It's minor shifts that will fractalize and, as they fractalize out, will grow in magnitude.

Your Mission: Love

We must, as a collective, choose love in every situation. We must cultivate a love culture – but not just any love culture. It must be a fiercely loving love culture where we accept each other in our totality, with zero judgement, and where we are kind and compassionate towards the world and its inhabitants – humans, animals, insects; Mother Nature in her entirety.

Love of a fierce nature is the order of the day. I cannot stress this word "fierce" enough. If you do not love fiercely, a constant barrage of negative potentials will eventually break you. You will crumble, react to another human being or event and your vibration will dip. You must love fiercely and ferociously to stay on track, to continue to elevate and be your Super-Human self. Fierce love is the geometric universal code, it's the fuel of our universe.

It is our mission on Earth right now to love in this way, fiercely and unconditionally. To love with the kind of love that goes beyond physical touch and human emotions. I am talking about a love that cannot be explained. A love that must be embodied beyond the body, in a state of elevated, vibrational bliss. It's the feeling when you leave your body and know oneness for the first time. I had a great spiritual teacher/guide when I started my journey and this human being showed me how to leave my body at will. It is a beautiful experience.

To be a master of dark and light you must love, unconditionally all facets of life, dark and light and in doing so experience the revelation when

you know that dark and light do not exist. That they are both vibrational spaces on a spectrum of light and beyond that light is sound. We are all expressions of the same source. We are the creator and the created, manifested into a myriad of forms, all playing a gigantic game. It's not so funny when you are under fire or living in a depressed state or seeing people killed, maimed, imprisoned, jumping from towers. You must ask, "Why is the game so cruel?"

We are all playing our roles perfectly. Some brave souls have sacrificed themselves to help others wake up, see the truth, and get back on the path. They incarnated for this specific mission. Other brave souls that committed atrocities are controlled, influenced in the human bodily form and that is why they do what they do. Surely no human being would ever blow up the Twin Towers, knowing they would kill so many and create so much fear. So, what made them do that? Who made them do that? How did they succumb to the pressure and tip out of balance? Were they no longer a master of dark and light? Were they even human?

All I want you to know now is that you are powerful, and you get to decide, in every moment, your next action. Take your time, create space through meditation and start to lift the veil on your own mind, body and the illusory environment that surrounds you. All of the trials and tribulations you have experienced in this reality have served you well. They have hit you, broken you, taught you, rebuilt you and polished you. They are a true blessing. They have taken you into the dark and light realms of existence and given you glimpses of your inner truth. Whether you have known this consciously or not is irrelevant at this stage. Just be aware and calm in all situations.

This new aeon, this new space we are creating as an evolving species, requires all of us to know that dark and light reside inside all of us. We must honour all of who we are, and the trick to mastering who you are lies in your ability to do it and not think about it. You see, when you think about it you put up all sorts of red flags. What do I mean? Well, inside of you lie "God" and the "Devil", but they are just words. Inside of you just lies potential. You cannot separate this potential because it's all energy. High- and low-vibrational actions are a possibility for every human. What you must do is learn to remember how to outwit the Devil.

The way you do this is to not tell him that you are coming. So, if you want to go to the gym, just go. If you want to eat clean and stay away from your favourite pizza restaurant, just do it and do not tell yourself that you are going to do it. You see, as soon as you tell yourself, "Right, I am going to do this today," there is a force that will tell you all the reasons why you shouldn't or why it will hurt so much or the other activities you will miss out on while you are at the gym or doing yoga or walking in the forest. So, make the decision to do something and then drop into your heart. This creates stillness from where thoughts are easily observed. You can see these thoughts, and continue moving towards your goals and dreams, without the inner dialogue. The voice in your head can be observed and paid zero attention. This is a skill; start developing it.

Imagine if you were a burglar and you were in a house stealing someone's belongings. You're filling up your bag with watches, money, jewellery and someone sees strange activity and calls the police, or you trip a silent alarm in the house that triggers a police officer to come to the property. The police are not going to be blasting their sirens coming down the street. They will shut them down way before they arrive; otherwise you, the burglar, will hear them and run, jump a fence and get away.

When you are making changes to your life, you must not notify the opposing forces of your decisions. You make it and then do it. You don't

think about it or chat inside your own head about it, otherwise you are opening up space for internal dialogue. The Devil and God start deliberating, and you know who comes out on top, most of the time, especially when you are starting something new. Outwitting the Devil becomes a necessity. So, don't put yourself in that situation. You are dark and light, the Devil and God, hot and cold, high and low, in and out. You are all things.

You must become a Jedi Knight and know that the knife can both kill another human being and cut bread and feed another human being. (Or maybe cut some fruit because Super-Humans don't eat bread.) But you get my point. You cannot run from your Shadow Side. You cannot stuff your Shadow Side down and bury it in the depths of your consciousness. You must embrace all of who you are. Our Super-Human Potential activates when we embrace and activate our wholeness.

Disciplining your mind, body and soul are mission critical to excel in the coliseum of life. Be relentless. Attack life. Move and lean into life. Don't wait for the tides to turn or the stars to align. Set sail now in stormy waters and keep sailing. Draw the Devil and God into the fires of your heart and utilize that balanced energy as your greatest commodity.

True Mastery

A lot of us, human beings on Earth that is, who are on this spiritual journey, are living with this pre-conditioned belief that to be spiritual, you need to be this vegan, rainbow-clothes-wearing fairy, living on the outskirts of modern society. Nothing could be further from the truth. While it is good to go into silence and meditate under a tree or in the woods or by a cliff, looking out across a vast landscape, this is not where the real spiritual work is done.

A true spiritual warrior, one who has cracked the code, lives in the trenches of modern society, deep inside the jungle – the concrete type – playing the game with a smile on their face, blending into the world seamlessly, unaffected by the daily dramas. There are people that are triggered by the simplest of things. Road rage is a classic example. I remember the days when I would still be thinking about the guy who pulled out in front of me when I was driving, hours after the event, seething, angry, discussing it with my partner that evening or my friend the next day – holding onto the emotion way after the event. I was one of those guys you would see smashing his steering wheel, screaming obscenities out of the window, often getting out of the car for a scrap. I see drivers today still acting this way and I smile.

Moving on and letting go is mission critical. Living in the thick of the action, surrounded by potential triggers and not being affected, is the only way to be. It's good to put yourself in among people, situations, and events, giving life the opportunity to test your new mettle, as you grow and expand spiritually. To start with, your armour will be dented and, every now and again a stray armour-piercing round may find its target and the rage or rejection kick in. Slowly over time the frequency of the armour-piercing rounds hitting their mark will lessen and eventually you can take off the armour because the rounds will either miss their target completely or dissolve into the cosmic fabric as you smile.

Once you reach this stage your armour becomes your awareness. You enter that present state of equilibrium, becoming your own master, not a slave to your external environment. You live from the heart and from within this mysterious cavern of harmony, life flows. Nothing bothers you. You feel at one with all things and you blend with your environment. You realize that everything is an extension of your own cosmic make-up and that you get to influence your reality. You step into your Super-Human genius selfless self and let your inner alchemist out to play, subtly changing your environment with your thoughts, feelings and emotions and observing everything around you, taking the charge out of every potential detonator.

Within you is the potential for all things, including so-called good and evil. You can hug and love and maim and kill. We all have the potential to unfold in every which way possible. A true master accepts this, harnesses this and uses the scope of wisdom lying within the epicentre of each physical cell, droplet of blood, bone fragment or bio-photon of light to choose that which will add value to the world and assist our planet in her own personal growth, so she can cleanse the home of her children (our physical world) and that of her celestial body, hovering in infinite space, playing holographically in a quantum world.

Observation is so important, as is non-interference and the ability to never explain your actions and decisions. Once you master these three elements, playing the game of life, in the thick of the action, is easy. All you have to do then is watch out for that good old, trusted friend, Mr/Mrs Ego, getting bored and wanting some mild stimulation, which always leads to the excessive kind if you let him/her out of their cage. On the other hand, when properly understood, your ego can be used to guide and assist you and keep you on the railroad track. When you observe your ego, you experience massive contrast and this contrast shows you where you are, where you could be and, more importantly, where you don't want to be or go.

The Wisdom of Acceptance

When we accept that the universe has a plan and that we will never truly understand the vastness of this grand cosmic play unfolding around us, and come to terms with the fact that we don't actually know what's best and that interfering with the natural flow always ultimately comes back to bite us in the butt, we enter a fluid stream that caresses obstacles in its path. Like water, we flow down the river of life, ebbing around the rocks, stroking them gently as we pass.

Acceptance in all situations allows the armour-piercing rounds to drop before their target, in this case you. You take a potential vibration-lowering situation and turn it into light, pure, dazzling, brilliant white light, and carry on moving. A true alchemist turns all situations into positivity, drawing and utilizing the energy. Now, when it comes to another human being passing back to spirit, there will always be emotions involved. We are in this human realm of physicality and emotions, after all, but when you can look at it from a spiritual standpoint, you realize there is harmony in death, beauty in the transition from one vessel to another or from one form to no form.

Maybe when we transition from our bodies, we also become so much more? We enter a vast and expansive cosmic dance, with no boundaries. Maybe death should be celebrated and not feared? When we accept all situations, there is zero judgement, no labelling and therefore pure observation. It's this observational standpoint that allows us to not interfere. When we look and judge, or look and label a situation as good or bad, we send signals into our brain and it communicates with our body and tells us to do more, to act, to step in and change the situation.

We must, as humans, start living in harmony with nature and nature's natural flow. We can remember how to build in harmony with the contours of the land, and that man and Earth can be two halves of the same coin, dark and light, blended together, working as a team, instead of man thinking we rule the roost and destroying the lands at will. Look at what happened in Thailand in 2004: greedy, money-hungry developers built their hotels on orange groves and too close to the shoreline and a tsunami came and Mother Earth reclaimed her land.

We live in a world of energy, playing the game of cause and effect. What you put out comes back to you, not because it's good or bad but because of the frequency, the energy you let out into this world. Every thought, feeling and emotion will be accounted for. Remember, you are in control of all three. So, start taking responsibility right now.

Once you have mastered non-interference and taking an observational standpoint, then comes one of humanity's greatest tests: the ability to never explain oneself. This is so tough for most people. As we grow up we are conditioned to please other people. We are taught that if we don't please others, they will not love us. This is a lesson that is taught without explanation. A child gets told off for doing things wrong and so the child, who only wants to be loved, does everything in their power to be loved, to feel love and to make parents, grandparents, teachers happy. This sets up a dysfunctional behaviour pattern and the child forgets who they truly are. The child grows up explaining their actions and reactions, thoughts and courses of action because they want to be accepted and loved. This is not a good and harmonious situation: when you feel the need to explain, you are not fully in love with yourself. When you do love yourself and you know yourself and you are living life by your own values and rules and not those of others, you really do not care what other people think.

For us to truly be at peace and master our own consciousness, we must not be influenced by what others think or feel towards us. If their behaviour towards us changes, we must not bat an eyelid. We must smile and go about our day in awe of our own magnificence. Stop being a people-pleaser. Love who you are and step into your own power as a sovereign being living and playing on Mother Earth's lands. She is happy to share them with us as long as we respect them; but if we don't respect ourselves first and foremost, how are we ever going to respect her?

Move away from the trance state that most humans are in, wanting instant gratification with zero or little effort. Realize that it takes effort to be extraordinary. It takes courage to be your very best version, to swim against the tide of the indoctrinated human herd. Remember, you are the most powerful being that has ever graced these Earthly shores, as am I. Let's be that force of nature. Let's flow and move with the universal tides. Let's be our own master and do what fills our hearts with bliss.

EXERCISE *Body Love*

I have an exercise I would like you to do right now. I want you to connect with your body, your organs, your bones and any sensations inside your body, positive feelings or painful feelings. Remember, pain isn't bad, it's an opportunity to heal. We will call this exercise Body Love!

I want you to close your eyes and sit or stand or lie in silence for 45 minutes–1 hour (or as long as it takes) and I would like you to do this every day for the next 21 days.

Start by opening your heart and feeling love. Open your heart wide, see and feel love, light, energy pouring out into your immediate field and surrounding you. Let it spill out for several minutes until you feel joy, bliss, divinity surrounding you and filling your space.

Next, I want you to scan your body, inside and out, with your consciousness. Feel every part of you, create space around every part of you and talk with it. Start with your feet. Bring your awareness into your feet, feel your feet and the space around them. Observe them from the outside and also bring your awareness inside them and feel them. Hold your awareness there and ask your feet how they feel, and then be. Let your feet communicate with you through feeling. If you feel any pain or tiredness or hurt in any way, shape or form, I want you to open your heart wider and love that part of you and continue to open your heart. Spend a few minutes loving your feet, being grateful to them and being with them.

Your energy follows your attention and focus. So, by loving your feet and any pain there, you will transmute it. The key is not to think. The key is to be and feel them.

You then do the same with your legs, followed by your hips, buttocks and groin, then stomach, then your back, then your spinal column and ribcage, then arms, then hands, then neck and throat and then your head and face.

Afterwards, you are going to focus on some internal organs. Firstly, your kidneys and adrenal glands, then your liver, followed by your gall bladder, pancreas, spleen, stomach, large and small intestines, heart and then lungs. Then talk to your eyes and your ears. Finally, you are going to bring your whole awareness up into the centre of your brain and back slightly (where your pineal gland or third eye is) and hold your awareness there.

The entire time you are going through this exercise, it's important that you breathe deeply. Long, slow, deep breaths in and out of your body. Ask the different body parts how they are feeling right now. Tell your body that you love it. Get to know how you truly feel. Not how you think you feel – go deep and truly get to "innerstand" your own vibration.

Your Body Is Truly Incredible

During this 21-day process, you will get to know your body better than ever. You will connect with you on a level you may have never connected before. Your body will appreciate the loving attention and your awareness will heighten. This is the perfect precursor to what is in store as we journey deep together. You are going to feel your body and you may be surprised at what your body tells you as you connect with it. It may communicate through feeling, or you may hear your body talk to you. Most of us take our body for granted and give it zero attention. I mean, when was the last time you sat down and had a conversation with your feet? Your legs? They carry you everywhere, yet you put on your jeans or trousers and socks and shoes and forget about them. It's time to reconnect – or maybe connect for the very first time.

There are going to be many other exercises I ask you to do as you read on. You can start them as you are going through this process, or you can do the twenty-one days and then come back and start the other exercises after. Personally, I recommend you do these twenty-one days and then start the rest, but it is your call. I am not here to tell you what to do. I can only speak from personal experience; what has worked best for me and my clients. Also, I am going to be sharing a plan with you at the end of this book. You may want to start this exercise now and forget about all the others until you have finished reading. Or you may want to dip your toe into a few. It's entirely up to you.

Spiritual Warrior

You are now taking the necessary beginning steps to change your subatomic nature, to be the light frequency you are inside this human vehicle. You are going to grow in courage and confidence and feel strong mentally, emotionally, physically, and spiritually. You will not only feel, but you will also *be* it. Your true warrior nature will rise to the surface as you begin to live fearlessly. You will realize, if you haven't already, that mediocrity is a disease and rising above it requires your true warrior nature to step into the forefront of your consciousness and lead.

Upon becoming a master of dark and light, a real Super-Human who lives by the code, embracing the fullness, richness and unquenchable taste of mastery, a man or woman steps into the space only a warrior of the spiritual arts can own.

Here I have listed the attributes of a spiritual warrior, what you are at the core of your being and what you are now allowing to rise within you. Read these carefully, print them off and hang them on your wall. These fourteen ways of the force are more important than the Ten Commandments.

Some of these ways may not sit with you right now and that is OK. As you go through this book you will know the truth and feel it deep within you, as one by one each and every one of them resonate.

1. A warrior is on permanent guard against the roughness of human behaviour. A warrior is magical and ruthless, a maverick with the most refined taste and manners, whose worldly task is to sharpen, yet disguise his cutting edges so that no one would be able to suspect his or her ruthlessness.

2. A warrior is ready to strike or defend, poised silently and calmly in the dead of night or the light of day when the situation, whether it be physical or ethereal, descends into their space. Aware and ruthless, the warrior sees everything: visible and invisible; to the warrior they are one and the same.

3. A warrior knows that on the precipice of adventure and mystical action, darkness and light become one. To run to or away from one or the other weakens the wise warrior's senses and leaves them open to manipulation.

4. A warrior will stand in truth, speak their truth and live their truth, in all situations, with no concern for the reactions of others upon hearing of his or her truth. The warrior is ruthless to the core, but with zero aggression in every moment; enforcing boundaries and knowing that controlled force itself is sometimes necessary, and aggression is a weakening of the soul.

5. A warrior is kind in combat, loving in war and happy in action, as the warrior sees no good or bad. A warrior fears nothing and loves even his or her own enemy, knowing

that the final strike will carve a lesson so deep into his or her soul that the warrior will be eternally grateful. The final strike is a blending of energies and a returning to the zero-point of creation, where the warrior and the enemy love once again. The warrior and the enemy, after all, are one and the same and are each other's greatest teachers.

6. A warrior will lead when necessary and listen intently always. The warrior's power lies in his or her silence as they glide, swoop or sail, stealthily, on their spiritual quest to open the hearts of many and raise the vibration of all.

7. The warrior knows there is no turning back. The warrior knows that they were placed in this space for a reason they may never truly comprehend, and they will give selflessly and receive graciously in all situations.

8. A warrior is strong and courageous yet humble and undistinguished, never seeking worth but knowing their worth deep in their crystal core. A warrior is ruthless and wrathful and impeccable in every moment.

9. The warrior distinguishes the weapon of choice, that of love, and uses it fearlessly, ruthlessly, and unequivocally, knowing that often love is harsh and it's the warrior's balanced and centred harshness that keeps him or her protected on their unwinding and otherworldly mission.

10. A warrior embraces danger in the same manner he or she would drink a glass of water. A warrior smiles in the face of adversity and the crumbling of the warrior's body is a choice that he or she makes when their work is done and the Earthly experience reaches its chosen exit point, and no time sooner.

11. A warrior knows not of death but transition. A warrior knows not of birth but transition. A warrior knows their sustenance flows from the ether and is not bound by Earthly pursuits of happiness and endeavour.

12. A warrior is a warrior because they chose this path while sat on a cloud of stardust, observing the multiple, infinite timelines, cascading and converging into the centre point of creation. A warrior lives by a code; that code is truth.

13. A warrior lives, embodies, and breathes in the code of this warrior life force to the depths of their cosmic spiritual DNA as he or she cracks open the fountain of knowledge that lies in the deep cavern of mystery, which humanity calls the heart, and the warrior knows as intelligence.

14. A warrior's temperament is that of a lion or lioness; the point of absolute stillness before they strike their prey, sensing their total surroundings, the crystal clarity of every vibration in the environment enables the lion or the lioness to act with absolute certainty, always hitting the mark. Discernment in every situation rises as the humble essence of the warrior's spirit lives to dance the universal dance and embody total light, showing his or her sisters and brothers how to create heaven on Earth as they walk the path of mastery.

You cannot transcend what you do not know. To go beyond yourself, into the mystical depths of your soul, you must first know yourself. Stillness is the key. What you discover may not always be pleasant – in fact I guarantee what you come face to face with will be challenging, and this is why going within is so difficult for most. It is however the most rewarding and fulfilling journey.

A journey filled with rocks, mountains, windy rivers, sunshine, and storms. A journey with no end, or at least one you cannot see, for now, while this long and breathtaking unfolding of multiple layers continues to reveal itself. You continue to slither through the undergrowth like a snake, rebirthing and rebirthing as you discover multiple versions of yourself, existing in the eternal now, across multiple time spaces, playing within numerous frequency bands all at the same time.

This journey is for the brave and ruthless spiritual warrior who knows they don't know yet, and in that simple "innerstanding" their entire universe opens up into a beautiful, sublime, yet crazy, chaotic, magical wonderland of eternal bliss.

One thing is for sure, the spiritual warrior will never get bored as they follow the infinite path to nowhere, bathing in light, rolling in darkness, climbing through storms and exploring, in dream time, the vast and expansive cosmic playground we call our universe, home to trillions of planets and stars. This is a trip. A real trip. Better than any drug on the planet. So, submerge yourself in life. Submerge yourself within yourself and buy a first-class ticket to this epic adventure called humanity.

In my life I have experienced the extremities of both dark and light and both have helped polish and carve and sculpt me. I recommend that each and every human being embraces whatever enters their space, with love not fear, and engages to "Innerstand" the lessons. There is gold to be mined from every situation. Hundreds of metres of rock may lie on top of the swimming-pool-sized gold mine and yet the woman or man keeps digging, knowing that fortune lies within the sweat, blood and tears and months (often years) of work to reach the prize. Seemingly tough situations (at face value) carry your greatest growth opportunities. Face everything head on and grow. Others will sharpen you. Remember, steel sharpens steel. A warrior will learn more from a strong, fast, agile, and fit opponent than from someone he or she kills in one single blow.

Others will show you parts of your human nature you may not want to see. Life is a mirror, and that mirror will keep showing up until you embrace, go within, develop, and grow. You are a warrior, beautiful soul. It's your time to expand and evolve, so accept and embrace life in all its glory.

Density Shift

This is such an interesting time on Planet Earth. As a species we are evolving rapidly. Consciousness is exploding in the hearts of many and our global vibration is skyrocketing. On the other hand, the world is getting crazier and crazier. Or is it? I see more control within the system every day, especially financially. Our cashless society could be catastrophic, as it may equal slavery. Or will it? Once there is zero cash and your money is all on screens and in the control of corporations (yes, corporations, because that is what banks are), and you can only access your money if you have this microchip, what will you do? Will you say yes or no? Ask yourself, what would my fearless inner warrior do in this situation? Say yes out of fear or embrace the unknown and say no? Or maybe your inner warrior is creating the alternative (to money) reality now, by planning and preparing, knowing the unfolding of events, as she or he has seen the future?

Maybe this cashless society is a good thing, and our beloved corporate bankers and those who believe they are at the top of the food chain, pulling the puppet strings, will be doing this for the good and grace of our human species and it will make life easier, having microchipped bodies to access our own money, as is already happening in countries including Sweden. Maybe you need to realize that it's on you and you only and that destiny is your hands?

On Earth and in our galaxy, there is a huge shift taking place. It's not a one-off in time. We have been experiencing huge density shifts for the last thirty to forty years. Recently, however, these shifts are getting stronger and more powerful. Spirals of light are streaming into our local environment, carrying light-encoded messages that are triggering us to awaken. The codes contained in the light are opening us up to knowledge and wisdom held on a subatomic, cellular DNA level and we are growing, expanding, awaking to deep truths.

Earth's Galactic History

Earth is an interesting planet. It's the heart (heart centre/chakra) of our galaxy. It was also originally dedicated to being used as a living library by the Seraphim/Lyran races, our galactic ancestors, and for 750 billion years wars have been waged throughout the galaxy and beyond, some of which have been for control of Earth. Because of its bountiful storehouse of minerals, crystals, gold resources and other metals, it was/ is the perfect planet to store information. High-vibrational beings decided that records from other planets, stars and galactic homes would store records within Earth and make it into this living library. Underground crystal cathedrals and crystal cities were created by these powerful, high-vibrational beings, to store information and create/harness energy.

Earth is also home to a Star Gate system that is extremely special. Through the Star Gate system here on Earth you can travel pretty much anywhere in the galaxy. Billions of years ago there were the Lyran wars. During these conflicts in space between extra-terrestrials that wanted free will and the Law of One to prevail and beings that wanted to rule with force and control, Star Gates in the cradle of Lyra were destroyed and our matrix became detached from the whole. From that point in time, our system was hijacked. These wars between extra-terrestrials are still being fought today on many planets, in many dimensions, and Earth is one of them.

Humans are the original guardians of Earth and humans carry the crystal keys that give us star-gate access. If human beings were not here on Earth, the Star Gates would close for ever. It is a failsafe mechanism that was deliberately installed by guardian races. The aim of those extra-terrestrials that want to control Earth was to keep us here; but they also knew they must make us stupid. It's why the majority of humanity is still asleep, walking around in a dream state, oblivious to the truth about their potential, fixed in an external, materialistic world. It was designed this way to stop humanity accessing this knowledge and wisdom. War has continued to rage over this planet (and others), between those forces who wanted control and domination and those beings who wanted peace and freedom. There are also many facets of the controlling forces, warring with each other here on Earth, in human bodies. This battle is still going on. It is being fought by us humans here on Earth and is mirroring battles that are playing out in the higher-dimensional playgrounds and throughout the entire multidimensional matrix. Most of us do not know it, as when we arrive here from other planets, stars, dimensional spaces, densities, or cycle back from Earth over and over, our memory is erased, blank-slated, and we have to figure it out all over again. We knew this before we came because we knew the importance of humanity, Earth and the major force it is within the galaxy. If Earth were destroyed, the galaxy would tip out of balance and there would be a chain reaction. Many other species would be affected and so you and I, along with many other galactic warriors, working to create peace and harmony, descended here on a mission. We are the galactic ground crew. The cosmic SAS.

Everyone thought 2012 was the end of the Mayan calendar but in actuality it was supposed to be the end of the world. Negative beings played around with Earth's mechanics (the planetary rod and staff) and planned to destroy Earth and in doing so, use its quantum energy for their own agenda. Powerful guardian beings prevented this happening.

The crystal cathedral and crystal city networks were encoded with huge energy patterns and strong frequency waves that would bombard our planet with light when we needed it. In August 2017 the crystal cathedrals were activated, and light started pouring up from inside the Earth as well as pouring down from the grand central sun and triggering major consciousness shifts at ground zero. January/February 2019 was another massive shift as the crystal city networks were activated. This changed our frequency again. 12D currents (flowing from the original primary light and sound fields) have been more widely available on Earth since 2012, although they were available before for those who knew how to access them through meditation and other conscious means.

The Krystal Spiral: Our True Timeline

The huge density shift on Earth has caused a huge ripple, within our time-space reality but also across multiple frequency bands or densities. Within the space we live on Earth, there are other realities, on different frequency bands, all taking place. They have their own atmospheres, moons, suns, and environments. Something incredible happened at the end of 2020. The suns, moons, and stars from each of these Earthly frequency bands all aligned, and another huge density shift took place. It was happening through the build-up to the winter solstice and continued on into the new year. Cosmic portals were opened, and massive waves of plasma energies came streaming in. This multidimensional alignment was huge for the positioning and continuation of humanity moving along our Krystal Spiral Timeline. This has created a huge shift in the collective along with the activation of crystal cities lying in the Earth, again on a different frequency. They have

created an elevated vibrational field and a huge consciousness explosion has occurred.

It's important to know that beyond our present frequency band, in this 3D/4D reality, fear, greed, and corruption are no longer a necessity for us (as souls incarnated in other realities) and so here on this plane of existence, the same goes for our soul's experience. It doesn't mean that fear, greed, and corruption do not exist in higher-dimensional spaces because they do, but for us as a species, shifting from this lower vibrational reality, a choice point on the Krystal Spiral Timeline is where we cross over and leave these behind; and those humans who choose will carry on, living the Fibonacci Timeline (imploding/limiting mathematics) where corruption and manipulation will thrive. Eventually those who choose this lower timeline will die and return to stardust and those who choose the connection to Source, and to activate their original blueprint, will create the potential to become eternal beings as they ascend. As I said before, all has its place and nothing is good or bad, just experience, and we must, as an evolving species, choose our experience within the cosmic framework being applied.

Many will hold on to what they know until the collective vibration forces them to surrender to unconditional love. Many will be pulled onto the new timeline, but some will stay. All potentials are available. The choice is with the Hu-Man! Remember, Hu (hue) means colour. We are colourful beings. There is so much choice in colour. Why would you go dark? Why would you go light? Why limit yourself when the spectrum of light/possibility is infinite?

What we can do as an aware element of our human tribe is activate our frequency templates/blueprints, lying within dormant DNA strands to further elevate our vibration and move this whole human experience into the next octave of evolution at a faster pace. We carry this power!

Fear and Other Feelings

In other realities, our quantum selves (because each one of us is a light source/energy/soul, having multiple other experiences) have been shifting out of many karmic/energetic pulses/patterns. We live in an energetic universe and if you give off a frequency, whether it be a mental thought, an emotional response, a physical action that is of a lower vibration, the waves of light/information/ energy flow out through the fabric of the cosmos and will return to you at some point. You are not being punished (which many believe, calling it karma); you are simply creating your reality. Your thoughts, actions, emotions are the building blocks that give you the creative quantum abilities to design your own reality. Most people are simply on autopilot, creating a reality full of chaos.

So, shifting out of karmic/energetic pulses/ patterns requires us to let go of fear in all other realities. There is a spectrum of emotions and love and fear are at the two ends of this spectrum. Any other emotion is a diluted version of one of these or a slightly varied vibrational version. Happiness, joy, bliss, ecstasy, are all responses produced by feeling love. Anger, guilt, jealousy, hatred, anxiety are all emotional responses produced through some kind of fear. That's what I mean when I say "fear" here.

The enormous energy wave that has been sent across our planet, through multiple densities/ realities, is gigantic. It has cleared so much trauma and now, here on Earth, we no longer need to play out the roles of human victims, living in a game that perpetually cycles drama through our daily lives. The opportunity is still there within the Fibonacci mathematics, but it's a choice for the aware human. Maybe, one day, after years of experiencing love, joy, and harmony, you forget what it's like to experience pain or guilt or fear or rejection, so you decide to have a lower vibrational experience, to remind you of why you moved away from it. Sometimes that contrast is priceless.

Because of the group collective and the massive manipulation that has taken place here on Earth, it's tough for most of the herd to see or feel beyond their feelings and their physical reality. But a Super-Human recognizes what is taking place at a subatomic level and goes beyond the thoughts and feelings of the mind and body and brings themselves into the space of bliss, joy, harmony. They make life a constant meditation, where they become the observer of their thoughts and emotions, and when this is done regularly, they take control of their consciousness. Life no longer triggers them, and they free themselves from the mental and emotional constructs of this game we call life.

It's important that you go beyond your body, beyond your thoughts, and start creating a garden of Zen internally, through the ways of being that I am going to lay down for you in this book.

The topic of human manipulation is vast, and I could write a series of books on this subject alone. This book, however, is about you becoming Super-Human, and I simply want you to be aware. Not to trust your thoughts, not to trust anything that anyone ever tells you, including me. I want you to take control by living from your heart space and feeling everything; internalize it and know it. If it's not your truth, let it go and move on. It's all just information, after all. You can choose to plug into whatever information streams you wish.

Just know that massive spirals of energy, galactic streams of information will be hitting this planet for many years and it's going to be an interesting time. Consciousness is expanding and our global family is elevating and unifying. We must distinguish between the truth of our heart and the manipulation of the mind. We must stay on the frequency of love, something you will find very easy if you follow the ways of being I share in this book.

Density shifts are never easy for any species, but for humans they are especially difficult because our bodies have become our masters.

What do I mean? Our bodies become addicted to the chemicals of trauma. It's why a woman will stay in a marriage where she is beaten, and if she does leave will find another man who does the same; because each time she suffers, chemicals are released, and the body becomes addicted to those chemicals. They can be near-impossible patterns to break. But by going beyond the body, by becoming quantum, you will create the perfect healing environment inside of you and any deep trauma, held within you, will dissolve.

When a traumatic event takes place, adrenaline is spiked into the cells; but, it has a shelf life. Like milk in a fridge that's been open for too long, it goes off and smells funny and tastes sour after several days. The adrenaline in your body does the same. If we don't let it go, release our emotions, then this toxicity lies there, waiting for another traumatic event to play out, and then this adrenaline compounds on top of the last lot. Eventually you become ill or suffer an injury or disease. This is simply your body reaching out to you to ask you to look inside and release these toxic emotions. The body, after all, is a highly advanced communication device.

The other issue here is that our body craves these chemical releases so much that it will do everything in its power to get the fix. A little like a crack addict needing his or her next fix, when the human being will often beg or steal to get their lips around a full pipe. When a traumatic event takes place, we often harbour it, think about it and play it over and over again inside our head. This is called a refractory period. The longer you stew over something, the longer this period goes on for. Sometimes it can be days, other times weeks, and into months and years in some cases. These chemicals are feeding the addiction. The longer someone is addicted (the longer the refractory period), the harder it is to break the habitual pattern.

Creating Reality from Our Thoughts and Feelings

As a species we are mental. Literally insane. We are like 9 billion mental patients living in a global mental ward. This is no exaggeration. Mental illness is defined as "any of various *disorders* characterized by impairment of an individual's thoughts, emotions, or social functioning, including schizophrenia and mood *disorders* such as bipolar *disorder*". When I googled "definition of insanity", I found this:

> **insanity.** *Mental illness of such a severe nature that a person cannot distinguish fantasy from reality, cannot conduct her/his affairs due to psychosis, or is subject to uncontrollable impulsive behaviour.*

If a person has a business disagreement and loses a large sum of money and then plays this event out, over and over in their head, for the next six years on and off, creating highs and lows of emotions, it creates a situation where they cannot handle their affairs and are subject to uncontrollable and impulsive behaviours. When a person plays something over and over in their mind, they trigger the emotional response and those chemicals are released over and over, poisoning the body and increasing the addiction.

What is even more crazy is this. We create pure fantasies to feed our addiction. Now, it's one thing playing an event over and over in your mind, years after it's happened; but it's another ball game altogether creating something that doesn't exist to feed the addiction. This is where we truly define the human species as an insane bunch fit for the asylum.

I am going to give you an example of what happened to me in meditation, not too long ago. Before I do, I want to remind you that I was fostered and adopted as a kid. My mother was mentally and physically traumatized during labour, my first foster-parents sexually abused me, my adoptive mother used to pull my pants down, bend me over the bed and hit me with a wooden ruler and my first schoolteacher (when I was five years old) pulled my pants down and smacked my bum in the middle of the class. So, rejection and lack of trust in women are patterns I have been working on since I embarked on this inward quest, and every now and again they surface. My refractory periods last only seconds these days, but every now and again the brain and body still search for those chemicals.

So, I was meditating, and I saw a thought. I observed it. It was of my girlfriend. Then I watched my head place my girlfriend in a bar. Next there was a guy. I knew I could have stopped this at any time by shifting my inner perspective, but I was not emotionally engaged so I didn't mind. I was simply observing and wanted to see how far the mind would take it. Next, they are talking, and he invites her home. I see them travelling in a car and then they enter a house, and he starts to kiss her. Now, I was simply observing my mind doing this. The thoughts, the images. It did all of this on its own because the body was desperate to experience the feelings of rejection and lack of trust. At this point I changed my inner focus. I then started laughing, I opened my eyes and was saying out loud, 'we are all mental, we are all mental.' I was at a tourist spot in Madeira at the time and the people around me, watching me laughing and shouting to myself, probably thought I really was mental.

And, they would have been a hundred per cent spot on! I think you will agree that creating something inside of your mind that doesn't exist, and allowing your body to feel the emotional response from it, is crazy. People have arguments with other people in their head, they are mean to people, get bullied, watch loved ones die, lose their job, imagine a car crash: all sorts of crazy events are created inside of our heads. The problem is that our subconscious mind doesn't know the difference between reality and what is going on upstairs, so we literally are creating our reality, mentally, emotionally, and vibrationally; and so eventually, with enough of those emotionally charged thoughts and images, whether positive or negative, we will make it real.

With this unveiling of the truth, and bringing deep-seated trauma to the surface, it's imperative that we observe our thoughts and emotions and not become them. We must step into our divinity and live authentically from our heart. We must be beacons of light and show others that we do not need to suffer. The age of the victim is no more. Be of service, love fearlessly, hug tightly, never be the first to let go, and use your heart and your vibration as your satellite navigation to keep you on the path of purity.

The faster we vibrate, the quicker everyone else will catch up with this multidimensional density shift. It's time to let go and surrender and totally trust in your heart-centred human experience. Time on Earth is getting REAL exciting!

I love you and respect you, you awesome warrior from the stars!

4

Preparation and Discipline

I have shared with you some of my personal experiences and demonstrated that there is much to remember, know and access, beyond this illusory veil. You know there is so much taking place energetically on this planet and I have only scratched the surface with you, just to open the door and plant the seed, to make you aware if you were not already.

In life, most people are never ready when their opportunity comes and so they dodge it, let it pass, often through fear. Fear of not being good enough, fear of failure, fear of succeeding and not being able to handle it, fear of loss if it goes wrong. Most of the best inventions, books, businesses, lie six feet under in the graveyard because people don't take action. It's sad but true. Each one of us carries wisdom, potential power and unique and magical gifts the world craves to experience, but fear stops most people sharing and expressing their truths, their authentic truths, which carry the energy of inspiration, joy, unity, and unconditional love.

In life, preparation is mission critical. We say some people are lucky, but there is no such thing as luck. Luck is when preparation meets opportunity. The problem is that a lot of our species take things for granted and have gotten lazy. If you knew that soldiers were coming through your lands and you and your family could potentially be tortured or killed, you would be ready. You wouldn't sit around idly, waiting for the inevitable. If you knew it was coming you would get up and take action.

Right now, the soldiers are already at your front door, they are inside your home, inside your bedroom. They already have your children captive.

They are not doing it through brute force, they are much more cunning and have them captive of their own free will. This is what's crazy about this planet right now. The technology we have at our fingertips is enslaving us. It's also incredible, though, because we get to communicate with our fellow sisters and brothers from across the water, women and men who we may have never met. There are positives and negatives in all situations.

Music is on everyone's phone. It's the biggest weapon of mass destruction, taking youngsters (and adults) out of their hearts and into their heads or into their lower false chakras (I will talk about false chakras later). Not all music is like this, of course, but the majority of modern mainstream music is.

Social media has become a way for teenagers to communicate, even with their friends who live a five-minute walk away. What happened to going out to play, jumping streams, hanging around, climbing trees, walking through the woods, kicking a ball about, cherry-knocking and doing the stuff kids did twenty-plus years ago?

What we must do as a species is embrace technology and utilize it to our advantage, to connect, share positive information to inspire and set people free – and then leave it alone. All the answers to all of our questions lie within our heart and once you become aware you realize that external information always guides you back to your centre. We carry lifetimes upon lifetimes of information in our subatomic structure and within the invisible (to the naked eye) field there is all the data (information) we require. Once our pineal gland, our third eye, is operating efficiently, and our heart and brain are in coherence, we can tap into this data.

We are supermen and superwomen who do not know yet that we are supermen and superwomen. Or maybe you do? We have a planet to elevate – I won't say rescue, but elevate –and in elevating the vibration of the planet, we will naturally lift it into new and inspiring, multidimensional heights where love is our number one commodity. To do this, we must look into our hearts and ask this question: "If the human species continues on this trajectory, will our children, grandchildren and great-grandchildren be enslaved in a mental prison (and eventually a physical prison), consumed by mind-numbing technology, eating dead food, playing video games that by then will be a part of our consciousness and not hand-held devices (we will be the video game and that this is not that far away if you look at the Metaverse being introduced by our old buddy Mark Zuckerberg) and paying half of our income for the new liquid gold, water?"

The answer is a gigantic yes.

We can, if we embrace this situation, take action and shift the trajectory massively by realigning ourselves with our natural and inherent gifts, connecting back to our planet and allowing the beauty of our green and blue ball to flourish and us as a species to thrive beyond measure, loving, creating, exploring and unifying as one divine intelligence, just like the ancient lands of Lemuria in its glory days.

We must become disciplined in our approach. Anyone who achieves anything in their life is focused, dedicated, and disciplined. The great thing is, to be a Super-Human is actually fun, transformative and exciting, as you expand on this journey. You do have to be disciplined but that does not mean the fun goes out of life. You simply have to dedicate yourself to do the

work, which isn't really work. You simply have to reallocate your time and be consistent. A lot of people choose to do new things, whether they be exercise or a business venture, and quit within a month, sometimes sooner. Starting is easy, following through and being consistent is where most people fail. I am going to be encouraging you to change your ways and adopt a new lifestyle. Instead of watching television, do qigong (not any old qigong but Star Magic style; as you will experience soon, it's a turbocharged version); instead of scrolling through Facebook, spend a little time doing some super-transformative breathing exercises, go to bed a little earlier and get up a little earlier so you can meditate and activate your pineal gland. These are three simple lifestyle choices that will change your entire perspective on life, kick-start a chain reaction of positive experiences, heighten your intuition and start the process of you becoming a Super-Human. I am going to lay out for you everything you require to be the very best version of you.

The ultimate word here is choice. You must be disciplined to make the right choices. Not the ones you are comfortable making, but the ones that will assist your human evolution, laying a positive and productive foundation for our next generation of Star Seeds.

People are lazy these days. It's a fact. The next generation doesn't understand hard work, dedication, effort. But once we start that inner journey, with discipline, we will discover our power, a formidable strength that is uncorruptible and infinite.

There is no immediate life hack that will take you to your end result. Why? Because there is no end result. Perfection doesn't exist when you seek out the very best. Why? Because there is always another level to strive for. Only by executing a life of discipline, geared towards a purpose or goal that you not only love but become healthily obsessed by and healthily addicted to, will you truly live, succeed, be happy and stretch the envelope of your human potential, as you progress, day by day, steadily on your mission.

Right Choices

We as adults, parents who are awake, have the opportunity to change the course of our entire human species, to create powerful, critical thinking, open-hearted, expanded multidimensional beings. What choice will you make? A few months ago, I was on a humanitarian mission in Cambodia with my friend. We did some awesome work assisting our fellow sisters and brothers. After we finished, we had a couple of days in the city of Phnom Penh before we flew out. As soon as we arrived in the city the energy was so heavy, full of lower vibrational forces. There were prostitutes, men and women from the ages of ten years on every street corner, loads of them, drugs and bars and the environment was intense. We hired a tuk-tuk and Lucky, the driver, kept offering choices. You want to go shoot AK47s or go to a temple? You want to go shoot elephants or go to a museum? We were bombarded with choices that would have led to completely different vibrational experiences. We chose the temples and the museums over the AKs and elephant hunts.

In life, you constantly have choices to elevate your frequency or lower your vibration; with every turn, conversation or action. The amazing thing is that we are all in control of our choices. Unfortunately, we are creatures of comfort and tend to stick to what we know. So, the majority of the time we do the things that keep us stagnant, keep us safe (or so we think), keep us comfortable, even if it's to the detriment of our health, well-being, mental clarity and the future of our species. Maybe you think I am exaggerating? Well, right now you get to make a choice. This is the point in this book where we get down to some action and have to make some very important decisions. This is where you decide to either close the book and go back to what you know, where you feel safe, your nice comfortable daily routine where no harm will come to you, or you decide to ride this magical wave, take off your gloves, saddle up, commit to this process and do what is necessary to elevate your vibration, expand your consciousness, become a high-vibrational Super-Human and unify with the rest of your brave fellow spiritual warriors who know that action must be taken, en masse, now, so we can alter the destructive course our species is on and take us all into a world beyond golden, a new dawn, a new age of human, the platinum and diamond age of the Super-Human.

People say to me: Jerry, you work too hard, you are obsessed, you are too full-on, how do you manage everything you have going on and still go to the gym every day? I seek out discomfort as I know it's the only way to grow fiercely. I am an untamed lion, a beast, and that is the way that I will stay. Having a savage mentality means you will never let yourself get comfortable, like pro athletes who retire, have made money and get lazy, stop training and put on weight. I am focused on my mission and no thing, no human, no human hybrid, no malevolent being, will ever stop me in my tracks. I stay hungry, like a lion on the hunt every day, wanting to go further, expand, grow, assist more of humanity on my quest with Star Magic. I detest mediocrity. In fact, I am shit-scared of mediocrity and stay as far away from it as possible. Most people are praised for their mediocre efforts and that is why they never excel, because mediocre only takes you to the bottom of the hill – halfway up it at best. The top of the hill for me is the warm-up. I know there are many hilltops beyond the first one and those hilltops will grow larger, into mountain ranges, with peak after peak. I will never stop climbing and once I reach the highest peak, I will just find a way to fly higher.

The process laid down in this book, the ideas, exercises and ways to unleash and harness your potential, are going to require you to focus, be disciplined and follow through. I have laid it all out, but only you can do the work. Remember this: discipline creates freedom. Failing to prepare is preparing to fail.

Apply the tools and you will be ready, prepared for anything and everything.

What are you going to do?

Self-Empowerment

Change can only be created by the one who is creating the change. Each one of us is our own saviour. No one is coming down from the heavens to rescue you, me or anyone else, and it's mission critical that you fully comprehend your own importance in the freeing of your mind, body and spirit. This adventure starts and finishes with you. You must take full responsibility and empower yourself.

When you choose this new way of being and start raising your vibration to that of a Super-Human, life may seem like it's falling apart for a little while. Friends, family members, your current life circumstances may change. Why? Because your frequency will change and so other aspects of reality that are not on your frequency will not interact with you, your life, your reality. We are playing a game, and all is energy. When you know how to control your vibrational rate, your thoughts and emotions, and live 24/7 in a place of Zen, the eternal now, the present moment, there is no room in your space for anything having a different energetic experience. It may seem a little messy for a while, somewhat chaotic, as relationships dissolve, business partnerships crumble, your interests shift and so your entire reality changes. It's a beautiful experience if you sit back and allow it to take place. The ego may fight for its illusory identity for a while, and that's OK; just be in a state of observation, take a non-judgemental standpoint and your old life will slide off of your back and your new life will rise from the cosmic fabric and become your new experience.

You will realize that you are the most important human being in your own universe and your love for you will increase, one-hundredfold plus. You will feel empowered, and you will fill up your own teacup with infinite, unconditional love. You will allow your teacup to overflow and spill out into your saucer, and it's from your saucer that you can give to others. You will, from time to time, retreat into silence when your teacup empties slightly, because you must replenish, in peace, raise your levels back up and then you can give to others. Functioning at 110 per cent is imperative. To be of service to humanity you must be overflowing. An empowered human being always puts their own energy first, enforces their boundaries and looks after themselves first and foremost, because they know that if their vibration dips, they will not be ready to assist others when needed.

For many years now, I have walked the planes of this Earth, travelled extensively, sharing what I know and remembering from others, my sisters and brothers of Earth. I used to be a criminal and now I live to share Star Magic, a healing frequency/modality/way of healing, with the world. I turned my life around, 180 degrees. If I can do it so can you or anyone else on this planet.

I have had many trials and tribulations and I know self-empowerment is the foundation upon which we can create and build a new world, for all of us to live in peace. When someone is offered power, they sometimes use it for the wrong reasons, or they become overwhelmed by it and crumble. There are others who build an indestructible Super-Human, carved from the fabric of their own adventures, and fearlessly carry a torch of inspiration to make this world a better place for all.

When a woman or man reaches deep into their own cosmic heart and journeys into the fabric of their own inner workings, a relationship is developed. This relationship is based on discovery and acceptance, a blending of multiple layers of human patterns and behaviours and spiritual consciousness and a gigantic realization, that nothing at all really matters. Not in the grand scheme of all that is. We realize our own significance and our own insignificance, and this is a true miracle.

When we step up onto this platform, we can truly build, grow, flourish. Some of the hard work has been done. The woman or man knows and accepts who or what they are and is ready to bring out their diamond cutting tools and start carving a master alchemist from the fabric of what they discovered. The journey is a continuous one, and that is the beauty of being a spiritual being having a human experience. Or should I say an extra-terrestrial being having a human experience? We are always carving, polishing, and refining our human selves, based on the ingredients in our soul's essence, interactions, and escapades.

The deeper we bore into our own consciousness, the more we find, the further we expand and the more ingrained it becomes, that we are all the same. We are light, information, playing in a holographic reality, and we know that love will melt away anything that does not serve us and allow our souls to bloom like an orchestra of bright flowers that have infiltrated a green field, letting off their fragrance and gracing the Earth with beauty. Our 9 billion population can bloom as an orchestra of light and that is what will happen. It is happening. That is my mission and the mission of many others, to see us rejoice once again as a global family.

So how does one become self-empowered? How does one become a master alchemist? How does one take a step back from the crowd, swim upstream and keep swimming against the tide of life that carries the herd, until they become the tide and move effortlessly through our worldly waters?

There are six mission-critical ingredients that one must live by to truly accomplish, flourish and stay focused on this path into the unknown and mysterious lands of exploration.

Self-Control

The first is self-control. This crazy human life with all of its twists and turns, created by people, situations and events, is a tricky road to navigate. We all want peace and harmony, abundance and happiness, but it seems being in the flow so one can experience all of this can be challenging to say the least. This human game, with its myriad of options on the emotional spectrum, its infinite daily choices and archaic, limited vocabulary, that is often misinterpreted by this thing we call perception, makes the game like no other. Without self-control it's easy to get caught up in everything happening around you and to engage in a destructive fashion. Of course, in certain situations you can be involved in a positive way. Well, one would think that; but we never really know what is for another's greatest growth, so non-interference, being the highest form of mastery, requires self-control. Self-control enables you to take a step back and observe all things, with zero judgement, perceiving each interaction from a neutral standpoint. Self-control gives you the stability to say no to things that are not conducive to your spiritual and human growth, such as low-vibrational food and low-vibrational people, two of our species' biggest distractions.

Right Thought

Right thought is next on the list. When we begin to choose our thoughts, the road to mastery is accelerated. The average human being has between 60,000 and 90,000 thoughts every day, swirling around in the background, creating so much static and noise. It's no wonder people lose their minds, make certain destructive decisions and get caught like a rabbit in the headlights, not knowing which course of action to take. To truly grow, we must choose to observe our thoughts.

This creates a much-needed gap between the human being and the thoughts in their head. The more you step back and observe the constant chatter, the more you realize how much nonsense goes on in your own mind.

A lot of the time the thoughts inside your head are other people's thoughts or thoughts sent into your consciousness by lower-vibrational beings, trying to bring you into a state of fear, which then gives them an opportunity to coerce you from behind the scenes on a subconscious level. Sometimes a contract is entered into between a human and another entity and the entity will live precariously through the woman, man or child in question or stay inside their energy field, siphoning energy and feeding when the human being is in a lower-vibrational state, nearer to the fear end of the spectrum, on the seesaw between love and fear. It's why we must choose love and live from our hearts every time. The head can be a dangerous place. This is why meditation is so important. Not the kind where you sit under a tree dressed in white, but the constant kind, where you are inside your body/heart, 24/7, 365, feeling your way through life.

Inside our heart we have 40,000 neurons that act like a mini brain. These neurons are what I would equate to a life compass. When you ask your head what you should do, you get mixed answers. The brain has a left and a right hemisphere and they function very differently. The heart however is not polar, like the brain. It is what it is and that is love, sovereignty and freedom. It is kind, compassionate and non-judgemental. If you ever have to make a decision, place the first three fingers of your right hand against your heart. When you place your hand on your heart, your awareness will go there and connect to the heart's neurons. You can then ask yourself the question at hand and your heart will assist you in feeling the answer, the best course of action. Connecting with your heart teaches you and helps you remember how to be present, be out of your head and not caught up in the bombardment of cyclical thoughts, thoughts from others, other beings or mind control devices that send waves through our airspace.

At Star Magic Facilitator Training Experiences and certain workshops, we remove the connection people have with these programmes and different entities, it's something we specialize in. If you have been to one of our Training Experiences, you will have witnessed some interesting sights.

So, it's imperative that you know how to live in your body and not react to life. When one lives inside the mind the potential to react is high. This is because there is a 0.25-second window between stimulus and response and so when you are in your head you react, quite often without even thinking about it, like a robot on autopilot. When you are living in your heart, you create space and clarity, and the triggers seem much further away. You observe the trigger through the space and can then make a calculated decision, either to carry on observing or to engage. You start responding instead of reacting. You will find that by continuing to observe, either the situation fizzles out or you get so much clarity that you either decide to walk away or to act with major precision and it all works out perfectly; when you connect consciously with the mini brain, the 40,000 neurons in your heart, your life compass, you start to truly master navigating this beautiful world.

Calmness

Calmness is a trait of every great leader. To be honest, people must step into their power and start leading themselves; but nonetheless, from the battlefield to the office, from the home to the football pitch, calmness is a crucial ingredient for the success of a relationship, war, sports match or business deal. Our emergency services are trained to stay calm; it would be no good them going into a panic on the other end of the phone.

Two people panicking is a disaster and in an emergency situation it will ultimately end painfully. When you live in your heart and observe your thoughts, you automatically hold a calm space and from here you can operate, conserve energy, and thrive in every situation. In a combat situation the calm fighter can last longer, picking and choosing their shots. In a relationship people press each other's buttons and it takes a calm and clear mind to take a step back, breathe and disengage as the egos will want to go to war. You can never fight fire with fire. We have all been in arguments and, once the situation has blown over, realized that it was pointless, but at the time you just couldn't back down. The ego becomes stubborn and cannot disengage. It requires a strong partner to smile and walk away and say I love you in the heat of the moment. When we do take this course of action, though, love melts away the so-called problem.

Action

Action comes next. Many people on this planet find it hard to take action and, even when they do, fade and dwindle and return to where they were very quickly. Maybe they are afraid of the hard work necessary, or maybe they are in fear of success or failure. Maybe in a relationship, the fear of rejection (something that has been huge in my life) stops them in their tracks. Maybe from communicating with the love of their life and letting them slip past, or maybe not opening up fully and showing their true self, their vulnerable side.

Others don't take action on a business opportunity or life goal for the reasons highlighted above, fear of failure or success. "What if I can't handle it?" "I will stay small and hide behind the curtains." As I mentioned previously, 90 per cent of the best inventions, books, ideas lie six feet under in the graveyard. It's because fear stunts some people. It completely crucifies others, to the point of deep depression and a life of misery. Personally,

I have a five-second rule. Once I decide to act, I do it within five seconds. After this the mind starts to chatter and comes up with a whole list of reasons you shouldn't move forward. Once you decide, you must act with focus, precision and with everything you have.

"Once" is a big word here. There are times when you know immediately that you must take action and there are other times when you remain in the stillness, centred, calm, feeling, pondering, until eventually something clicks, and you reach a conclusion. This is when you act, when you know, 100 per cent this is what you must do. Once you do decide to take action, you must not think. Do it with all of you. With your heart, your soul, with every fibre of your entire being. Solid action will enable you to blaze a new trail, for others to pass through, as you carve your own soul journey from the fabric of life.

Discipline

Discipline is next. Once you are on the path, following your heart, listening intently to the universal communication, the faint whisper in your ear, the signs in your daily life, you must exercise discipline. As your light strengthens, you will draw attention. Energetic attention. A force will come into play from time to time to test you and challenge you. To offer you an experience that will tempt your cells into a course of action that is not congruent with your values, who you are and your spiritual/life mission. It could be a simple meal that will throw your training out, or a glorious money-making scheme that takes your attention away from your mission. Either way you must say no. Exercise, nutrition, business, relationships, they all require discipline. If you want to be a Super-Human, then discipline is a must.

Our children these days are often growing up in a world that is handed to them on a plate and so the sense of working hard, creating and growing their interests and setting life goals to fulfil, is being lost. Their inner drive is not robust. As parents we must inspire by example, motivate through our own personal endeavours and be awesome role models for our kids. Executing focus, discipline and determination on a daily basis is where it's at. Too many people want things right now. Some things manifest very quickly, and other things take a little time. To truly build your life force energy, raise the electricity levels in your body, and be able to run this frequency, takes consistent daily practice. To build muscle, be fit and healthy requires the same. To be happy takes discipline. To remain undistracted in a world full of every possible distraction requires you to remain disciplined and steadfast in your approach to life. We live in a world where the mould of mediocrity is often accepted; while others around us may blend into that mould, we can use discipline to break it, sustain it and continue to grow.

Love

Love is the sixth ingredient. Not "unconditional love". Love is love. You either love or you don't. I know I have mentioned unconditional love, but now we've had this conversation, love will be love. Loving with zero conditions is easier said than done for most and actually requires practice. It's something that we are, and so it should be easy and flow naturally, but we have been conditioned to judge, blame, ridicule and shirk responsibility and so get caught in a crossfire of emotions, thoughts, and lower-vibrational actions.

Now, it's important to ascertain the kind of love I am talking about. It's not the "I love you my dear" type of love that you think about and talk about and say to a loved one. Love itself goes so very deep. It is infinitely greater than bliss, joy, and ecstasy. It's a love so pure, a love cradled in freedom, a love that has no words and has infinite amounts of joy, bliss and ecstasy flowing through it, under it, around it. This love is natural to us but has been forgotten because our emotional

spectrum keeps most of us locked between extreme fear and a little bit of fear. Every now and again we move over to the love end of the spectrum, but rarely all the way to the end.

With practice, you can develop this love and cultivate it. Once you get a glimpse, a taste, you will keep striving to be there always, in a blissed-out state of compassion and gratitude and love for all things. And even "a blissed-out state of compassion and gratitude" are still just words, I am using to try to describe the indescribable. This love is a love experienced beyond the physical vessel; but once you have experienced it, you can develop it and get close to it while still being inside this incredible super human avatar vessel.

The first five ingredients lay the foundation for a woman or man to love. When someone is doing or saying something that could potentially offend you, or maybe a stranger bumps your car in a car park, you can exercise self-control, choose alternative thoughts (not the barrage that will land in your head at the time, placed there by your trusted old friend, Mr/Mrs Ego), stay calm, take a measured form of action and be disciplined to follow it through (as Mr/Mrs Ego will continue to bombard you with other ideas) to the end. Loving another in all situations is a must. It doesn't mean you have to agree with them or support them in their endeavours, but that you have to love them for who they are and see the light beyond the physical form. See the essence of creation. You will see your own light inside and realize that we are all one light, one stream, one energy, all playing this game as different versions of each other in a great big play.

The more you love the more love will flow back through your life. We are a human family, a cosmic tribe, and we came here to help each other expand, so let it be. Flow and enjoy, moment after moment as you travel these earthly planes, interacting with other energies in your space and observing the human cloak, going about its daily tasks, trying to figure it all out. We are all the same beautiful soul, and this planet is an awesome training ground to bring you into equilibrium. Surrender and allow it. All is divine and flows effortlessly. Love is the underlying fabric that blends it all, seamlessly, together.

Electromagnetic Beings

We are physical beings on a solid Earth, trying to figure out how to play this game, and at the same time we are like the sun: electromagnetic. We thrive off of light and sound because we are it. We are powered by frequency and can soar, just as we can be controlled and subdued by frequency. Right now, on Earth we are in a frequency war.

There is high- and low-vibrational energy everywhere. They can both run through the same space (on different information or light streams, different mathematics) and on different frequency bands. Your own vibrational frequency determines which frequency band you are tuned in to.

My mission is to give the human race the opportunity to set itself free, and there is a unique elixir, a combination of musts, that you can weave into your human existence, such as meditation, exercise, the consumption of high-vibrational foods, time-restrictive eating, sun-gazing, fasting and more.

One more of these is qigong, an ancient tradition that I have been practising every morning for several years and something we do plenty of on our Level 2 Facilitator Training and a little of on our Level 1 Facilitator Training. All of our Star Magic Infinity Members have been shown the Star Magic way of qigong. This way of doing qigong is different. We have taken the best from the best and brought in a little high-vibrational Star Magic frequency to create something magically powerful. A second-to-none version of this ancient tradition.

So why is it so important? In our bodies we have what is known as the mesentery, sometimes referred to as the second brain. The mesentery is a fold of membrane that attaches the intestine to the abdominal wall and holds it in place. It assists with internal knowing, your "gut instinct", and is also like a battery that stores chi/life force or energy.

Also, we have 75–100 trillion cells in our body and every cell carries an electrical charge along with an intricate network of nerve fibres and nerve endings.

During a qigong practice, which consists of slow hand, arm and body movements, deep controlled breathing and visualization, one brings oxygen and light into the body. It clears your cells, vital organs, and meridians (energy channels), packs your mesentery with high-vibrational energy, unifies the total cellular charge from every cell and activates your electrical energy in an incredible way. In a nutshell, it fills up your battery, and this energy can be used to revitalize your organs and amplify your personal frequency. It can also be used to charge your physical body and your light body and spirit body, so you can prepare your mathematical structure for ascension.

The way we do our qigong (Star Magic Style) also has a profound effect on the activation of your pineal gland or third eye. We use breath and movement to create pressure that will bring cerebral spinal fluid (Christ/Kryst) up through your thirty-three vertebrae (Jacob's Ladder) and into your twelve cranial nerves (twelve disciples), which creates the activation (resurrection). The process stimulates, nurtures, and nourishes your nervous system in a unique way; in the brain, your *medulla oblongata* (responsible for internal knowing and accessing quantum information) and your *substantia nigra* (responsible for molecular change) will also be stimulated in a major way. Your energy levels will go through the roof. You will also increase dimethyltryptamine (DMT) levels, switch on your lymphatic system and tap your DNA. The reason for me using biblical terms is to show that the resurrection has nothing to do with a man rising from the dead, but is simply about a human being activating their third eye and realizing their power, their wisdom, that they are God, Infinite Intelligence, the universe. This is why we are constantly stimulated externally, because going within is the pathway to us accessing our *multidimensional abilities and certain forces want them forgotten, by us, for ever.* (Just to be clear, there was a resurrection that took place but it wasn't Jesus that was resurrected. It was someone else pretending to be Jesus, but that is another story that doesn't quite fit here.)

We will connect you to the electromagnetic (male/positive) frequencies from the stars and the magnetic (female/negative) frequencies from the Earth. Knowledge comes from light and information, which is electromagnetic, and your energy comes from your connection to the ground, magnetic. Your intention (electrical – Star based) infused with your emotion (magnetic – Earth based) offers you the recipe for a galactic recalibration of information streams and energy and a reordering of such that can and will manifest.

This Way will totally amplify your energy field, with the process connecting your alpha transmission centre/In-point (ATC) – a cosmic gate located anywhere from 12–15 inches up to 3 metres (it's always in flux) above the crown of your head that controls the flow of light/information/cosmic energy from the stars and allows it to flow safely through your system – to your omega transmission centre/Out-point (a cosmic gate located a few metres below your feet, in empty space, that births your frequency into the Earth; again the distance below your feet varies as this transmission centre is also in flux) and opens the flow of cosmic information, from the stars to the Earth, grounding you into the planet in 5D and above, and turns you into the planetary guardian (a woman or man, living on Earth, taking high-vibrational light streams and grounding them in to the planet to assist with ascension) you came to this planet to be.

This is one phase of preparing your body for these off-planet frequencies; the second phase is nutrition and the third exercise. All help you to create a solid physical body, ready for light code execution into the Planetary Grids.

Humans and Evolution

Human beings are mission critical in the evolution of our planet. You might say "But the planet would do just great without us." And while that is true, she would thrive without humans being present, the planet would not evolve in a way it can with humans. Humans are destructive creatures when out of balance but when in balance are some of the greatest quantum architects in the universe. Mother Earth could spit us off her body at any time she pleased, but she signed up for this just like we did. She has created the playground for us to learn/remember. She is like a giant nursery and a nursery teacher for children and we are the children running around the nursery, playing, making friends, having fun, having arguments, learning skills, how to communicate and interact, and she is holding massive space for us. When we, as humans, power up our physical bodies and our light bodies to work in harmony, and can handle the full force of the multidimensional energies available, we will amplify Earth's new frequency code.

Something to point out here is that Earth may be returning to stardust in the next 200 years (unless the guardian races can undo the damage done to her rod and staff). She is holding space for her children (us humans) to give us time to figure out how to ascend our physical bodies, or at least our consciousness, out from this time-based matrix, before she returns to stardust. At present, Earth will not be ascending like us humans. She has chosen a different path. There are extremely powerful beings assisting Earth in holding her mathematical template in place, so we have the opportunity to ascend, as the darker forces wanted to destroy Earth years ago. As previously mentioned, this was so they could steal the quantum energy that would be released during the downfall/destruction. You see, the battle for energy is not just on a human level but on a planetary, galactic, and universal level. It also goes to show the complete lack of love of these forces, desperate for quantum energy; they would not bat an eyelid while destroying a planet and 9 billion humans.

The energies are becoming less solid, non-geometrical (yet still geometrical) and are instead becoming a Krysted Spiralized Geometrical Code of Energies/Light. These Krysted Spirals will flow out from the Earth's Krystal Reservoir through every human and vice versa. The more inner work we do and the better equipped we are for these galactic energies, the faster we amplify the Krysted Light throughout our beloved planet. We are the gatekeepers that will unleash the Krystal Spiral Timeline, through our own Krsyt Light. I see these frequencies in the space. I have done so since 2013, after I wrote my book *Into The Light*. That process activated something deep within me and for the following nine months I spent two hours every day in Egyptian Mystery schools learning/ remembering how to use the code that became Star Magic Healing. This code is a constantly moving, consistently shape-shifting, fluid pattern of geometry that moves through space, ebbing and flowing, changing shape and at the same time maintaining a consistent formula through its mathematical structure. The Krystal Spiral (we will discuss this later on) has always been there, along with another spiral that most human beings have been connected to, because of the mass manipulation on a level of frequency.

Star Magic Qigong and Evolution

I have a two-hour Star Magic qigong routine. Within it there are six exercises, which, when combined in a certain sequence, will fill you up with light/energy, bring you into a deeply present state, activate your third eye, open your heart, raise your vibration, switch on your lymphatic system, activate your DNA, elevate DMT levels, charge your electrical nature, bring every cell of you into a unified state, switch on those kundalini energies that everyone talks about and so much more, including the activation ignition of your multi-density light body, your Spirit Body and the expanded mathematics of what you truly are. The clarity of vision and self that this will bring into your world is beyond words.

These six exercises alone will supercharge you. All you have to do is follow this routine. Maybe start off by doing it once or twice a week and gradually increase it until you make it a consistent daily practice. Progression in all things is key. Rome wasn't built in a day: start off slow and build upon it. Or, if you are like me, you will do it daily from the start because you find that the benefits are unrivalled. We all have our own path. But you can control the levels you go to. You can take it easy and charge yourself mildly, or you can and charge yourself to the maximum every time, consistently pushing the envelope to see how far you can take it. There are no boundaries.

Remember, this routine is deeply healing and very expansive, so your body and consciousness will go through some adjustments. You may experience ascension symptoms: headaches, dizziness, sore muscles, kidneys, liver and other bodily components, because you are healing, amplifying, and recalibrating, mentally, physically, emotionally, spiritually, and most of all energetically. You will be releasing deep trauma (which can be painful) as well as activating important elements of your internal and multidimensional workings.

EXERCISE 1 *Charge Your Mesentery*

1. Start standing, with your feet somewhere between slightly apart and shoulder-width apart, whatever feels comfortable for you. You can always readjust after practising and seeing what feels best for you. Have a slight bend in your knees to take any pressure out of your lower back. Ensure your posture is nice and tall. Head up, shoulders back, chest out, spine straight. In an optimal scenario you will be barefoot, on the Earth. If you have to do it inside, then that is OK, you can still energetically plant your feet in the Earth and connect. Go quantum.

2. You are going to press your feet into the ground and feel like you are sat on a horse, pressing your toes into the Earth/ground and pressing inwards against the imaginary horse's body. Feel like there is a force pushing back against you (your knees/inside of legs) and you are gripping the horse tightly while pressing your toes and feet solidly into the ground. It takes some getting used to if you are new to this, but with a little practice it will feel natural.

3. Now you are going to fire-breathe for thirty-six breaths. Short and sharp for a quick warm-up. Fire breathing consists of breathing in through your nose, down to the pit of your stomach and back out through your nose. You are going to do this hard and fast. In and out is one breath. As soon as you have completed the first set of thirty-six breaths, you are going to focus on the centre of Mother Earth. Right in her centre there is a large merkaba, her heart.

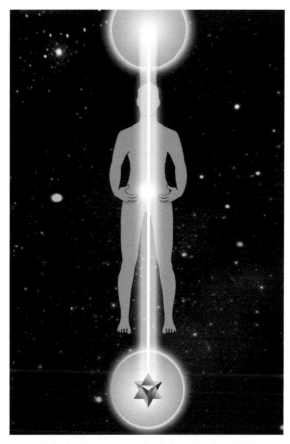

1. Light flowing into your body from Earth and Sirius

Please look at the illustration. That is you, stood on the Earth, on your imaginary horse, feet pressed firmly into the ground. Your hands are in that starting position. Now focus on Mother Earth's heart, her merkaba, and draw the light from her bottom tetrahedron. The light is a platinum colour. Visualize it flowing up through the rocks and minerals, through the surface of the planet and into your perineum. Now focus on the star Sirius, the Dog Star. (Remember Sirius is everywhere. You don't need to get logical and think of its exact location. We live play and dance in a quantum/holographic reality. Set your intentions to connect with Sirius and see/feel/know that connection.) Visualize an electric pink light, flowing down from Sirius, through Mother Earth's atmosphere, through the skies, into your crown. See both of those lights ever so bright and strong.

Next, I would like you to squeeze your buttocks, your perineum, genitals, and pull all of your stomach muscles towards your spine. You will squeeze these areas and release these areas as prompted throughout the routine. It's the squeezing/tensing/tightening/pulling and releasing of the muscles in these areas (along with your focus and breathing) that will push and pull the cerebral (spinal) fluid up your body. You will also be encouraging energy to rise. It will take some getting used to, but after a week of this you will be a pro and it will keep getting better and easier and it will feel more natural. Be focused and disciplined like the Super-Human you are.

We've looked briefly at the mesentery, and we use it in this practice too. You can visualize it as a thin square battery. That is what I do and simply entangle this image with the mesentery through my intention. Or some people visualize it as a sphere. It really doesn't matter; the key is your intention. If you know you are sending qi/energy to your mesentery, then you are. Even if I see it as a square, the light/energy that builds as it's filled up through the routine, becomes spherical, expanding out beyond the square.

You are also going to hold the tip of your tongue on the roof of your mouth throughout this entire process. There are exercises where it's not possible to hold it there and you will soon figure them out, but for the majority it will be possible, so keep it there. It opens up a unique energy channel through your body.

Now you are going to breathe in, pull the platinum light up from Mother Earth (which is already flowing into your perineum), into your mesentery (where the qi is stored) and as you do, your hands will gently move up in a slow motion. They will reach your shoulders or slightly higher (whatever feels comfortable) as you complete the in-breath. See illustration 2.

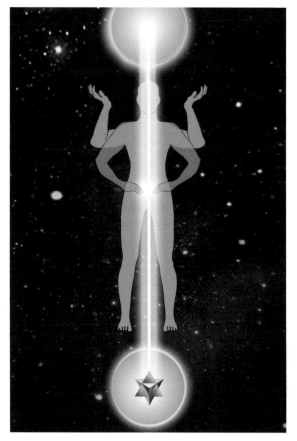

2. Pulling and directing the light from Earth and Sirius into your mesentery

You will then let go of the squeeze, breathe out slowly and, as you do, turn your hands over (palms down) and bring your hands back down to the starting position. As you do you are pulling the light from Sirius down into your mesentery. That is one repetition. You will then squeeze again, pull in your stomach muscles and repeat. You are to do this thirty-six times. Remember, your focus and intention plays a huge role in all of this work. You are building the energy in your battery/mesentery, breathing and becoming present, bringing magnetic Earth energy up and electromagnetic Star energy down, and also starting the movement of energy towards your brain. As you inhale, the sutures of your skull slightly open up and your sacrum, the bone at the base of your spine, flexes back, the spinal fluid drains and when you breathe out/exhale the sacrum flexes forward and the sutures close. So, by exhaling and inhaling and engaging the squeeze, you start to push the cerebral spinal fluid up through the spinal column and towards the brain. This is very important, as you will see moving through this routine, because it is the beginning of you activating your pineal gland. We are going to do two separate stand-alone exercises for activating the pineal gland later in the book, but there is no point wasting this wonderful opportunity to activate it some more during the qigong exercise.

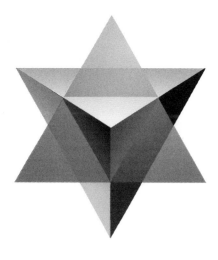

3. Merkaba

EXERCISE 2 *Activate Your Merkaba Field*

The second exercise is a beautiful continuation of the first. You will notice they all flow on from each other seamlessly. Even if it feels awkward at first because it's new and you are reading at the same time as practising, it will become second nature.

Now you have started to charge your mesentery and build that battery and amplify your cosmic and your Earthly connection. Mother Earth's merkaba field is also connected to the Earth's grids, so information starts to flow more freely in a myriad of ways. Your feet are still pressed into the Earth and by default, energy is now flowing from the Earth, through your feet, up through your legs and into your body as well as that platinum Earth frequency charging your mesentery. Remember, you are an extension of the Earth, just like a tree. At this stage I want you to amplify this experience and visualize roots flowing from the soles of your feet, way down into the Earth. Feel those roots getting strong throughout the duration of this Star Magic qigong routine.

This exercise is to activate your merkaba field (an energy field around the outside of your physical body) and bring it into perfect balance. There are many merkaba fields within your body and light body structure, but for now, we will just focus on this one (see illustration 3).

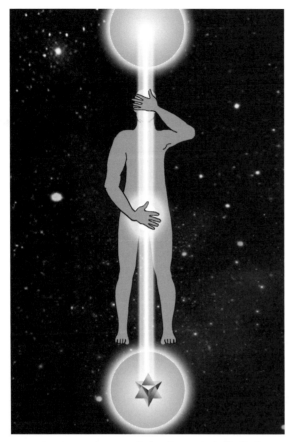

4. Starting position: Right hand over the ball of light (now located above your perineum) and left hand over the forehead

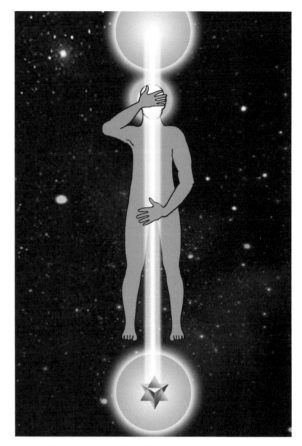

5. Reversed position: Hands now reversed and the ball of light in and around your head

At present you have light stored inside your mesentery. I want you to move that light (see it as a sphere) down (with your mind/intention), several inches into the space above your perineum. Now you will place your right hand in front of the area of the ball of light and see electrical energy flowing from your hand to the ball and vice versa. Your left hand will be over your forehead, in line with your pineal gland. Your fingers can be closed or open. I sometimes have them open and sometimes closed. Just whatever feels right in the moment. Remember, the energy is still flowing from the Earth and Sirius into your body/mesentery. This will not stop. You can check from time to time if you like, and keep seeing it get stronger and brighter. The tip of the tongue is still on the roof of your mouth.

What you will do now is move your right hand to the pineal gland and left hand to just above the perineum where the right hand was, so they reverse positions. The ball of light will track the right hand. So, the energy is moving up into the brain and back down and through the central channel.

Your hands must cross over your heart every time. This means that the bottom hand is always moving faster than the top hand. There is a reason for this.

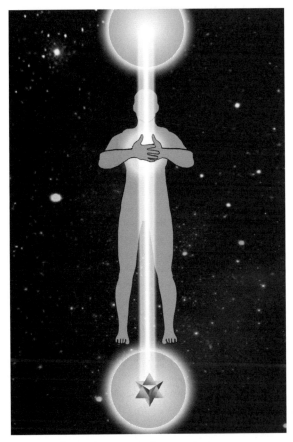

6. Hands crossing over the heart each time you move the ball of energy/light

on the body) from the heart to the pineal gland. Your movement, intention and electrical energy communicate with the heart to fire up your merkaba and bring it into a balanced spin ration.

Before you start this movement, you are going to be doing the same as in the first exercise: squeeze your perineum, genitals and buttocks and pull your abdominal muscles back towards the spine and, as you breathe in and move the hands, the ball of energy moves up into your head. You let go of the squeeze at the top, breathe out slowly through the mouth and bring the ball of light back down. As the ball of light moves up, I want you to track it with your awareness, all the way up into your head. Once the ball of light reaches the perineum area again, after you bring it back down, you squeeze and repeat. You will do this thirty-six times. Up and down is once. Remember your hands must cross over your heart every time and both hands must hit the finishing position at the same time. This means that the bottom hand always travels faster than the top hand. The last point to remember is that the hand going up always stays closest to the body. So the right hand goes up on the inside and down on the outside.

I know right now it seems like a lot to remember, but once you get this routine down it will become the cornerstone of your life.

The bottom tetrahedron (female) of your merkaba field moves twice as fast as the top one (male) when operating effectively. The merkaba field can be out of balance at times because of the game we are playing on Earth. Lower vibrational forces attack this field of energy to destabilize you. As the hands cross over the heart (transmission) centre every time, the magnetic heart frequency is pulling information from your mental and physical bodies and communicating with your merkaba field. It's also important to know that the distance from your root centre to your heart centre is twice the distance (mirroring the twice-as-fast speed element of the two tetrahedrons. In effect, the rotational particle spin rates in the bottom and top tetrahedrons, are in equal proportion to the distance between the points

EXERCISE 3 *Activate Your Spinal Column*

The third exercise, again, beautifully leads on from the second. Right now, that ball of qi is just above your perineum. You have also been continuously running energy from Sirius and the Earth into your mesentery, as well as energy pouring up through your imaginary but very real roots. First up, bring the qi/energy from your perineum area back up into your mesentery and merge these two sources of energy together (mesentery, which has been continually filling up, and the sphere).

At this point the light in your body will be a brighter, bigger ball of light. Stronger, more intense. If you still yourself, you will feel it. You will feel electricity building inside your body and on the outside, all around it. At this stage I start seeing trillions of tiny little electrical streams flowing out from the ball of light into every cell in the body. There is this huge electrical conversation and energy exchange taking place. Remember, you have electrical charge in every cell of your body.

Now it's time to amplify that connection and really switch your body on. Next you will place your hands by the sides of your body. Squeeze the perineum, genitals and buttocks and pull the abdominal muscles back to the spinal column and breathe in deeply. As you do, you will bring your hands and arms up into a cross position and stretch out your chest. This opens the heart. As you breathe in, feel and see light being drawn from all around the outside of your body, into your mesentery.

Maybe you can see and feel the light in your breath, also charging your mesentery? I see and feel the light from Mother Earth flowing up, the light from Sirius flowing down, and I see light flowing in through my nose as I breathe as well as a field of light flowing into my body from all around. All charging my mesentery. My cells start to crackle with energy. Visualize it powerfully and with a supercharged intention.

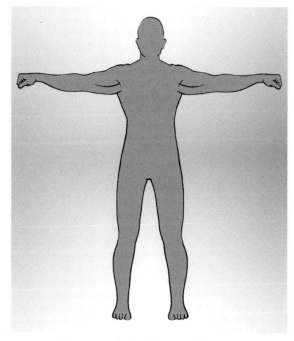

7. Arms expanded and chest and heart open after breathing in

Next, once your belly and lungs are full of oxygen, you are going to breathe out really fast and contract your entire body and pull your arms in (see illustration 8).

You will naturally let go of the squeeze as you do this, and your tongue will leave the roof of your mouth as you breathe/blow out hard and fast with tight lips. As you do this, you start to pump energy up through your body and into the brain. The spinal column and central nervous system really get activated. Then, re-engage the squeeze and tongue and go again. Repeat this nine times, then close your eyes and be still.

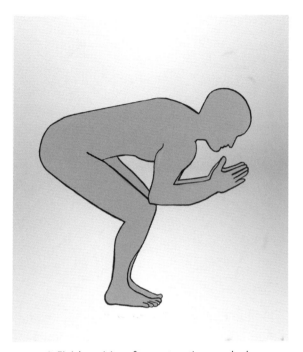

8. Finish position after contracting your body
and breathing out

Feel the energy running up your spinal column, through your back. Around your hands, face – everywhere. There is subtle energy everywhere. You will feel the energy running from the Earth, through the roots and up into your body. The energy still flowing from the Stars and Earth into your mesentery. You will do four sets of nine, with a thirty-second break (one minute if you like but I usually go for thirty seconds as it keeps the intensity going) in between to tune your consciousness in to those subtle frequencies. Feel them in your spinal column. Feel them in your space. Feel yourself merging with the space or maybe the space merging with you. There really is no separation. The thirty-second to one-minute break is to really tap in and feel. Be still and experience what is happening inside your body.

EXERCISE 4 *Charge Your Cells*

The fourth exercise, again, flows on effortlessly from the previous one. With your hands by your sides, focus on the ball of light in your mesentery. Keep your hands where they are. As you breathe in, see the ball of light drawing in more energy/light and as you exhale, see the ball grow with its newly drawn-in energy. You will breathe in and out and as you do, the ball will grow.

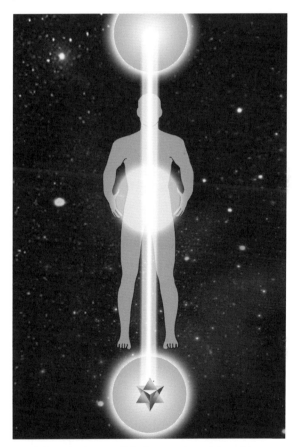

9. Drawing in more light/energy through breathing,
the ball of light growing larger with each breath

It will grow out past your physical body and start pushing your hands up. Eventually your hands will be out almost straight, resting on top of this ball of energy, as you and the ball of light become one. This requires zero energy, and it will be comfortable to have your hands resting on it. No sore shoulders. You must go beyond your body.

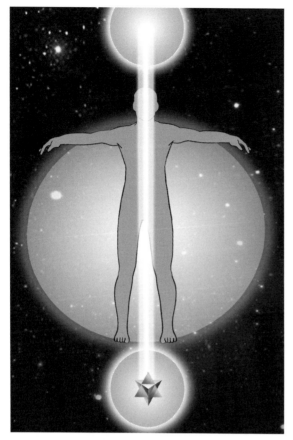

10. Ball of light full-grown and hands and arms resting on top of it

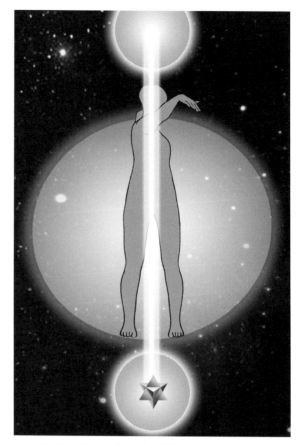

11. Twisting to the right while you are squeezing and holding the breath in

You are light – remember this. With practice you could rest your arms on this ball of light for hours. Your hands are supported by the energy. It should feel like you have a broom handle across your back. There can be a slight bend in your elbows and your hands are loose.

Next, you are going to squeeze your perineum, genitals, and buttocks, pull your abdominals back towards your spine and make sure the tip of the tongue is still placed on the roof of your mouth. Then take a long deep breath in. As you breathe in, you will focus on that platinum light from the Earth and see it flow all the way up into your crown. Note: it will still be charging your battery as that is in full motion. Both things will be happening. You will bring all of your awareness up to your crown, following the light as you pull it up.

Once the light hits your crown, bring your awareness into the centre of your brain and back slightly, exactly where your pineal gland is. Hold your breath and keep your focus here. Now, while you keep squeezing and pulling in your abdominals, turn your body from side to side with your arms out, maintaining the position.

The squeeze, the pull, the breath hold and the turning, along with your focus on your pineal gland, is going to send/pull/twist/encourage the cerebral spinal fluid and the energy, up your spinal column and into the area of your pineal gland.

We will talk about this in a lot of detail later in the book. For now, simply trust the process. You will feel the benefits anyway and they are colossal.

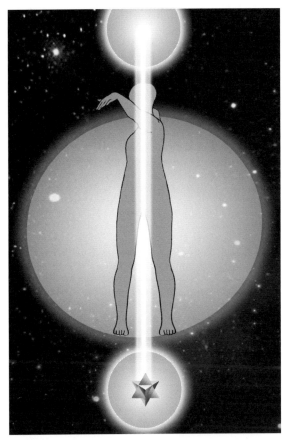

12. Twisting to the left while you are squeezing
and holding the breath in

I actually count my turns and try to beat the last one. Eventually you will get 100 turns and more, but if you are only getting thirty or forty turns to start with, that's OK. It's not easy for some people, especially if you don't do any breathwork already. Soon you will be a Jedi breather. Build and build and build. Be consistent and the results will speak volumes.

Once you have completed three sets of the in-breath, you will do the same but with the lungs emptied of oxygen. So, you breathe out everything – and I mean everything. Squeeze your perineum, genitals, and buttocks, pull your abdominals back towards your spine, raise your arms, pull the light to your crown, awareness on your pineal gland, keep squeezing and start turning. It's much harder with no oxygen. Get as many turns as possible, let go of the squeeze, breathe in (not out this time, for obvious reasons) and regulate your breath. When you do this, as before move your hands up and down. Here, on the first breath in you will bring your hands up, whereas in the previous exercise with the out-breath you brought your hands down when you first breathed after holding. Once your breath is regulated, repeat the process two more times, trying to get more turns each time. Push yourself.

When you really push yourself on this, your entire body will get hot, it may well vibrate from head to toe and you may really have to fight to control the first in- or out-breath and not to blurt it out. This control, when you really want to take a deep breath, amplifies your frequency.

You don't want to get to the point where you blurt out your breath because you are about to pass out. But you do want to get to a level where you feel a little lightheaded but are still in control. When you control the breath out, it should be very, very difficult to let it out slowly. Remember this. It's a marker for you. As you practise and get used to this, you will go to extraordinary levels of vibration.

You are going to turn as many times as you can. Count the turns, keeps squeezing. Once you get to the point where you cannot hold your breath any longer, you will let go of the squeeze, breathe out and as you do, lower your arms. Do it slowly. Ensure you do not blurt out your breath. Control it. The controlling of the breath and the slow release is mission critical. You will then breathe in and out several times until your breath is under control. As you breathe in raise your hands and as you breathe out lower them, in synch with the breath.

Once your breathing is regulated (and that should not be easy if you really push yourself on the turns/twists and the breath hold), re-engage the squeeze, pull in the abdominals, raise your arms and go again. You will do this three times.

It should not be easy to regulate your breathing. If it is, you are not pushing yourself. I have seen women and men have some huge experiences at this stage of the routine. Bodies shaking, massive downloads of light, biological upgrades taking place, kundalini energies firing up through the body. Please note: each time you bring your arms back up, you just lift them up to the ball. The ball remains so you do not have to breathe in and lift the hands/arms up with the light like you did at the beginning of the exercise.

Once you have done three sets of the exercise holding the breath in and three sets holding the breath out, stand still for two minutes and feel your body. If you really go for this, the energy shooting around your body will be amazing. I want you to really push yourself but (again to drill the message home) don't get to the point where you blurt or spit your breath out or breathe in really fast on the out-breath part of the turning routine. The breaths in and out MUST be controlled. You will find your rhythm as you move through this.

After you have rested for two minutes and tuned in to your body's rhythm, frequency and the subtle energies (which become much less subtle as you progress), I want you to focus on your battery/mesentery and the ball of light there, connected to all the other cells, energy crackling. I want you to do three minutes of fire breathing, pumping that energy in and out and seeing the light from your battery send charges of energy to every cell and every cell responding and sending charges of energy back to the battery. No need to squeeze and release during these three minutes.

Now it's time to move to the next exercise.

EXERCISE 5 *Connect to the Cosmos*

You are going to adopt the standing tree position below.

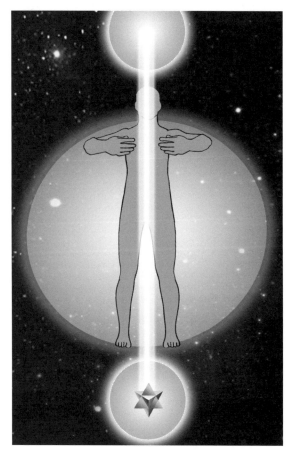

13. In standing tree position

Your body is going to be upright. Check you're riding that horse and your knees are pushing in against the force of the saddle and your feet and toes are pressed into the ground. Your spine must be straight, and your hands and arms will be in a loose position as per the illustration above.

Your shoulders and upper back will pull forwards slightly and the tips of your fingers will be in line with your heart and pointing towards each other. The energy from the Earth and Sirius are still running into your mesentery.

Now, I want you to feel the point of the back of your heart centre on your spinal column. This is the point where your upper back and arms will pull slightly forward from. This action opens up important energy channels. As you adopt this position you will feel it. Next, I want you to see and feel the light flowing up through the roots in your feet, up your legs and into your perineum. Both streams of light from both feet will meet here. Then see and feel the energy flow up until it reaches the point in your spinal column (at the back of the heart) where your upper back and arms are pulling forwards from. See the energy/light flow to this point, split into two streams and flow down both arms, out through both hands, through all the fingers and both thumbs and then flow into the opposite fingers and thumbs. The energy will circle around (in both directions) and keep flowing up through the roots as you push your feet firmly into the ground. You are now in the perfect position.

Now you will squeeze your genitals, perineum, and buttocks, and pull your abdominal muscles back to your spine. Breathe in, see the light flow up to your crown, bring your awareness around your pineal gland, hold for thirteen seconds, let go of the squeeze and chant as you release the breath. You are going to chant seven tones. These are the first seven audible harmonics that flow out from creation.

Ka, Ra, Ya, Sa, Ta, Aa, La – the first letter of each spells Krystal, referring to the Krystal Spiral.

While you chant Ka, Ra, Ya, Sa, Ta, Aa, La – the separately, ensure that all of your attention is on your pineal gland. Once you have chanted Ka, all of your breath will be out. You can then re-engage the squeeze and repeat chanting Ra, then Ya and so on. Repeat each tone separately and three times through. So, you are chanting twenty-one times in total.

When you chant, it's the A sound that connects you to Source/God/Infinite Intelligence. Every time you chant, you must have your attention/awareness on your pineal gland.

As you go through this process keep checking on the flow of energy through the roots of your feet, Earth, and Sirius. Visualize it. It's a lot to take on at first but once you have done it daily for a week, you will get into the swing of it, just like everything. Practise!

To finish, lower your arms and draw the ball of light (that's been there since the start of the previous exercise) from around you back into your body. Visualize it flowing back in, stronger and brighter, and pack all of this light into your mesentery. Once it's inside you, be still and send light to your lungs, kidneys, liver, gall bladder, pancreas, heart, stomach, spleen, large and small intestines, and adrenal glands. You can also send it to your throat and your brain. Share some love with these vital bodily components. Even though you are drawing the light back inside you, your energy field will still be amplified and so you will feel the energy around you as well as inside of you.

Now, the same as the previous exercise, I want you to focus on your battery/mesentery and the ball of light there, connected to all the other cells, energy crackling. I want you to do three minutes of fire breathing, pumping that energy in and out and seeing the light from your battery sending charges of energy to every cell and every cell responding and sending charges of energy back to the battery. There is no need to squeeze and release as you do this.

EXERCISE 6 *Opening Up the Energy Channels*

Now, we will move onto the sixth and final exercise. Just like the previous one, this position opens up your energy channels in the most incredible way.

You will adopt the position in the illustration below.

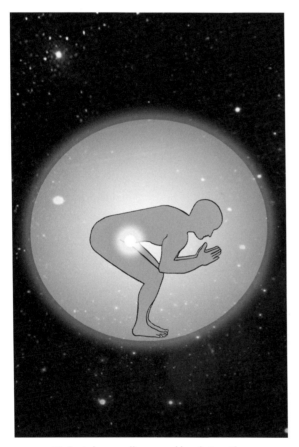

14. Feet, knees, elbows, and hands together, bottom pushed back and flat back

In this position you will move your feet for the first time. Bring them together. Your knees will be touching, your butt sticking out, your back flat and spine straight and your wrists and elbows together. Put the tip of your tongue on the roof of your mouth and hold this position for five minutes. It will be tough at first. Your legs may burn, tremble and shake. Just ride it out. Focus on breathing deep and slow and empty your mind. This position opens the energy channels inside your body in the most incredible way and truly activates you. You will feel it.

Once you have finished, lie down on the ground and stay still for as long as you wish. This is where you reap the benefits of your hard work. Now the body will do what it's designed to do best: self-heal. Be still, feel, observe. You may find you drift off or start journeying. Enjoy the process. Surrender and let your body do what it wants to do. Your body will now start to recalibrate. In this space deep healing will take place. You may journey, dropping into deep meditation. Just be and allow. You've done the hard work, now kick back for as long as you want. There are times when I have things to do and I will go and do them; other times I will lie there for twenty minutes, or sometimes an hour or more.

This routine may well take you 1 hour and 15 minutes to 1 hour 30 minutes to start with, but as you get used to it you will reduce the time. It usually takes me 50 to 55 minutes when I am in beast mode. It will radically enhance your life. It's a good solid process that will transform your life and your energy. Create the space and do this. Your frequency, state of mind and heart will change. You will be a much more energized, calm, and centred human being. Your electrical nature will start to show up in so many ways. You are an electrical being: know this. You are now taking massive steps to becoming a Super-Human. You are opening yourself up to more information, light, more energy. You are now going to start operating like an electromagnetic being who came from the stars, with unique abilities. Follow this process, starting once or twice a week and build it up to every other day, and eventually it will be more important than brushing your teeth and taking a shower. Or, as I said before, make it a daily must from the get-go. You are awesome, and I respect you for choosing this path!

5

Super-Humans and the Body

The Power of Cold

Once you have rested after your morning qigong routine, I want to introduce you to something else. Every morning, without fail, I have a cold shower. If you are not used to it, and you love getting under that warm water, then the thought of diving into cold water instead might be daunting. But if you are on this mission, you may already be aware of the importance of loving the cold.

I first discovered the importance of the cold around twelve years ago. I owned a mixed martial arts and fitness centre in New Zealand. Every Friday we would fill up a great big plastic bath with water and buckets of ice. The bath was an old container with the lid cut off. You could fit four people in there, real comfortable. We would sit with the ice water up to our chins for ten minutes. It took inflammation and bruising out of the body and totally rejuvenated us. After a week of boxing, Muay Thai, circuits, sparring, wrestling, pad work, sprints, and weights, it was the perfect way to end the week. Once you got out of that ice bath you felt brand new.

The Russian Systema, a Russian fighting system tip a freezing cold bucket of water over their head, first thing in the morning and last thing at night. There are so many benefits to exposing your body to freezing cold water, such as elevating your immune system, lowering cortisol levels, and increasing your metabolic rate. It also brings you into the present moment because you are focused on your breath and the cold. Other benefits include increased alertness, improved skin and hair, elevated libido, boosted fertility, improved circulation, drainage of your lymphatic system, activation of your central nervous system; it speeds up recovery after exercise, relieves depression – and believe it or not, while cold showers wake you up, they are also great for putting you to sleep.

I want you to start introducing cold showers to your daily routine. Once you have finished your qigong routine, jump in. Now, you don't have to start with freezing cold. And I am only suggesting you start with 20–30 seconds. Or maybe you will find you are like me and go straight in for a few minutes. The choice is yours.

If you take the second option, get under the cold, wash yourself, breathe deeply and slowly and move around as if you were in a warm shower. Don't stand there thinking, "It's cold!" Breathe, move, wash yourself as you would if it were warm water and get out. Do not run the warm water after. You will actually find that when you get out, you'll feel warmer than when getting out of a warm shower. If you do decide to go straight into the cold, you can always do it for 20–30 seconds and build up daily. I generally do it for approximately five minutes.

If you want to take it slower, that is completely cool too. Remember life is a series of stepping stones. What matters is that you keep stepping. As long as you are, then you are progressing and bettering yourself each day. You are the only one you need to overcome. The only competition is with you, after all.

You can start off under lukewarm water for 15–20 seconds and then gradually increase the cold; slowly turn the dial so your body adjusts and acclimatizes. And then go colder. Once the water is as cold as it gets, stay there for 20–30 seconds. The next day 30–40 seconds. And so on. After a week or whenever it feels right, go straight to cold and then start building up your time.

It is much better to shock the body with the cold and breathe through it. The adrenaline spikes faster and the adrenaline awakens the body. It peaks, and then it brings the cortisol levels right down. Personally, I am always trying to shock the body wherever possible. I am always challenging my body. I do it with exercise, with everything. I try not to prepare my body by deciding what I will do. So, I often change things up and mix them around. I will be going about my day and drop down and do thirty push-ups or pick up a kettlebell and do some Turkish get-ups.

Cortisol and Cold

Stress is one of the biggest killers in our world and chronic diseases are caused by oxidative stress and the continuous presence of cortisol, which is a stress hormone. The controlled adrenaline rush in our body during a cold shower brings the cortisol right back down after the experience. Cortisol is a big problem in modern society because we have a lot of stress, and it doesn't go away, because we keep on going. Our mind says, "Oh I have to do this! I have to do that! and that! and that!" The cortisol won't stop. So, when you take a cold shower, the fight or flight system breaks down as the adrenaline shoots up and drops back down. And all the stress hormones go down with the adrenaline. If you are operating at Super-Human levels, stress never comes into your life because you utilize the potential stress energies in a different way, but none the less, cold showers are the best for Super-Humans and Super-Humans in the making.

It's very simple. You will feel a lot better, much more calm, peaceful and tranquil. You will go from sympathetic nervous system activity to parasympathetic nervous system activity, which is the system that's activated when you're resting and digesting. You come off the accelerator and onto the brakes. The body appreciates this big time!

Super-Humans' Golden Nectar

The most sacred liquid that you can feed your body is your own urine. It's the only liquid on the planet that contains all of the information on your own body.

For almost the entire course of the twentieth century, unknown to the public, doctors and medical researchers have been proving in both laboratory and clinical testing that our own urine is an enormous source of vital nutrients, vitamins, hormones, enzymes, creatines and critical antibodies that cannot be duplicated or derived from any other source. Urine can be used for healing cancer, heart disease, allergies, autoimmune diseases, diabetes, asthma, infertility, infections, wounds and on and on – yet we're taught that urine is a toxic waste product. This discrepancy between the truth and public information regarding urine is ludicrous. But remember, healthy people don't make money for Big Pharma.

If you have been, like most people, trained from your earliest years to regard urine as a mere waste product, the thought of using it for its healing powers may seem shocking. Yet urine therapy has long played an important role in the holistic medical traditions of societies all over the world. It is mentioned in the Ebers Medical Papyri, an Ancient Egyptian medical papyrus of herbal knowledge.

Urine is not a dirty and toxic substance. Medically it is referred to as "plasma ultra-filtrate". It is a purified derivative of the blood itself, made by the kidneys, whose principal function is not excretion but regulation of all the elements and their concentrations in the blood. Urine can be compared to leftovers from a meal, and this metaphor may help us understand why our bodies excrete elements that are valuable to our health and well-being.

Nutrient-filled blood passes through the liver, where toxins are removed to be excreted as solid waste. This purified "clean" blood undergoes a filtering process in the kidneys, where excess water, salts, vitamins, minerals, enzymes, antibodies, urea, uric acid and other elements not usable at that time by the body are collected in the form of a purified, sterile, watery solution – urine. The function of the kidneys is to keep the various elements in the blood balanced. The important elements in the blood are not filtered out because they are toxic and harmful to the body, but simply because the body does not need a particular concentration of an element at that specific point in time. It is this regulating process of the kidneys that allows us to eat and drink more than our bodies need at any one time.

Urine is considered to be an invaluable source of nourishment and healing that perhaps has been too controversial or not financially rewarding enough for it to be talked about or maybe too healing and so the pharmaceutical companies hide it as best they can and so it's not encouraged as a potent medicine. One's own urine, a living food, contains elements that are specific to one's body alone. The body is constantly producing a huge variety of antibodies, hormones, enzymes and other natural chemicals to regulate and control its functions and combat imbalances that one may not be aware of.

Clinical studies have proved that the thousands of critical chemicals and nutrients found in urine reflect the individual body's functions. When re-utilized, these chemicals and nutrients act as natural vaccines, antibacterial, antiviral, and anti-carcinogenic agents, as well as hormone balancers and allergy relievers. The information that urine contains therefore cannot be duplicated or derived from any other source. Just as nature produces no two people who are exactly the same, there are no two urine samples in the world that contain exactly the same elements.

Multiple sclerosis, colitis, lupus, rheumatoid arthritis, cancer, hepatitis, hyperactivity, pancreatic insufficiency, psoriasis, eczema, diabetes, herpes, mononucleosis, adrenal failure, allergies and so many other ailments have been relieved through use of urine therapy.

I remember when I decided to try it, I collected my morning urine in a glass and stood in front of the mirror psyching myself up to drink it. I brought the glass to my lips, drank it – and started laughing. I was expecting it to taste horrible, but it was alright. And after drinking it a few times you actually start to like it.

The middle stream of fresh, warm, morning urine is the most potent, and drinking it mixed with fresh juice can make it easier, although it is best not to mix urine with other foods or drinks or to take it within an hour before or after eating. Personally, I drink it straight. I collect my urine in the morning and drink after midday when my daily fast finishes. I keep it in the fridge until then. I only drink my first morning cup, but I know others who loop their urine. They literally carry around a container, catch it all and consume it. It's called looping for obvious reasons.

Urine may be used as eye drops and ear drops, in footbaths and even as an enema. As nose drops it can help loosen mucus and clear blocked nasal passages. Gargling with it is helpful for a sore throat, and inhaling it relieves sinus and respiratory congestion. Taken internally, it has a laxative and diuretic effect, as it cleanses the digestive tract.

Ingested and/or rubbed into the skin, urine purifies blood and tissues, provides useful nutrients, and sends the body a signal about what is in or out of balance. This last effect is called (oral) autoimmunization.

As I said, it's the only liquid on the planet that contains all of the information on your own body. It's also free and readily available. Why would you not drink it? It's the Super-Human's Golden Nectar.

Feet: Give Them Some Love

Every day we wake up, shower, put on our shoes and socks and go through our day. We have these amazing feet that carry us everywhere, yet when do we pay them any attention? When do we give these incredible components of our physiology some love?

I spend five minutes every night before bed gently massaging my feet from top to bottom as I tell them how grateful I am for them. When you love your feet and massage them, messages are sent to all parts of your body through the nervous system, by what are known as reflexes. This is where the name reflexology comes from.

Reflexology, an ancient tradition, involves applying pressure to and massaging certain areas of the feet. Its aim is to encourage healing and relieve stress and tension. The hands and ears can also be used, but we will be focusing on the feet, as each part of the foot links to all other parts of the body.

The arrangement of the reflexes has a direct relationship to the area of the body they affect. For example, the right side of the foot is linked to the right side of the body, while the tips of the toes correspond to the head. The liver, pancreas, and kidneys connect to the arch of the foot, and the lower back and intestines towards the heel.

EXERCISE *Massage Your Feet*
In a session, a reflexologist will apply pressure to certain reflexes. The aim is to stimulate energy flow and send signals around the body, targeting areas of tension. Reflexology aims to holistically restore balance to the body. I want to encourage you to be your own reflexologist. Every day, start at your heels and work up to your toes. If you feel any sore points (which indicate stuck energy),

massage them out until the soreness has gone. As you massage, feel gratitude for your feet, which carry you everywhere. You will be surprised: once you start developing this relationship with your feet and body your energy will be stronger, and you will feel cleaner and lighter and more vibrant.

As you work you may feel hot or cold flushes and energy through the body, as all parts of the body are linked. It's normal. You will start to understand your body and how all of it is interconnected at a very deep level. Spending a little time with your feet is the perfect Super-Human bedtime ritual.

The Platinum Light Body

We are children of the Stars. Young humans with ancient souls. We carry divine wisdom encoded into us, by ourselves, we came down to Earth to be the experience of our very own creation. As humans, we haven't even scratched the surface of our own inherent, natural abilities stored in the cosmic blueprint of our DNA. We haven't accessed a fraction of the potential in those little crystals (that we activate by performing the qigong routine in the last chapter) in the centre of our brain, nestled inside that pine cone/the pineal gland, or third eye.

Our pineal gland is so much more than a gland. It's a Star Gate with built-in access codes to enter our cosmic nervous system that runs through every power grid, ancient site or cosmic generator, that's ever been created, across multiple timelines, densities or frequency bands. The key to accessing these codes lies within the crystal mainframe of Mother Earth and her magnetic energy, along with the codes contained with the electrical light streams and magnetic pulses from our celestial star families, planets, moons, suns, stars, and planetary, galactic, and universal Star Gates.

The electromagnetic spin points hovering, vibrating in our platinum light body are the trigger/access points to multiple frequencies or bands of information that contain ancient knowledge within our cosmic light body. This is an extension of our light body; they are essentially one and the same, but at the same time very different. Both are a part of you, and both are accessed by light codes. The frequency and vibration of the encoded light determines the level of access. Imagine that one set of codes gives you access to the first three levels in a building (your light body) and another set of codes gives you access to floors 4–7 (your cosmic light body).

When the light body and the cosmic light body integrate fully, the fabric of the cosmic web will be interwoven through an intricate stream of light encoded data streams. The pineal gland is crucial in this process.

These light encoded data streams will birth the new dawn, moving beyond the rebirth of the golden age, into the platinum age and diamond age. Or maybe there will be no rebirth and instead we will collaborate as a global community and create something new and exciting and supersede anything this magnificent Earth has ever seen. This time around it will be phenomenal. Beyond anything the human brain, with its current functionality, could comprehend. We are already there. There is no past or future. We are simply playing our parts perfectly as galactic frequency enhancers, grounding these ancient extra-terrestrial light streams into the Earth.

We have around our physical body a complex web of spiralized geometry, encoded into streams of light, which is what I call the platinum light body. I started seeing this back in 2016, around clients and people in my workshops and trainings after I had taken them through certain activations. After taking many groups through many light encoded activations during meditation, I started to realize what triggered the activation of this platinum light body and what didn't and how it affected people emotionally, physically, mentally and spiritually.

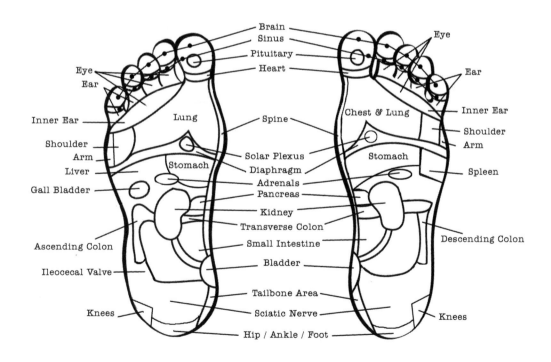

15. Reflexology chart of the feet

Everyone who I took through the activation (and please remember, no one can activate anyone else – I simply take people through a process where they activate themselves, and anyone who says they will activate your DNA is completely insane. No one can do it for you. It's a personal choice and personal mission) saw huge growth and acceleration in their life and mentally they had so much clarity. However, there was an adjustment period (generally lasting between two weeks and four months) when their physical bodies, including the brain, had to recalibrate to these new streams of data. That process generally lasted between two weeks and three or four months but did go on longer for some and to be honest, once the process is initiated, it's a constant stream of changes. A huge acceleration occurred partly due to a huge purge taking place, as old emotions rose and deep trauma healed. Physically they became stronger and healthier, much calmer and focused on life generally, and on their life mission. Accessing and living in the present moment became natural. The ego let up, and being the observer of their life, instead of being wrapped up in the daily drama, became easy. To activate this light body, there is a process, which we will go through later on.

Illustration 16 shows the structure of the activation chamber within your platinum light body. You will see your physical body, surrounded by a merkaba, then an octahedron and an icosahedron. You will also see the body's natural toroidal field. Around the outside is your activation chamber, consisting of thirty-six tubes of light on the outer shell that feed into eighteen streams of light at the top and bottom. These eighteen tubes of light feed into the in and out points, the alpha and omega, which we will discuss shortly. There are other components such as the Kathara Grid that also fit into this structure and we will add thosein later on.

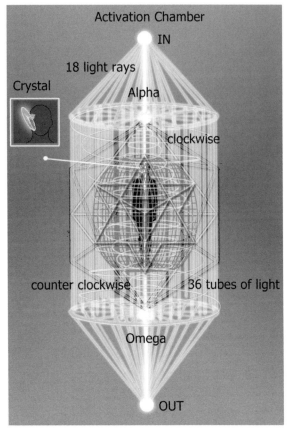

16. Activation chamber and some components

The size of this fluctuates from an average of around 12 metres in height to much larger, and sometimes a little smaller. In many people I've seen it contract and expand, but it generally returns to its natural size of 12 metres from the alpha to the omega.

We are multidimensional beings and there are many of us in the same space at the same time. What that means is that, within the quantum field, there are many of these structures around multiple versions of ourselves. So, there are multiple Jerrys and each one has this structure. As all of the structures spin they create a powerful field of energy.

It's important to know that the merkaba field, the octahedron (and also the icosahedron components), while they look solid, are constantly in flux and are moving in and out of form, due to the new Krystal Spiral Earth Codes. Everything is moving into a fluid state.

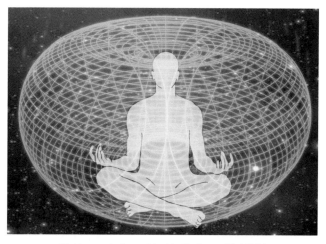

18. Human being sat inside their toroidal field

Through meditation, certain breathing techniques, by using the qigong routine, you activate your body's own toroidal field, naturally amplifying it (see illustration 18).

Energy flows out from your crown, up through the empty space (which, as you can see, isn't that empty), then loops back around, underneath your body and back up through your perineum, creating this doughnut-like shape. We also have a smaller toroidal field inside our heart, and the planet has a large one too.

As our platinum light body comes online, multiple versions of our platinum light body spin (constantly) and create a larger toroidal field around you.

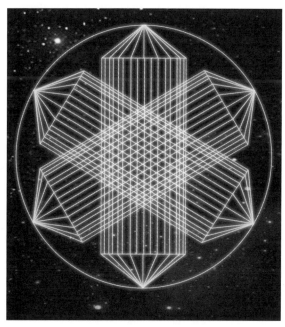

17. Front view of activation chambers

The above illustration shows what you would see from a front-on view if you focused in on this image. Actually, you would see many more activation chambers than this in the same place, but if I were to depict them all you wouldn't be able to make anything out.

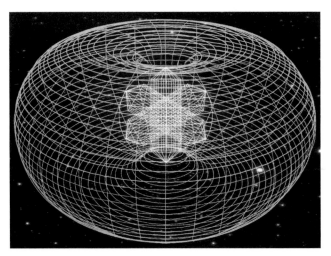

19. Multiple activation chambers spinning and creating a larger toroidal field which expands and contracts in unison with the activation chambers

In illustration 19, you can see that cosmic light travels down from the stars, through the in-point (alpha transmission centre) of the activation chamber and out through the out-point (omega transmission centre) at the bottom. We are actually giving birth to light codes and assisting the Planetary Grids. The alpha is male and the omega female. The sperm travels down (from the stars, and the flow of light is controlled by the male transmission centre) through the womb (the human body) and out through the vagina (the omega transmission centre) and into the planet. It's important to note that within the body's energetic field, there are multiple transmission centres that further control the flow of cosmic energy.

Our mission on Earth is to take high-vibrational light and ground it down into the planet. We essentially are the conduits that are giving birth to new frequencies on Earth and recoding Earth's ancient architecture. Light/information is flowing into our galaxy from other galaxies and universes and these new spiralized fractal patterns/geometries of light are changing us on a subatomic level. As they flow into our nervous system (which consists of 45 miles of electrical wiring), the information contained in these streams flows into our body's cells and triggers a response. Our DNA responds, the mitochondria in our cells respond and the codes contained within the light open access points within our cellular structure, which contains ancient knowledge and wisdom.

The bridge between us as humans accessing this information is our platinum light body. Running these codes also takes control of our epigenetic overlay. Epigenetics is where the environment can affect the cells and we can change our environment physically and mentally and metaphysically, thus creating cellular change. There are also negative epigenetic overlays installed into our energetic fields by negative beings that want to feed off of our low-vibrational energy, and by doing this work you will resemble the epigenetic overlays to their original order, so they work in harmony with you.

Ombromium crystals

You will notice in Illustration 16 that in the activation chamber there is a crystal in the right-hand side of the head. It functions like a satellite dish – it picks up signals. Every human being has one.

Four years ago I was at my computer writing another book when suddenly I disappeared into the screen and ended up on a planet called Bevricon in the constellation of Boötes. I met some incredible beings (which looked human but were not) and visited some healing and recalibration chambers. The beings showed me these crystals and told me they are called ombromium, an off-planet crystal you cannot find on Earth. They showed me that these crystals lay dormant in our heads, ethereally and that they will start to activate when humanity is ready and moving through the 50–100Hzt frequency range (5D and higher).

We are tapping higher than 5D harmonics constantly, as we expand and contract our Light bodies and amplify the rate or vibration and oscillation, the speed at which light moves to and from the centre point. And when we enter these higher frequency bands, we trigger the protocol of the ombromium crystal being activated. It's a little like off-planet plasma light hitting our cells and activating more strands within our twelve-strand DNA template to access our full cosmic Krystalline light body structure.

The pineal gland and this little crystal are both receivers; the crystal is like the pineal gland on steroids. I shared information on this a few years back on a YouTube video and people contacted me saying they had experienced pain in this area but when they went for scans at the hospital there was nothing there.

It's true: when this crystal activates, it can be painful. The pineal gland and ombromium crystal communicate with the brain and rewire certain neural pathways. So, if you experience any pain in the right-hand side of your head, just know what is taking place.

Transmission, Transformation, and Transmutation

As these potent, reality-changing frequencies pass through our nervous system and light body structure, we ground them down into the planet. Up above our head is the alpha transmission centre, a part of our extended 5th-density light body. The off-planet frequencies flow through the ATC (which is male and is responsible for controlling the ebb and flow of cosmic information flowing into our space from the stars) through our platinum light body, through our human nervous system, out through the bottom of our 5th-density platinum light body and out through the omega transmission centre (OTC), which is female. The ATC is approximately 12–15 inches to 3 metres above our crown (always in flux) and the OTC is approximately 3 metres below (but can be a little less as they are also in flux). The light body

expands and contracts. Remember, everything is in flux and moving.

As these frequencies flow through the male ATC and the female OTC we are giving birth, through the omega and into the planet. These codes are helping our species ascend into higher vibrational octaves of light. The role we play in this is mission critical. Humans are like the cord between the electricity supply and the kettle. Without the cord, the water would never get hot. Mother Earth needs us just as we need her. We are all playing our roles in this cosmic game.

Once a human being is attuned and working with the platinum light body daily, the light body becomes aligned to the cosmic platinum and diamond ray (which actually looks a translucent electric-blue colour but has diamond and platinum light codes within it), an information stream containing coding, essential for ascension. This starts to build the spiritual foundation to realign us with our original blueprints: what we are beyond our physical form.

Ascension is a shift in the energetic spectrum of frequency patterns held in a dimensional space, which, when absorbed and activated into the layers of the planetary and human bio-energetic field, activates its DNA Silicate Matrix template/blueprint instruction set, through various codes and coding.

This catalyzes a chain of events that creates a complete transformation and transmutation of various patterns and programs held in the energetic templates/blueprints of the human soul's journey within a cycle of evolutionary time.

When activated, these patterns begin to shift, re-emerge and clear from the layers of experiences coded into every cell and memory pattern held as an energetic vibration within the body's architecture. This part of the biological ascension process may manifest physical, mental and emotional ascension symptoms. However these symptoms arise, just know that you are ready and can handle the process. Embrace and befriend and you will transcend, quickly and efficiently. Resist and you will stifle the natural flow.

There is an entire ethereal crystal grid network that creates all things. It's like a gigantic hard drive, streaming data. The whole game is based around control of this architecture and once you know how to unplug from certain data streams and into new, empowering and uncorruptible data streams, new experiences will show up in your reality, ones that will fill you full of joy, bliss, harmony and strength. Once you are plugged into the cosmic energy flowing into your space in geometrical spirals or waves of magic and your platinum light body is activated, your entire world will transform, naturally. The whole codex of humanity is changing. The structured geometrical nature of our reality is becoming a fluid spiralized reality where the geometries flow. I first noticed this in 2013 when I started seeing moving code in the empty space that flowed and morphed. Whenever I look at anything, between me and whatever I look at, I see code. The entire universe is mathematics and geometry. When I look at the sky I see the code, it's always there.

Doing your qigong, Star Magic style, bringing in the coding contained within the light streams from our Earthly and cosmic grids, rebalances our inner mathematics and realigns us with our original template/blueprint and our source code, which is the foundation for success in this evolution of your soul and Super-Human spiritual abilities. As we know, we are electromagnetic beings, and it's the platinum light body that fires up, bringing about this change. You will bring so much light through you that your body's frequency will elevate universally, and the amount of qi stored in your mesentery will furnish you with the opportunity to change and seriously amplify your life. Qigong is the foundation but there are other tools you are going to need to incorporate. You will need to live a Star Magic

Super-Human lifestyle. And this is important to hammer home. It's not a hobby, it's not some drop-in-and-out-of pursuit that you do here and there, it's a lifestyle. You become this way of living.

The light is intelligent and will naturally connect you into the krystalline grid networks and the planetary architecture so you can embody the new frequency-encoded architecture of our invisible but very real world, and be hosted much like a computer on an upgraded server. Make the best choices: feel your way, listen to your heart. The process is different for everyone.

Spiritual Nutrition

As I travel this world, I meet many healers, spiritual teachers, gurus, who are overweight, carrying massive energetic burdens, unfit women and men who eat GMO food, smoke, drink and simply could not run a mile or maybe not even walk one. So why does this matter?

I've come to realize that we must be fit, strong and healthy, mentally, physically and emotionally, to be able to take these off-planet frequencies, embody them and ground them into the planet effectively.

When people who are not physically fit facilitate healing, they can get away with it to a certain degree. For example, facilitating the healing of small number of people from the comfort of their home or centre. But if these people step it up and try to go to a new level, healing larger groups of people over a weekend or a longer workshop or training, their bodies will rapidly decline. Holding space for a lot of people takes a certain stamina. It's the same when it comes to the real work (running these higher-frequency streams) and the reason we are here on this planet that we are looking at in this book.

I met an older/wiser lady (ninety-five years young) in Turkey, who runs a huge spiritual organization. When it was time to leave, she got up from her chair and her assistant brought in a Zimmer frame. Surprised, I asked her what had happened. She said, "Jerry, I've been communicating with the cosmos for eighty years, it's destroyed my nervous system. If I did all the stuff you youngsters do these days such as yoga, qigong, exercise, ate well, I truly believe that I would be OK. If I knew about nutrition and how to look after my body, things would have been different."

This really hit home to me. I knew it anyway and was on this path, encouraging the Star Magic Tribe to eat high-vibrational foods and exercise, participate in qigong classes and truly prepare their bodies, physically for these galactic changes, but this was great confirmation. Methods like exercise routines, eating high-vibrational food, meditation, among other things, are crucial components in preparing your body for ascension. I am not interested in half measures. I am interested in pushing those illusory boundaries and seeing how far we can take it. Warriors prepare for battle. We are planetary guardians fighting (with love and awareness as our weapon and shield) to create peace and harmony on this incredible planet.

Food

As a kid, I would eat a big bowl of sugary cereal with milk and eight tablespoons of sugar, and sometimes go back for seconds. I ate convenience food like ready meals for dinner. I used to suffer with terrible migraines. I couldn't see, they were so bad. I used to carry a loaded plastic case and be ready to fire a syringe into my leg with the press of a red button. The worst migraines, the ones where I was puking, would disappear in minutes, once I injected myself.

Every morning when I woke up, I would take eight to twelve painkillers before I did anything, just in case I got a migraine. I realized much later, after I'd started eating really clean, that it was

the sugar being expelled from my body that had caused the migraines; every now and then as an adult I would fall off the clean wagon and eat sugar, and, guaranteed, a couple of days after, I would get a headache. It was my liver kicking out the toxicity, which often passes through the brain before it leaves the body.

I had no body fat as a young kid; even though I was eating rubbish I played every sport going and was always out running around with my mates. When I got to thirteen years of age, I stopped getting taller and got fatter. I remember undressing one day and seeing three rolls of fat. I was so embarrassed and devastated. I started running five to ten miles every day. I still ate a bad diet, but at least I lost the body fat. I share this so you know that I have been on a journey with food and exercise.

I recommend you listen to your body when it comes to food. We are all different and must operate our physical vessel from a unique standpoint. Personally, I feel a predominately plant-based nutritional plan is best. We must eat photons (sun-drenched foods that are alive) and drink electrons (water). Some people say raw is best, but I know others whose bodies respond better to vegetables that are cooked – lightly, not destroyed by too much heat. I eat fish here and there and have started eating eggs again recently, after my body started to crave them. Your body knows what's best. Listen to it.

I use a raw protein blend, which contains all of the trace minerals the body requires; this is important as soils are so depleted these days. Topping up on minerals and vitamins is important. Selenium, zinc, magnesium, potassium, copper are a must, as are omega 3, vitamin D3, a good stem cell supplement, seaweed products, all of which you can find in any good nutrition shop. I take a multivitamin and add turmeric, spirulina, wheatgrass, moringa, and maca to my shakes every day.

I predominantly eat fruits, vegetables, and nuts, and use plant-based protein powder. As well as this I drink at least four litres of water per day and a glass of my own urine, as discussed previously. There are days when I take no supplements. There are times when I don't take some of my supplements for several days. Again, with supplementation, listen to the body. It knows what it requires but you must be still enough to hear/feel/know the communication.

I fast for eighteen hours every day, from 6 p.m. to 12 noon the next day. This gives my body a chance to recover and utilize the energy for more important things than breaking down food. There is also a metabolic enzyme that is triggered once you put anything into your body that is not water. This enzyme has a lifespan of twelve hours as we are diurnal creatures. Food or light activates them. Once you go past twelve hours, any food that goes into your body isn't utilized correctly, as the enzyme stops working. The longer you can make your fasting window the better. Research shows that time-restricted eating/fasting enables us to reset our circadian rhythm, meaning better digestive function, detoxification, enzyme and hormone production. There are many additional benefits, such as *improved sleep, improved blood sugar control, weight loss and an overall better sense of well-being.* Logically it makes sense – by eating within a specified window we are allowing our body time to rest and repair. We are giving our pancreas a chance to rest from producing digestive/metabolizing enzymes, and enabling our digestive and detoxification organs to work only when they are required to.

Studies also show that fasting lowers anxiety and depression, reduces blood pressure and insulin resistance markers and increases the activity of liver enzymes. As well as my daily fast, I do a 24-hour fast weekly, a 48-hour fast monthly, and twice a year do a five-day fast.

Fasting activates AMPK (a protein and cellular energy sensor) in response to stresses that deplete supplies of cellular ATP (the cell's energy currency) such as low glucose, hypoxia and exposure to toxins. This activates autophagy, a process by which components inside of cells (including proteins) are degraded and recycled. Autophagy is important for cellular and tissue rejuvenation. It removes damaged cellular components, including misfolded proteins linked to Alzheimer's and other diseases.

AMPK is "considered to be a major therapeutic target for the treatment of metabolic diseases including type 2 diabetes and obesity signalling pathway and inhibits mTOR," (a protein, originally discovered in yeast, that controls cell growth and metabolism in response to nutrients, growth factors, cellular energy, and stress). As a central controller of cell growth, mTOR plays a key role in development and ageing and has been implicated in disorders such as cancer, cardiovascular disease, obesity, and diabetes, which in turn activates autophagy. This only begins to happen naturally, however, when you substantially deplete your glucose stores, and your insulin levels begin to drop.

By forty-eight hours without calories or with very few calories, carbs or protein, your growth hormone level is up to five times as high as when you started your fast. Part of the reason for this is that ketone bodies produced during fasting promote growth hormone secretion, for example in the brain. Ghrelin, the hunger hormone, also promotes growth hormone secretion. Growth hormone helps preserve lean muscle mass and reduces fat tissue accumulation, particularly as we age. It also appears to play a role in longevity and can promote wound healing and cardiovascular health.

By fifty-four hours, your insulin has dropped to its lowest level point since you started fasting and your body is becoming increasingly insulin-sensitive. Lowering your insulin levels has a range of health benefits both short- and long-term. Lowered insulin levels put a brake on the insulin and mTOR signalling pathways, activating autophagy. Lowered insulin levels can reduce inflammation, make you more insulin-sensitive (and/or less insulin resistant) and protect you from chronic diseases of aging including cancer.

By seventy-two hours, your body is breaking down old immune cells and generating new ones. Prolonged fasting reduces circulating IGF-1 levels (IGF-1 is a hormone found naturally in your blood. Its main job is to regulate the effects of growth hormone (GH) in your body. Normal IGF-1 and GH functions include tissue and bone growth) and PKA (an enzyme playing a key role in a number of cellular processes) activity in various cell populations. IGF-1, or insulin-like growth factor 1, looks a lot like insulin and has growth-promoting effects on almost every cell in the body. IGF-1 activates signalling pathways including the PI3K-Akt pathway that promotes cell survival and growth. PKA can also activate the mTOR pathway.

You can see where this is leading – pressing the brakes on IGF-1 and PKA through nutrient restriction and fasting can turn down cellular survival pathways and lead to breakdown and recycling of old cells and proteins. Studies in mice have shown that prolonged fasting (greater than 48 hours), by reducing IGF-1 and PKA, leads to stress resistance, self-renewal and regeneration of hematopoietic or blood stem cells. Through this same mechanism, prolonged fasting for seventy-two hours has been shown to preserve healthy white blood cell or lymphocyte counts in patients undergoing chemotherapy. At seventy-two hours of a fast, studies have shown that the immune system is completely reset. When people come to me with cancer, I have a protocol and a part of that is fasting to reset the body and support healing.

The best part about fasting is the refeeding stage! It's important to break your fast with a nutritious, balanced meal; this will further improve the function of cells and tissues that went through a clean-up while you were fasting.

You should include plenty of vegetables, plant fibres and plant fats such as broccoli and avocado, with healthy proteins and some whole grains or legumes too, if you choose. (Avoid sugar and processed/packaged foods – at all times, but after a fast even more so.) Learn what works best for your body, and what *you* feel best eating following your fasts. You can see now why fasting is mission critical to restore your body's internal components, for rejuvenation and growth. Activating these benefits is a must for any Super-Human. Remember it's about potential. We all have infinite potential. So, do everything in your power to activate it.

My day normally starts at around 5 a.m. I do cardio-vascular exercise in the morning (a jog, after my qigong, meditation and breathing exercises. I am going to share with you my weekly regime later) and weights/boxing/ circuit training around 11 a.m. Once I finish at 12.00 p.m., I start eating, and finish eating at 6 p.m. This works well for me. When I travel I sometimes adjust my schedule and when I have long online trainings I have to adapt my schedule but I always follow the same plan. I move it forward or back several hours.

It's important that you experiment with your body and work out what's best for you. Start with a twelve-hour fast and slowly increase it. Eventually you may eat for one to two hours per day. Some of the best bodybuilders on the planet eat for one hour a day, straight after training. And they pack serious muscle. Gorillas and rhinos eat leaves, and they are the most muscular beings on the planet. I'm not suggesting you go 100 per cent plant-based, as that is not for everyone, but there is massive nutrition in sun-drenched foods. In 2013 I went fully vegan and after several years I really started to notice my body deteriorating with the intensity of my workouts. I felt great for the first two years but then it changed. I continued for a while and then started introducing other sources of nutrition. It really isn't for everyone. I met a guy in LA at the Conscious Life Expo. He'd been vegan for thirty-plus years. His bones were so brittle. He said when he falls or bumps his body, things break. I suggested he started eating other foods and he said he can't because he had stuck the vegan label on himself. He put the label before his health. That is crazy! When it comes to eating and fasting, there are human beings that move around in a really high vibratory rate due to only consuming plants, fruits and vegetables and they become very ungrounded. This again is not a good choice. You are not 100 per cent in control of your consciousness when you are like this, and there are other energies playing around in the space that will take advantage of the fact that you are buzzing like crazy, match that frequency (the one you are on in your high state) and potentially download frequencies into your body and your light body that are not conducive to your spiritual growth and your ascension. Being fully present is important.

You came to Earth to be extraordinary, so be extraordinary in every which way possible. Eat clean. Train/exercise. Meditate. Elevate your frequency and expand continuously. Most of all, listen to your body.

Exercise

We are awesome beings here on Earth and if you want to truly thrive, exercise is a must. I know people will tell me they are happy not exercising. Others will tell me doing exercise is not necessary to thrive. I call that bullshit. These are people who have either never tried exercise or have never pushed themselves to the point where it hurts and it's tough and you smash through those barriers on a consistent basis, getting fitter, healthier, stronger, sharper, getting dopamine hit after dopamine hit, feeling awesome about yourself.

Taking the body into the red zone (pushing yourself/your body to the point of extreme pain), keeping going and making the red zone your comfort zone and then moving up a level into the next red zone is a phenomenal feeling. Seeing how much you can get from your body is rewarding. Your body is capable of so much, yet most people never stick at their exercise regimes long enough to find out what's possible. They quit. Why? Because it's painful when you start and the body gets sore; but once you commit, decide, choose, focus and exercise discipline and the body and mind know you will not quit, that you are relentless, they will stop being stubborn, surrender to the pain and start adapting, changing, growing, getting stronger. You will tear muscles open so they can grow and develop. Your lung capacity will elevate, and you will be able to run longer and faster, sprint quicker.

There really are no excuses for not exercising. There are so many levels at which one can engage in physical exercise; all I am suggesting right now is that you do a little more than you are doing. If you are doing nothing, then walk. If you are walking, then jog. If you are jogging, drop down from time to time and throw in some push-ups and burpees. If you are circuit training, try some yoga and swimming as well. If you are a wheelchair user, get some small dumb-bells and exercise your shoulders, biceps and triceps. If you can't afford dumb-bells, get two tins of beans and use those. The point I am trying to make is, wherever you are you can do something, and if you are doing something, you can do a little more.

Mix it up. If you are lifting weights and doing cardiovascular exercise seven days a week, try dropping to five days; box one day and do yoga another. It's about variation and progression.

Sometimes to improve you just need to rest or do a lighter or different activity. Our body adapts to its environment, so shock it. Do different things. Get your pushbike out and cycle for 25 miles at 4 a.m. Really mix it up.

When I run there is no thought, just space, and when there is space, the magic flows. There is room for communication, both subtle and extremely direct and powerful communication.

Jogging on an open road, meditating, qigong, are all ways to tap into the creative energies, often suppressed or drowned out by a busy mind. When you quieten your mind, you open a floodgate of universal intelligence that can often bring forth gifts from positive (and negative so maintain your discernment) beings, playing in other densities or frequency bands, willing to share knowledge and wisdom that you can use to create greatness in your life and positively affect your sisters and brothers of Earth. You tap into the light and information streams that carry vast amounts of spiralized geometrical data. With an open heart, connected to your pineal gland, this data can be translated into ideas, inventions, books, and developed as skill sets to trigger transformation.

When I exercise, I am so present that ideas flow from the invisible world. So, exercise gives you the opportunity to build muscle, get lean, strengthen your core, strengthen your mind, enhance your endurance, build mental focus and clarity and generally make you feel super-awesome. It's important to note that exercise doesn't have to take a long time. Fifteen to twenty minutes of non-stop circuit training, when you put the effort in and go hard, is better than walking or jogging slowly for two hours on a treadmill. Every day I train hard and three to four times a week I take myself into the fires of hell to carve my soul into a beast that can handle life. When you take yourself into the deep dark holes mentally and physically, nothing in life can

shake you up. For me some of my favourites are 100 calories for time (as fast as you can) on the Assault Bike, 2 miles for time (as fast as you can) on the treadmill, 2 miles on flat ground with a 55lb bergen (same weight the SAS carry) for time (as fast as you can) and carrying two 25kg plates for 5 kilometres for time (as fast as you can).

I want to give you some options for beginner, intermediate and advanced levels of fitness. I am going to throw in three short challenges for beginners and seven circuit options for intermediate and advanced levels. You will also find a list of exercise descriptions for those who are new to exercise or don't know these specific kinds. You can also look these exercises up online.

Remember: be relentless and execute daily and, at some point, training will become a healthy obsession, a beautiful addiction, a must.

Beginners

These challenges are for those of you who have not exercised before or have not exercised in a long time. You require zero equipment. Just you.

Challenge 1

(Please note waking time can be adjusted. Early is all that matters)

DAY 1: Wake up at 6 a.m. and walk for 10 minutes.

DAY 2: Wake up at 6 a.m. and walk for 15 minutes.

DAY 3: Wake up at 6 a.m. and walk for 20 minutes

DAY 4: Wake up at 6 a.m. and walk for 25 minutes.

DAY 5: Wake up at 6 a.m. and walk for 30 minutes.

DAYS 6–14: Wake up at 6 a.m. and walk for 30 minutes.

DAYS 15–21: Wake up at 6 a.m., walk for 25 minutes and jog for 5 minutes, slowly, but faster than walking.

DAYS 22–28: Wake up at 6 a.m., walk for 20 minutes and jog for 10 minutes.

That is your 4-week challenge. Once you have accomplished this, move on to Challenge 2.

Challenge 2

DAY 1: Repeat Challenge 1 from days 22–28 but jog for 15 and walk for 15. In the afternoons or evenings, you will need to set aside 20 minutes to do the following bodyweight circuit:

1-minute squats. 1-minute jumping jacks. 1-minute sit-ups. 1-minute push-ups (do them on your hands and feet if you can; drop to your knees if you need to). 1-minute lunges on your right leg. 1-minute lunges on your left leg. 1-minute plank (break it into 2 x 30 if you need, or 4 x 15 seconds, but just do it).

The same goes for each of the exercises. Get through them. Jog slowly for 3 minutes (we call this active recovery) and then repeat one more time. When you are working for 1 minute on each exercise, there is no hurry. Just keep moving at this stage. Do your very best.

DAY 2: Repeat **DAY 1**.

DAY 3: Repeat **DAY 1**.

DAY 4: Repeat **DAY 1**.

DAY 5: Repeat **DAY 1**.

DAY 6: Repeat **DAY 1**.

DAY 7: Rest.

DAYS 8–14: Repeat day 1 and then do 20 burpees at the end of your afternoon or evening workout.

DAYS 15–21: Repeat days 8–14 and then jog for another 5 minutes at the end of your afternoon or evening workout.

DAYS 22–28: Repeat days 15–21 and do 90 seconds of plank at the end.

Now move on to Challenge 3.

Challenge 3

DAYS 1–7: Repeat Days 22–28 from Challenge 2. On the morning run you want to be aiming to jog the full 30 minutes now. If that is easy, increase the run to 45 minutes.

DAYS 8–14: Repeat days 22–28 from Challenge 1 and as soon as you finish in the morning you will do 30 burpees. In the evening. Repeat Days 22–28 from Challenge 2.

DAYS 15–21: Keep the morning routine the same. In the afternoon you are going to do the following. 10 jump squats, 10 burpees, 1-minute wall squat. 1-minute plank. 10 plank to press-up (5 each side). 10 leg raises, 10 leg extensions, sprint 20 metres and back 3 times as fast as you can. Rest for 90 seconds–2 minutes. Repeat 4 times.

DAYS 22–28: Repeat Days 15–21 and add 100 jumping jacks to the end of the afternoon workout.

If you are new to exercise or haven't exercised in some time, this plan will get you started in the right direction and then you can follow your heart, what you are guided or feel drawn to from there. You will be so happy you got off the couch and went for it.

There are no excuses. If you start work at 6 a.m., get up at 4 a.m. and go to bed earlier. Make it work. Be ready for whatever life throws your way. After this three-month plan you can join a gym, do cross-fit, yoga, swimming, a martial art or a combination of different things. Remember, it doesn't have to take hours. The routines above take less than 1 hour and 15 minutes a day and they will transform your world. Do them. Start today, now. Don't put it off. The opportunity to make excuses, to take the easy road, will flow into your mind regularly. People, events, food: they can all be excuses. Stamp them out. Crush them and stick to your game plan.

Intermediate to Advanced

I am combining these two together because they are in the form of circuits and if you already train/exercise, you will know that any circuit training session can be reduced or amplified by reps or time. So, I will leave it to you to decide whether you want to reduce it or amplify it. I recommend you do one bodyweight circuit session a day and have one day of rest in the seven. You can mix them in with your other trainings. They are short and sweet (well maybe short and tough, but go hard or go home, beautiful soul), so get them done. I am going to share seven circuits. You can pick and choose.

Circuit 1

WARM UP: 100 jumping jacks

Followed by 20 burpees, 20 jump squats, 20 push-ups, 50 plank taps, 20 mountain climbers, 20 v-sit-ups, 20 leg raises. Rest for 30 seconds–1 minute. Repeat 6 times.

Time yourself. Next time try to beat that time.

Circuit 2

You will need a bar, climbing frame or tree branch for this.

WARM UP: 1 minute of burpees

Followed by 30 plank to press, 20 squat thrusts, 20 pull-ups, 30 jumping lunges. Repeat 6 times with no rest. Finish with a 5-minute wall squat followed by a 3-minute plank.

Time yourself. Next time try to beat that time.

Circuit 3

WARM UP: 50 jump squats

Followed by 20 super-burpees (burpee with a tuck jump), 20 (10 each side) Turkish get-ups (add weight as required), 20 sit-ups, 20 leg extensions. Repeat 5 times with no rest (the sit-ups and leg extensions are your active recovery).

Then 50 mountain climbers, 50 push-ups, 50 jump squats and 180 ankle taps (no break) followed by 2 minutes plank to finish.

Time yourself. Next time try to beat that time.

Circuit 4

You will need a field/park/or any space where you can run 30 metres.

WARM UP: 50 jump squats.

Followed by 20 push-ups, sprint 30 metres, 15 push-ups, sprint 30 metres, 10 push-ups, sprint 30 metres, 5 push-ups, sprint 30 metres, 5 burpees, sprint 30 metres, 10 burpees, sprint 30 metres, 15 burpees, sprint 30 metres, 20 burpees, sprint 30 metres.

Then for your active recovery, 20 sit-ups, 20 leg raises, 20 v-sit ups, 90 seconds plank. Repeat once more.

Time yourself. Next time try to beat that time.

Circuit 5

WARM UP: 50 jump squats.

Followed by 10 minutes burpees. That's it. Great way to kick-start your day.

Count the repetitions. Next time try to beat the amount of burpees.

Circuit 6

You will need a field/park/or any space where you can run 40 metres.

WARM UP: 100 jumping jacks

Followed by 20 star jumps, 20 sumo-squats, 20 jump squats, 20 push-ups, 30 Russian step-throughs, 20 crocodile push-ups (10 one way and then 10 back to the start point), 20 mountain climbers, 3-minute wall squat, 90-second plank. Then sprint 40 metres, jog back slowly and go again. Repeat 8 times.

Time yourself. Next time try to beat that time.

Circuit 7

You will need a bar, climbing frame or tree branch for this. Plus, some open space to run.

WARM UP: 30 burpees, 30 jump squats

Followed by 20 push-ups, 10 clap push-ups, 20-star jumps, 20 pull-ups, 20 jumping lunges, 20 close-grip push-ups, sprint 20 metres, 30 mountain climbers, 20 jump squats, 10 v-sit-ups, sprint back. 100 Russian twists (active recovery). Repeat 5 times.

THEN TO FINISH: handstand position against a wall or tree (in empty space if you are able). Hold for 30–60 seconds. 5-minute wall squat, 3 minutes plank.

EXERCISES

Squats

Start with your feet slightly wider than shoulder width, toes pointed slightly outwards. Lower your buttocks towards the ground, nice and deep, and then push back up again.

Jumping jacks

Start with your feet together and your arms by your side. You will jump your feet outwards, wider than your shoulders, and your arms will rise up to and above your shoulders. You will then jump back to the starting position.

Sit-ups

Lie on the floor. Bring your feet/knees up towards your buttocks. Place your fingers/hands on the sides of your head (not behind) and pull your upper body towards your bent knees. Go all the way up and then lower your upper body down.

Again: do not put your hands behind your head and pull it forwards. It's no good for your neck.

Push-ups

(Do them on your hands and feet if you can, or drop to your knees if you need to.)

OPTION 1

Place your knees on the floor. Place your hands on the floor in front of you, then lower your chest towards the ground. Just before you get there, push back up.

You will need to play with the distance of your hands; you do not want them too close to your lower body, otherwise when you lower your chest to the ground, your butt will be stuck up in the air.

Your hips and chest must be lowered towards the ground together, with your back straight, not bent.

OPTION 2

Same as option one but your knees will be off the ground so only your feet and hands are touching the ground.

With both options you can increase and decrease the width of your hands to hit the chest slightly differently. Play with it.

Lunges

Stand with your feet together. Step forward with one leg. A nice big stride. Keep the forward foot planted. Now lower your back knee down towards the ground. Just before it gets there, push it back up several inches. You want to push off your front foot and back toes and you will feel the muscle working on your back thigh, in the quad area. You want to make sure that your front knee does not go over your toes. If it does, readjust slightly. Work one leg and then change sides.

Plank

Place your elbows and forearms on the ground, your toes together and also on the ground. Your body must be straight. Squeeze your legs, core, hips, abdominals while you are in this position. Do not let your hips drop. If you cannot hold it, rest for a few seconds and then go again.

Burpees

Start standing. Feet together. You are going to bring your hands to the floor, kick your legs back, lower your chest to the ground, push back up like a push-up and then bring your feet towards your hands and jump as high as you can in the air.

Super-burpees

You will do the same as above but instead of jumping at the end (after you have brought your feet back towards your hands) you are going to bring both knees up towards your chest as you jump.

Jump squat

Start with your feet slightly wider than shoulder width, toes pointed slightly outwards. Lower your buttocks towards the ground, nice and deep, and then jump up as high as you can.

Wall squat

Find a wall. Place your feet 30–60 cm in front of it. You will need to play with the distance depending on the size of your body and length of your legs. Now go into a squat position with your back straight against the wall. Hold this position.

Plank to press

Get into the press-up position from above. Now lower down onto one elbow and forearm and then the other until you are in the plank position. Now go back to the push-up position, keeping your toes on the floor and knees off the floor. Now do one push-up. Then lower yourself down to one elbow and forearm and then the other and return to the plank. Repeat.

Leg raises

Lie completely flat. Keep your legs straight and lift them up to 90 degrees, then lower them back down until they are two inches off the floor. Then raise them up again.

Leg extensions

Sit on the floor. Place your hands behind your buttocks for support and lift your feet off the ground. Now extend your legs and bring them back in again. You want to be leaning back slightly. If you can release your hands from the ground too, maintaining balance, then do it.

Plank taps

Start in the plank position as above. Now reach out as far as you can with your right hand and touch the floor. Bring it back and then repeat with the opposite hand. Ensure your body is straight and your hips don't sway when you are reaching.

Mountain climbers

Start off in a press-up position. Now move your left foot towards your left elbow. Keep your back straight. You don't want your bum sticking up in the air. This is your starting position. You are now going to alternate your feet. Keep your hips down as low as you can. Keep repeating and squeeze your core/abdominals as you work.

V-Sit-ups

Lie flat on the floor. Bring your arms up over your head so they are flat on the floor and pointing away from your head. Now bring your legs and upper body off of the ground together. You want your fingers to touch your toes in the middle. Your body is creating a V-shape. You then lower your legs and body down, but your shoulders, middle and upper back and feet do not touch the ground. You then raise yourself back up, keeping the pressure in your abdominals/core.

Squat thrust

Start off in a press-up position. Now take some body weight on your chest and arms and bring your feet up between your elbows and your hands and kick them back again. Keep your back straight. You don't want your bum sticking up in the air.

Pull-ups

Hold onto a tree or pull-up bar or climbing frame. Hang with your body straight. Your hands can vary in width and you can play with this to work your muscles differently. Now pull yourself up until your chin is in line with or above the bar and then lower yourself down.

Jumping lunges

Start in the lunge position as above. Now jump from one leg to another. Back and forth.

Turkish get-ups

Lie down flat. Place your right hand facing towards the sky. Now get up and make sure your right hand is above your head the entire time. Once you've stood up, lower yourself back to the floor until you are lying flat with your right arm still pointing towards the sky. That is one rep. Repeat. You can start adding small weights to the hand above your head. The more weight you add the more you will have to engage your core/shoulder/chest and mind.

Star jumps

Stand with your feet together. Bend your legs and touch your toes. Now spring up powerfully and extend your arms and legs into a star position. Land back in the same position as you started with your feet together. Spring from one repetition to the next.

Sumo squats

Exactly the same as a squat but you will start with your feet wide, like the stance of a sumo wrestler. Feet pointed out more. Squat deep towards the floor and push back up.

Russian step-throughs

Start with your feet together, crouching down and your fingers/hands on the floor. Lift your left hand and kick your right leg through until it's straight and your right heel touches the floor gently. Return to the start position and then do the opposite side.

Crocodile push-ups

Start in a push-up position but with one hand forward and one back underneath your pecs (chest). Do a push-up, then reverse the hand position by moving the hand that is back in front of the hand that is in front. You will have to shuffle your feet and toes and move forwards as you do this. All the time, keep your back straight and hips stable. You are walking forward like a crocodile. Then do another push-up with the other hand in front and the hand that was first in front now behind. Keep walking forwards, maintaining the position of a crocodile. Back totally straight.

Clap push-ups

Start in the push-up position. Lower your chest towards the ground, push up with force; your hands will leave the ground and you will clap your hands together before your hands touch the ground again, ready for the next push-up.

Close grip push-ups

Start in a push-up position. Now move your hands together. Your thumbs and forefingers should be touching. Now do your push-ups from here.

Russian twists

Start sitting. Lean back slightly and lift your legs (80 per cent straight) off of the floor. Touch the floor by your left hip with both hands and then touch the floor by your right hip with both hands. Keep your legs as still as possible. Add a medicine ball/dumb-bell/kettlebell to the mix, or any kind of weight you wish.

Handstand against a wall

This is what it says on the tin. A handstand against a wall. Place both hands on the floor, 10–15 inches away from the wall, then walk your feet towards your hands and kick up until your heels are resting against the wall. Maybe you want to chuck in a press-up from this position, then lower your body and push back up. Work towards doing it with zero support.

Time is not an excuse; these routines are short. Go through the different options and try them all out. They will hit your entire body, including the heart and lungs. This isn't all you should do. This is to mix in with your existing workouts. Add in a swim once a week also. On your days off training, go for a gentle walk. Active recovery is a must. The body needs rest, and it also needs movement, so get the balance right. This is important. When you start exercising or step up your existing levels of exercise, the body gets sore. Don't be one of those people who rests because you are sore. People say they have over-trained. No, you just got your lazy arse, off the couch and are feeling it. Breathe, go and workout again the next day. Now, you *can* over-train. I have done it and when you do it's tough to pull yourself out.

It happened to me in 2007/8. I was training real intensely. Seven days a week, twice a day on some days. My healthy obsession tipped out of balance. I was like this for over a year with no break. This is not respecting that your body needs to rest. I started to notice my attitude changing slightly. It was so subtle: my workouts were deteriorating; I was doing some crazy circuits and beating my times, and then my times slowly dropped. I decided to take two weeks off and do nothing. I did get that spark back, but it took me a while to get back to full capacity. It's important to rest, fully. There are times when your body is just sore and you should push on, and times when it actually needs rest. When you commit, you will figure it out.

As you can see, this spiritual journey is also a human journey. We are in these physical bodies and our physical bodies are an extension of our Spirit, which is an extension of our Soul. We must look after them and make them as strong and robust as possible, so we can utilize them fully in a physical capacity but also so we can run high frequency through them. I recommend you stretch your body for 15–20 minutes after every workout. Not before. You want to stretch when the body is warm, not when it's cold; stretching cold can increase your chance of injury. Or, warm up a little and then stretch. I have found that if I keep my hips, glutes and hamstrings super-flexible, the rest of my body is OK. I still stretch every body part, but these areas are high-priority for me. Search full-body stretching routines online if you are unsure. Just like with exercise, ease into it and slowly build it up. Slightly deeper, a little longer.

These exercise routines/circuits are mostly all bodyweight routines, so you can do them at home, on holiday, on your travels, most of them in a hotel room or prison cell (let's hope that isn't necessary but you get my drift); you can do them anywhere. For those where I say you need a bar, a tree branch will do. So money and time are no excuses.

Be a Super-Human and work on all aspects of who you are. Remember you can increase or decrease your repetitions, increase or decrease exercise or rest time. Everything can be added to or subtracted from. Once a week, have an iced bath. Submerge for ten minutes. (You may want to build up to this.) Get a truck or tractor tyre for your garden and, every now and then, go out into the garden and flip it 150 times – again, you're shocking the body. Or get a sledgehammer and hit the tyre for a few minutes.

If you're walking through a park and you see a pull-up bar, go and do as many pull-ups as you can and then hang on for as long as you can. If you see a tree, climb it. Get the body used to moving in different positions. A game of football, a tennis match, a game of squash; they all activate your body in a different way. Maybe try a sky-dive one day, or a bungee jump. Taking your body out of its comfort zone is the only way to grow. You will develop, expand, become stronger – mentally, physically, emotionally and spiritually. Trust this process. Trust yourself and build resilience, speed, power. You are training to be Super-Human. Your body must be strong in order to handle these new light frequencies coming to Earth and you want to be prepared mentally and physically for whatever comes your way. Remember this!

Headstand

There are so many different types of exercise; ones that make you sweat and breathe deeply and others that are more controlled and activate the body in other ways. The headstand is the perfect example of the second type. The headstand has many benefits, both physically and mentally. It is one of the most activating things you can do for your body.

You can do your headstand near a wall for a little support or just in open space. Make sure you are not near any tables or objects in case you come out of the pose quickly and in an uncontrolled fashion, as you are learning/remembering.

I like to go up into a headstand and then breathe deeply into my belly, incorporating different types of breathwork, ones we will cover later in the book. For now, start practising your headstands; you can incorporate the breathing later.

Here are some of the benefits:

1. Balances the heart and the circulatory system. When we invert the body, gravity helps to bring the blood in the veins towards the heart.

2. Breathing and the circulatory systems are strengthened.

3. The brain, spinal cord and the rest of the nervous system are provided with an increased blood supply, rich in nutrients.

4. Any condition of the nerves, eyes, ears, nose and throat can be improved.

5. Awesome for relieving constipation.

6. Increased memory and intellectual capacity.

7. Improved concentration, willpower and focus.

8. Stimulates a physical and mental feeling of harmony and balance.

9. Reduces fluid retention in the legs.

10. The thyroid gland, pituitary gland and pineal gland are stimulated. As a consequence, the other endocrine glands are coordinated and stimulated.

11. An increase in blood pressure has a positive effect on the brains, eyes and ears.

12. Mental fatigue, depression and fears dissolve.

13. Stimulates the central nervous system.

14. The baroreceptors are stimulated, which allows the body to regulate blood pressure better.

15. Positive effect on the heart.

16. Strengthening of the back, shoulder and arm muscles.

17. Blood circulation and the lymphatic system are stimulated throughout the body.

18. Improvement of digestion and secretion of toxins.

19. All vital organs are stimulated.

You can do your headstand near a wall for a little support, or just in open space. I repeat, make sure you are not near any tables or objects in case you come out of the pose quickly and in an uncontrolled fashion.

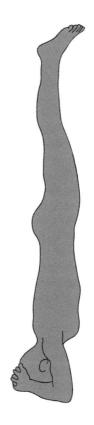

20. Head stand position

Basic instructions

1. Sit on your knees and bring your arms to the floor under your shoulders.

2. Keeping your elbows there, bring your hands closer and interlock your fingers to form a cup.

3. Place the top of your head on the floor, with the back of your head held by your cupped hands.

4. Keeping your head and your elbows there, straighten your knees and lift your hips upward. Keeping your weight on your elbows, walk your feet toward your head, keeping your knees straight.

Keep walking until your hips are directly over your shoulders.

5. Slowly lift one foot at a time off the floor, bringing your knees in toward your chest. Hold this position for one breath, pushing your elbows into the floor.

6. Keeping your knees bent and together, slowly straighten both legs to the ceiling. Focus on a point, keep pushing your elbows into the floor, and breathe slowly and deeply.

Coming out of the pose

To come down, keep one foot toward the ceiling and, with control, lower the other foot to the floor. Lie still and relax for a while. Five to ten minutes. Just feel your body and the energy inside it.

If you have any head or neck injuries, then please be careful. Take it slow. I used to spend time, before attempting the headstand, simply putting my head on the floor with my hands next to it. A hundred per cent of the weight in my hands and my feet, with the top of my head touching the floor, 0 per cent weight on my head. Slowly adjust the weight to 95 per cent and 5 per cent. Move your head back and forth and side to side, real slow. You can do this for 20–30 seconds and slowly increase/shift the weight adjustment until your neck feels stronger and can take more weight. Eventually you can be on your toes and head with your hands off the floor. When you feel ready, move into your headstand.

This is a Super-Human must. Spend some time upside down each day. Be inverted. It's beautiful. You will feel amazing afterwards. It's like a drug. One that has no detrimental side effects.

Oxygen – the New Coffee

When most people get tired, they reach for a coffee or a sugary snack. What I am about to share with you is better than any coffee or sugary snack on the planet. I am going to give you another option to focus and energize you. A healthy choice that knocks coffee out the park and out of this universe. This healthy choice is oxygen – but oxygen consumed in a specific way.

Most people do not breathe properly. They breathe shallow, short breaths, and this is not healthy. When you breathe into your chest you activate your fear receptors, but when you breathe into your belly, you activate calm receptors. Breathing creates electrical activity in the brain and this activity starts a chain reaction, creating emotions and chemicals. In turn we feel a certain way, and then we often behave/act a certain way as a result. For example, if we breathe shallowly, we feel fear, our body contracts, we tighten and hunch forward and look to the floor. This in turn makes us feel anxious or depressed. If we breathe deeply and slowly, we feel calm, we expand as a result, our chest opens, our shoulders go back, we look up and feel confident, focused.

If you have never really paid too much attention to your breath, for the first ten minutes of every day for the next week, when you wake up, stand or sit on the edge of your bed, with your back straight. Close your eyes and breathe in through your nose, all the way down to the pit of your stomach, and back out slowly through your nose. As you go from your ten minutes of focused, slow, deep breathing into your day, keep bringing your awareness to your breath. Being aware of and maintaining this slow deep rhythm will change your life. You will be calm, and your frequency will rise as you create space in your body, mind and life, by simply being still and aware enough to not let the thoughts in your head run you. You will become less reactive (and eventually non-reactive), non-judgemental, relaxed and focused on the elements of life that will nurture and grow you.

Once you have changed (after a week of practice, maybe sooner or maybe a little longer) to a deep rhythmic breathing pattern, I want you to start a breathing routine that consists of three different types of breathing that will elevate your life to a whole new level. We touched upon these during our qigong routine, but I want to give you another, simple 4.5-minute breathing routine that will expand you gigantically.

The three breathing methods are *fire breathing*, *holotropic breathing* and *pressure breathing*.

Firstly, to remind you, fire breathing is where you breathe in and out through your nose, hitting your belly deeply with each breath. You can put your hand over your belly button as a target for the breath. Pressure breathing is where you breathe in through your nose and pull the light from the Earth up through the body to the pineal gland in the head and hold it before releasing. Holotropic breathing is where you breathe in through your nose down to the pit of your stomach, and then forcefully out through your mouth, with a kind of shout/roar. With all of these breathing methods, you must squeeze your buttocks, genitals and perineum and pull your abdominals back towards your spine.

You can do this routine at any time during the day; we are going to utilize it as a replacement for those times whenever you would usually reach for coffee or a sugary snack. It's an awesome reset and so energizing. It can freshen you up and focus you for the rest of your day's activities.

EXERCISE *Breathing Espresso*

The first thing you are going to do is stand with your feet shoulder width, a slight bend in your knees, squeeze your perineum, buttocks, genitals and pull your abdominals back to your spine. Keep the tip of your tongue on the roof of your mouth for the first and second exercises (you won't be able to do that for the holotropic (third) breath, however).

Place your right hand over your navel (this is to be used as your target for each in-breath) and then fire-breathe for thirty-six breaths. In and out of the nose, hard and fast.

After thirty-six in- and out-breaths, you will focus on Mother Earth's heart, her merkaba, down in the centre of the planet, and see her platinum light flow up into your perineum and collect. Then from there, pull this light up with your in-breath, all the way up to your crown. Your focus will follow the light up your spine, through your central channel and up to your crown. Bring your awareness to the area of your pineal gland, which is in the centre of your head and back slightly. Remember, where your attention goes your energy follows.

You will hold the breath for a count of thirteen seconds and then let it out slowly, letting go of the squeeze down below as well. Repeat this process two more times (three times in total). This is pressure breathing.

You will then do thirty-six hard and fast holotropic breaths. Breathe in through the nose, down to the pit of your stomach hard, and then out through the mouth hard, with a little noise (shout). I recommend squeezing and pulling for 6 in- and out-breaths and let go for 6 in- and out-breaths and repeat through the process. This is one cycle.

Repeat this three times.

At the end of the three sets be still for one minute and observe your body. Then continue with your day.

Each cycle takes about ninety seconds, so if you are focused, this whole thing will take 4.5 minutes. It takes you five minutes to drink a coffee when it's hot, and it costs you money and has no real benefits. This short and sweet breathing routine will activate your whole system, re-energize you and offers you so many more benefits. We don't need to discuss them at this stage but we will cover them later. For now, experience this by trying it. If you don't drink coffee, replace your green tea, soda, whatever you reach to for a pick me up. If your breathe is already your pick me up, then, boom, you are ahead of the game.

You can utilize this breath before you go back to work or into the gym or a business meeting, or maybe to turbocharge your frequency before you get home to the family. You can use it as a tool to boost your energy so you can carry on, being focused and productive. When you get home to your partner or family each day, they want you switched on, especially if you have children.

Another option, instead of moving straight on with your day, is to let the one minute of silence at the end go on. You could lie down and just let your body recalibrate and do what it wants to do with all of this extra light and oxygen, in an activated state. You will feel amazing if you surrender, let go and just be. With your eyes closed you can see the truth, geometry, patterns, a kaleidoscope of magic and information. Feel the energy moving around your body and just allow, accept and enjoy and feel total bliss.

This tool will give you huge energy, deep cleansing experiences and consciousness upgrade after consciousness upgrade and it takes 4.5 minutes and it's free. It's the new coffee, baby!

Meditation

Meditation is a must, for everyone. I want to get very clear on meditation and what it is. Many people have their own perception of what it is; and it has become tainted by so many variations, meditation products and different theories that people have got confused and shied away, thought it will take over their life, thought that it's too hard (because every time they try their mind chatters non-stop) and only for dedicated monks or spiritual or religious people.

Meditation is something every human being can do. It can take a little practice, but everyone is able to do it. Firstly, you do not need to wear white clothes or dress like Mary or Jesus (however they truly dressed. No one really knows because for all we know, Mary wore pink yoga pants, a vest, had dragon tattoos and had her hair in dreadlocks and Jesus wore a leather jacket with black shades and ripped jeans and they both smoked weed, consumed magic mushrooms and lit up bars, nightclubs and brothels back in their day). You can wear what you want. You do not have to be under a tree or on a mountain, carry crystals, burn incense or bow to any religion, spiritual pursuit, mystical deity or be any particular thing whatsoever. For your information, once you get good at it, life becomes one constant meditation.

There are different styles of meditation that we are going to work towards – which really is a terrible way of saying it. Because you don't have to work towards anything, you simply have to do nothing and be, and that involves going nowhere. The aim is to turn in; remember, you are an infinite being, created from sound, vibration and light and you are it all. We simply have to peel back the layers and enter that space of nothing or no-thing, beyond thoughts, actions, feelings, into a place of darkness and stillness. Here in the space, you can connect to the frequency that created our world, our galaxy, our universe and multiple other universes beyond this one. It's a space full of energy, powerful cosmic energy. You can call it the field, a place, a sacred space, the womb of creation. From this empty, dark space all things are possible.

The four styles of meditation that work best based on my personal experience and my work with thousands of clients, are as follows:

1. *The Constant Meditation*
   Used all day every day.

2. *The Deep and Expansive Meditation*
   Used to journey, heal and collect data.

3. *The Creative Meditation*
   Used to construct and create your life.

4. *The Guided Meditation*
   Where you are guided by someone who will take you on a journey or simply guided you into the still expanse of your own human vessel.

1. **The Constant Meditation**
Used all day every day.

When you practise meditation, you create space. You start to feel like you are observing life, your thoughts and your emotions. It may seem a little strange to say that you can observe your feelings or your emotions, because when you are angry or sad or hurt, you feel those feelings. There is, however, a gap that starts to arise, a subtle gap, yet extremely powerful and profound once you access it. When you start to meditate you become still. At first your mind wanders, your body becomes agitated, the conversations start inside your head about what you didn't do earlier or what you must do tomorrow or the relationship with your boss or parents or spouse that is a little rocky right now.

The mind will do anything it can to distract you from the present moment. You see, in the present moment the ego has no power. It can only exist in the future or past, when it associates with an event that's taken place previously in linear time or an event it creates in your head, which will take place in the so-called future. For example, it creates an event where you arrive home and find your spouse has left you because of an argument that took place earlier that day. In real terms, the spouse will not leave; but the mind creates these scenarios. And the subconscious mind doesn't know the difference between what's going on internally and externally, so when these scenarios are created internally the body starts to get its fix of chemicals released through imagined (but very real for the body) trauma.

The more you meditate and observe your mind, the more you realize that you and your thoughts are not the same thing. Most of the time, we "become" our thoughts as the mind gets up to its mischief, creates an illusory scenario, the chemicals are released, and the body gets its fix. Once you become an extraordinary observer, you will watch the thoughts in action and then change focus. Remember, wherever your focus and attention go, your energy follows. So, focus on peace, happiness, connection, on a life where every situation is one that you thrive and expand in.

Once you get to this stage, life will become a constant meditation. In every waking moment, you are fully present, fully aware of your environment, the people in it, the situations and events unfolding, and you simply observe all things. You look but you don't label, you observe, and you don't judge. Once you take those labels and judgements out of the mix, you dissolve the opportunity to create a connection between the thoughts/labels/judgements and your body.

We all have, or have had, some issues with fear, anxiety, hurt, rejection or whatever drug we are addicted to. But the beautiful thing is that we are changing as a species, as a family. Our awareness is heightening, and our consciousness is expanding. So much of our own energy (around 80 per cent according to science) is wasted on unnecessary thoughts/thinking. In other words, thinking uses our energy/life force. When our mind is still we conserve and build energy. Wouldn't you like to have all of that energy (the extra 80 per cent) at your disposal to be used for other things? You can do this, now. You can make life a constant meditation, be free, free to love every human being as a sister or brother, playing this interesting game we call life.

To practise constant meditation, I simply want you to go about your daily life and observe yourself.

Watch how your mind talks about other people, situations, events. Watch how it mentally attacks, blames, defends, so naturally. Once you catch it, smile, laugh (another Super-Human activator), and continue observing. The more you watch, the faster the labels will disappear. If you look at a tree, just look at it without saying it's a tree, out loud or in your head. If you see someone in a red jacket, don't say "oh, that's a lovely jacket" or "a hideous red jacket," simply observe them with no thought. Everything is energy. Everything is equal. Go about your daily life. If someone honks their horn in traffic at you and gives you the finger, smile, open your heart, say "I love you" and immediately focus on what's in front and where you are going and being present as you flow and move. When you breathe deeply and consciously, you enter a constant state of meditation.

You do not even have to close your eyes. In our Star Magic Healing workshops and trainings, I encourage people to try guided meditation with the eyes open and in a standing position. The experiences can be profound. No thoughts, no images, no nothing. This is meditation. Separation from the attachment to the thoughts or feelings is meditation.

2. **The Deep and Expansive Meditation –**
   Used to journey, heal and collect data.

The deep and expansive meditation is my favourite. This is where the lid is blown off the proverbial box and you enter a deep and expansive void that has no top, bottom or sides. It's an infinite labyrinth of nothingness and within that nothingness, magic is conjured from the deepest and darkest threads of the cosmic fabric. You see, light is what most spiritual seekers seek, but the truth is that light is the tip of the iceberg. Beyond light there is darkness, vibratory fields of empty space that contain knowledge and wisdom, wrapped in a kaleidoscope of musical notes that emit no sound, yet are profoundly rich, more exciting than the most flamboyant orchestra on the planet. This kaleidoscope of musical notes

floats through a web of spiralized geometrical shapes that have no solid form, are totally invisible and yet carry a spark of energy so powerful and bright that one cup of this energy could power the entire universe for all of eternity.

When you enter this dark, empty void, it is just that, a dark empty void, and once you submerge yourself (surrender) into this void it's like floating on a magic carpet. You lose sense of your arms, legs, body. You forget about time and you drift and float. Other times you race through space, faster than the speed of light, maybe flying over oceans and mountain ranges and then all of a sudden the mountain turns into a mouth and you fly through the mouth into an electric pink tunnel, surrounded by mystical beings who wish to share knowledge and then before you know it you are nosediving into a street lamp, wondering if you will survive and as soon as you hit the street lamp, five metres above the busy London tarmac, it becomes the softest velvet sky and you are floating once again, going nowhere, just a barrage of spiralized geometrical shapes flow through the centre of your mind and your heart is expanded, everywhere, connected to all things and no-thing at the same time, feeling an overwhelming love for the mystical totality of the universe. It makes no sense logically but, in this space, logic is obsolete. The universe is communicating with you through mathematical equations, patterns, codes and spirals of light that your soul knows all too well and translates them for you upon your return to Earth.

Other times you can be in this void and all of a sudden you are up high, looking back down at your body, and then see yourself as a child. You are in three different spaces at the same time. You are an observer of both your physical body now and you as a child, watching, learning/remembering. In this space there will be something for you to take from it, grasp or "innerstand".

When you go into a deep expansive meditation, you must go in with no motive, no expectation, no aim or goal. When you truly let go and surrender to the experience, it will take you to the most magical places and show you the most extraordinary things.

So how do you get there? How do you enter this void? And once you do, upon your return, how do you "innerstand" what just happened?

There are different ways to enter this space. Through the heart space (or heart chakra as some people like to call it) and the crown, which are both exit points and entry points. Other times your immaculate presence in the moment of surrender can cause the space in your body to expand and your body to dissolve, and you become pure consciousness; you feel like you are in many places at the same time (and that would be true, because you are a multidimensional being, existing in all places at once. Once you get past your body and thoughts you truly know this. You don't believe it, you know it. Believing is for Super-Humans in the making. It's a stepping stone. Seasoned Warriors Know the Truth!).

You must get used to being. Just being still with no thoughts or emotions, no body, no pain, no past, no today, no nothing. This is easier said than done, because we know the little voice in the head starts chattering (moaning and playing up like a child) when it gets no attention and remember, it can only get its attention in the past, so the present moment is utterly scary for the ego. So have a little sympathy, and instead of battling it, wrap it in cotton wool and love it and then bring your awareness, your attention onto your breath.

Breathe really deep, long, slow breaths (through your nose), all the way down to the pit of your stomach, and let them out slowly, through your nose. Start to move your awareness around your body. Bring the awareness into your chest and look at your heart, feel it beating, love it and

be grateful for it. Then move your awareness down into your stomach and observe your vital organs and see the space that surrounds them.

You can then move into your hips, legs, feet, observing your body and realizing that you and your body are two completely different things. You are moving around the inside of it, but you are not it. Maybe you go one step further and realize you are the awareness of your awareness that is observing your body.

As you look around your body, you may just find that you start drifting and enter this empty void and forget about your breath and body. This happens to some people but not everyone, and either way is completely normal.

Bring your awareness back up into your chest and look forward and see a window or doorway, an opening. This is your entrance into the void. Feel how empty it is, see the darkness, the expanse, the infinite space that goes on and on and on. Don't focus on it but give your awareness a gentle nudge towards it and just let go. Let the portal in your heart take you and it will. You can say to yourself: I surrender to this experience and am in the hands and heart of the universe. I am open, ready and willing to experience whatever is for my greatest growth. Say this and let go, be, allow, accept.

You can do the same thing with your crown. Practise and feel what is best for you. Others journey within. They find space in their body and the space expands. As the space expands you get lost in it and float. That space becomes infinite, and it unfolds. Everything is inside that space. All potentials and all possibilities. Again, be, surrender and become the space and let it naturally happen with zero expectation.

The other option is to bring all of your awareness into your head, into the centre of your brain and back slightly, where the pineal gland is nestled. Feel the energy field of your pineal gland expanding. As it does, see and feel the space that it creates and go into this space. Feel and be in this space. Feel the infinite space go deeper and higher, growing 360 degrees in all directions. As it grows feel yourself floating and let it take you. Surrender to the experience. Again, you can say mentally: I surrender to this experience and am in the hands and heart of the universe. I am open, ready and willing to experience whatever is for my greatest growth. Say this and let go, be, allow, accept.

Have no judgement! You will learn/remember, "innerstand" at a deeper level, go to depths of love that can only be felt beyond the human experience. When you do go to these depths of love, there is no turning back. When you experience the world of spiralized geometry, the kaleidoscope of colours and patterns that make total sense through feeling and not thinking, you will never be the same human being again. As you go through the process of stilling the mind, creating the space and being, you have to be determined. Your body and mind will do everything it can to get you to come back (or stop you going, even though there is nowhere to go), get up and check your phone, think about anything and everything, that isn't the space you are becoming. Make your body sit like a dog. You are the boss. If you feel pain in your body when you enter meditation, use it to go deeper. Never run from it, move into it. The same with noise. A bird, a car a noisy neighbour. Use the sound and go into it. Everything is an opportunity to go deeper. They are tools, not hindrances. Change your perception. The ego will want to get annoyed at the noise. Watch it trying to instigate trouble in your head and then smile and say we are going into that noise, into that pain. And go!

Now let's turn our focus to the second question: Upon your return, how do you "innerstand" what just happened? This is a great question and there most certainly is a wrong and a right way to go about this. One thing you must

never do is to try and "innerstand" the spirit world or language of light, the geometry, the code, literally, with your analytical mind. Instead, let the information be absorbed into your consciousness. Feel and let it be. It may translate into a human/logical "innerstanding" during meditation, or once you are back in your body, you may continue to absorb the information and feel what the message/s or communication means, and your feelings will translate this into an understanding – or "innerstand"ing – that you can articulate and then share.

Like anything, it takes a little practice. And there will be times when information will come through that seems like complete nonsense. But the information is working on a deeper level.

When you are in deep meditation and the colours, patterns, data is flowing into your consciousness, you are beyond thought. Allow it to flow and trust that you will be able to translate/understand/"innerstand" it without *trying* to translate/understand/"innerstand" it.

3. The Creative Meditation –
Used to construct and create your life.

The creative meditation is one where you exercise a little more control and at the same time surrender to the experience. You want to set your experience up and then get lost within it so that once again, you lose track of time and space. This meditation is utilized for creating and manifesting. You start off as usual, breathing deeply, centring yourself and becoming the flow within the present moment, with no thoughts, labels, judgements, just in the space as an observer.

As you breathe and still your mind, bring your awareness into your heart and rest it there for several minutes. See how spacious it looks and feels.

You can then expand your space by feeling it grow. Grow it in all directions. Feel the space opening up and sink deeper into it. You feel lighter and calmer, and the space becomes darker and darker until you are floating in a void. You are there in empty space, just being.

You are now in the quantum world, in the womb of the universe, the womb of creation. You are connected to an energy, full of code, that has the capacity to create planets, stars and universes. It's in this space you are to set about creating your life. You can start to see the business you want to create, or have already created, thriving. You see your relationships, your health, you travel in this space to exotic or favourite destinations that are on your bucket list, you live in the house and drive the car. You don't just visualize; you actually live it in this quantum space. You do this until this inner world becomes realer than your external environment. You feel and experience everything as though it's happening in real time. Remember, your subconscious mind doesn't know the difference between the inner and the outer world; it communicates with the body, your cells are affected by their environment and now the environment is what you are living in this meditation. So, your cells are being imprinted with this reality.

The creation of this internal reality, infused with the positive emotions of what it would be like to live that reality now, signals the expression of genes that tell the body that this is the reality it's living in. This is epigenetics, which we looked at earlier. The environment affects the body but this time the environment is not external and real, it's being created internally. When you do this regularly, and live it every day in your mind, data is being exchanged in the quantum field and people, situations and events are being orchestrated in your favour. The entire universe and everyone and everything is gearing up to create for you. It's incredible. Everything and everyone become unconscious agents of the universe, working to create your most extraordinary version of life.

When you engage in this inner world, you may get thoughts trying to distract you. Your body may be restless and try and get you to move. Be patient, keep doing the work, keep creating the inner world and live in it.

When you do eventually return to your body and start feeling it again, it should feel strange because you were so immersed in your inner reality. This is when you are catalyzing massive change. You are starting a process of reconstruction, recalibration and activation after activation as a newly inspired chemical process takes place inside your body, one that has and will continue to have positive and lasting results.

A lady called Wendy joined our meditation library and followed the process. She got a new job within a few months that doubled her income, stopped drinking alcohol (which she had been doing since she was eleven years old) and completely changed her life.

A man named Rob had stage four cancer. Rob started at one of our two-day events and then joined the meditation library. He created a new life within and connected with the Star Magic frequency. Within sixteen days, his tumour had gone. How is this possible? Well, Rob was bullied at school and felt a huge lack of self-worth. His family environment now, was one where he was bullied by his wife and children. He had become detached from the source of all creation, love. After engaging in the meditations, morning, noon and night for a little over two weeks, his health was back. This happened because his inner world changed. He connected with the truth, that he, Rob, was/is a sovereign being and that no one can affect his emotions/thoughts and cause him to react in any way, unless he so chooses. Rob became responsive and stepped away from being reactive.

When you do the work, nothing stands in your way. When you are dedicated to the cause and disciplined in your approach and follow the Star Magic way, you will shift, big time.

I have many stories from clients about this process, ranging from the disappearance of tumours to holes in hearts mending, eyesight being restored, their businesses booming when they had been about to throw in the towel and many, many more.

There is no time in the quantum field: everything is now; so when you go into this space, you liberate huge amounts of energy, and all of this energy goes instead towards creating this new life.

Once all of the B.S. vanishes, that once wasted or misdirected energy is fully at your disposal. This new life that you are creating is a life that exists, a possibility out of an infinite pool of quantum possibilities, in the sea of spiralized geometrical energy, waiting for you to tap into it. Remember, if you see it in your mind it must exist. Your imagination is reality.

So back to your meditation. Stay in this space for as long as you can. You may find that when you come back into your body and your awareness is back in your reality (for the time being while the new one evolves), two hours have passed, or maybe it was only fifteen minutes but felt like three days because so much happened. When you go past your body, your thoughts, emotions and your environment, you enter the quantum field and here you have a blank canvas. Think of an artist. She or he will never paint on a dirty canvas; but when you are in your daily life, with thoughts, emotions, a body, an environment, these distractions are like dirt on your canvas, hindering the masterpiece you are about to create. When you go into meditation, bringing your awareness into your body and then looking around it, realizing that you and your body are two different things (even though your body is an extension of your spirit and your soul), and you see and feel the space all around, and you go into that space and become it, you are going past the dirt on your canvas (your mind and body) and the

empty space and the empty space becomes your clean space of creation. You have access to all of the paintbrushes, colours, pencils an artist would require and you start creating.

When you go to these deep spaces and return, you will bring back a new perspective on reality, on life. You will start to integrate the quantum with the physical and the physical reality of matter will become brighter and lighter and carry an underlying essence that you now see rise to the surface and invigorate your reality. When you bring a whole new shine and exuberance to your world with nothing but the chemicals you chose to release, such as compassion, love, joy and ecstasy, you truly deserve to have the Super-Human stamp on your chest. Why? Because you have activated the heart to such a degree that this force is now showing up everywhere – and you manifested/created this. You should be proud of yourself for this achievement. You have activated the most powerful compass there is: your heart. It will light up your world and guide you and all you must do is listen and take action.

Meditation. Meditation. Meditation.

4. **The Guided Meditation –**
   Where you are guided by someone who will take you on a journey or simply guided you into the still expanse of your own human vessel.

Years ago, I would tell my kids the most elaborate stories. We would wake up in the morning and go on these magical adventures. We would shrink into pixies, travel through trees and pixie communities, ride on dragons, meet mythical creatures, go to other planets through vortexes and have the most incredible time. I didn't know at the time, but I was learning/remembering how to guide others through meditation. One day I was invited to speak at a Mind Body Spirit festival, and I took the audience on one of these journeys. They loved it.

Since then, I have done thousands of guided meditations and every single one of them has been different. You will never come to a Star Magic workshop and experience the same meditation. Why is that? Because you cannot dictate the energy at play. Each workshop has a new audience, new space, new energy, new frequency and when you truly "innerstand" energy, you know that everyone in the room is playing a vital part in the experience and each soul in the room is communicating energetically and telepathically to add their frequency and what their soul requires to experience to heal, to the mix. You could come to eight Be Super-Human workshops and the results will happen but how we get there will always be different. I never plan a workshop. I never plan a meditation. I have an idea of where we are headed, and the rest unfolds in the moment. This is True Mastery. Real Alchemy.

I recommend everyone adds guided meditation to their meditation practice. We have hundreds of them on our website, ranging from five minutes to three hours. The incredible thing about guided meditation is that, during the meditation, you can download certain codes and frequencies into the individual or the entire audience. We are all bio-computers, and we download data 24/7/365. During a guided meditation I can plug you in to new data streams to create healing, abundance, beautiful relationships, health . . . you name it. The list is endless.

If you haven't yet experienced a Star Magic Guided Meditation, then head over to Infinity on the Star Magic website and get stuck in. There are meditation programmes to add to your Be Super-Human Routine that I will share with you at the end of this book. I don't need to cover this aspect of meditation in too much detail, and all you have to do, is simply decide. Do I want to try one of Jerry's Guided Meditations or not? If you do, you know where to go.

If you have the right guide, your mind and heart will be blown wide open, and you will expand exponentially. I warn you though, Star Magic Meditations are like entering a world of fantasy that is very real. You will have the opportunity to connect with beings from all over the universe and beyond and you will get to know how a Super-Human really lives.

12, 9, 6, 3 Preparation Strategy

Once you are tapped into the field and have been for some time, you can access the quantum world in a heartbeat. For those who are new to meditation or healing, though, I have a very simple breathing exercise to bring you into the present moment and activate you, ready to heal or meditate.

I call it 12, 9, 6, 3 and 12–6.

The majority of people can go too deep before a healing session using the 12,9,6,3 protocol and so the 12–6 protocol is better as it calms your mind without taking you too far. Those with a very active mind, however, may want to use the 12,9,6,3 protocol before healing to really calm that mind and get into the perfect state for healing.

Before meditation, you want to go deeper and get really tuned in, so the 12, 9, 6, 3 is perfect. Again, we are all unique and so you have to play with it and find your sweet spot, and be aware that this may change.

EXERCISE *The Process for Meditation*

- Sit up straight, lie down or stand.
- Breathe in and out (deep and powerfully through the mouth) twelve times.
- On the twelfth breath, breathe out and hold for as long as is comfortable.
- When you need to breathe, breathe in, and hold it for as long as is comfortable.
- You then repeat with nine, six and three breaths, holding out and in at the end of each of them for as long as is comfortable.
- Doing this before a meditation sets you up perfectly for a beautiful journey.

EXERCISE *The Process for Healing*

- Sit up straight, lie down or stand.
- Breathe in and out (deep and powerfully through the mouth) twelve times.
- On the twelfth breath, breathe out and hold for as long as is comfortable.
- When you need to breathe, breathe in, and hold it for as long as is comfortable.
- You then repeat with six breaths, holding out and in at the end of each of them for as long as is comfortable.
- Doing this before healing sets you up perfectly to tap the field efficiently.
- Use these protocols as stepping stones if required. If you feel you have moved beyond needing them, then leave it. Or you may want to experiment with it anyway. You are the boss. Trust your heart and listen to it, beautiful soul!

Sexual Energy

The most powerful energy that we can access and utilize to our advantage is sexual energy. It can be harnessed and used to rejuvenate and heal our body. First, it's worth posing two questions: what is sex and is it good for us, and why do we want to have sex in the first place? Well, that's more like three questions, but two are in one.

There is nothing wrong with having sex; however, quite often we want to have sex because of animal instincts and quite often it's a means to an end. We feel attracted to another human being, and we want to have sex, connect and work towards that incredible sensation we call an orgasm, experience it, together if possible, and then lie there for a minute or two in each other's arms before moving on with our day and life. At the start of a relationship, it's all new and exciting, but as the relationship goes on it becomes less of a novelty; it turns into the norm and is taken for granted and a quick kiss, I love you darling and up most couples get to continue with their day.

My grandad always said to me when I was growing up, the secret to a good marriage is to have sex at least three times a week and never go to bed on an argument. He was married to my nan for sixty-three years before he died of cancer at the age of eighty-seven. My nan continued on until she passed back to spirit on her ninety-seventh birthday. She even went out and found another fella and was back in the saddle. Used to make me chuckle. My grandad's advice is good advice. The going to bed without making up first is as solid as it gets. You change the energy: go to bed in love and so wake up in love. I speak to many women and men who struggle in their relationships, and many go to bed on an argument, leave for work the next morning still enraged, and when they get home the next day they still are not speaking. Quite often sex is a way for them to get over it but, in my opinion, having sex and thinking you are reconnecting, when the vibes are low, is not a cool idea.

When we have sex, there is an exchange of information or energy. In life in general, we exchange light/light codes, simply by being in the same room and often when we are apart if we are thinking about someone, consciously or unconsciously. When we touch skin to skin, we absorb other people's energy. Even just shaking hands with someone, energy is absorbed. Eating food with other people, you can absorb their energy from around the table and ingest it. If these are true, what do you think happens during sexual intercourse? Huge downloads of data occur. Once one human being enters another, there is a massive energy exchange.

Even having a one-night stand leaves an energetic imprint in the other human being that will last for ever. The reason for this is because that human being doesn't know it's taken place and so it stays. It's like leaving a virus on a computer: it's silent and doesn't show any signs, while it's stealing information in the background and sending it elsewhere.

Now you are aware of all this, you can go into meditation to remove any energetic imprints, stored on a cellular level, from any past relationships.

EXERCISE *Transmute Stored Cellular Memories from Relationships*

Close your eyes, get comfortable and breathe deeply. Bring your awareness into your body. Now, focus on one body cell, enlarge that cell and see space around it. Separate it from all of the others and know that this cell contains the same information that is held in every other cell. Grow this cell until it looks like a large football, maybe two by two metres, and then ask that cell to show you any past relationships that you are storing energetic blueprints from. Be still and wait to be shown or to feel, like you are looking into or feeling into a screen, the past relationships in your life.

One by one, look at each relationship, open your heart and show/feel love and compassion for this situation. See a golden and electric green light flow out from your heart and place this code into the gold and green light. The code is **DCB8686** and it is programmed to transmute this light/information/stored energy into love/ high-frequency light and shift it from your consciousness. Do this for each relationship that surfaces. Remember, a one-night stand can leave the imprint of another human being too. Remove that virus also.

You may see relationships where you didn't have sex and simply talked or hugged; or maybe a business relationship where you spent a lot of time together. You may see both women and men; don't be alarmed. Accept the process and move on.

OK, back to where we were. Jumping into bed to fix something is only going to make a situation worse, because those ill feelings you were carrying have now deepened and have been drilled into your partner on a subatomic level. You may have sex and feel great in the relationship for twenty minutes, a few hours or even days or weeks, but that pain will resurface. Communicate verbally, talk it through, share your feelings, dissipate the emotion and then – once your vibrational frequencies are high, and aligned – then have sex. Or maybe you will want to make love.

From now on we will discuss this subject in a different way. Until now I have used the word sex to describe this energetic exchange, but I feel that where we must take it is "making love". Sex is animalistic and even though it's amazing at times having animalistic sex, it's not where we want to go as a Super-Human. Animalistic sex is often quick and is all about the end result, the orgasm and ejaculation and that release of energy. The question is, where does this energy go? The answer is it shoots straight out of the top of your head. You reach that point of climax, the energy shoots up through your body, out of your crown and into the cosmic fabric. For you it's wasted, but not for others. There are other entities, beings that most of us cannot see, that will take your sexual energy and use it for themselves, but this is a whole other subject matter entirely, which we may touch upon later.

What is important for you to realize and "innerstand" is that you create massive amounts of energy when you make love, and when you ejaculate and have an orgasm (the wrong way) you lose it. You feel an incredible feeling for a short period of time and then it's gone. This energy is sacred. Why would you throw it away? Well, we have been conditioned to believe that we have sex to reach an end goal. That is ejaculation and the orgasm and sometimes procreation. We have not been taught to make love to energize at a level that will raise our consciousness, elevate our vibration, exercise self-discipline and reach heightened states of ecstasy that we never knew were possible, and connect so deeply to our partner that we fall in love deeper and deeper each time we make love.

What I want to share with you first is a way of harnessing your own sexual energy and using it to heal yourself. And then I will share with you a way to connect with your partner at an extraordinary level and use the sexual energy you create between yourselves to heal, connect, expand, manifest and evolve together in your relationship to new, heightened states of awareness and expanded states of consciousness.

Before I do this, I want to highlight this particular point. Ejaculation and orgasm are two completely different things. What we want to do is separate the two. We want to orgasm without ejaculating. We also want to harness the vital life-force energy that is released during orgasm and keep it; but not only keep it – direct it.

When people ejaculate, they lose energy. And as we get older it takes longer to recover after ejaculating. I have read many different theories from different traditions and they are all slightly different. What I know is we are all unique human beings so, as with everything else, you must play/experiment and see what works for you. I have spoken to many women and men about this, and every man says that after abstaining from ejaculation for a period of time, their energy levels increase, more and more so as time goes on. Women have given me mixed feedback. Some women say that they become energized from ejaculation; but the majority say they feel more energized not ejaculating. As I am not a woman, I will have to leave it to you to experiment yourself. What I can tell you is that women who have practised the ways I am about to share say that by following this protocol, their energy levels go through the roof.

I say to every man I meet, stop masturbating and refrain from sexual intercourse for forty days and let me know what happens. The results are amazing. People look and feel different. They think differently and are more emotionally stable. I have suggested the same thing to women and again I have had mixed feedback, but the majority have said they feel more energized. It takes discipline because men think about sex every three seconds on average and women every six seconds, so you have to commit and go for it. What I know from personal experience is that not ejaculating gives me so much energy. It builds and builds. When you start harnessing your own life force or qi by holding onto the energy you create through orgasm, your life is going to change.

Harnessing Sexual Energy with Masturbation

Firstly, let's discuss masturbation. It's easier to practise on your own as the temptation to engage with your partner is out of the equation and you can fully focus on you. First, lie down and get comfy and start to pleasure yourself. Take your time. As you do, I want you to bring your awareness into your heart and open your heart. Focus on it and imagine a golden light, a powerful energy flowing out from it into your space. It's like a golden flower, blooming and opening and pouring its sacred essence into the space. Really feel the love flowing from your heart and continue to pleasure yourself to the point of orgasm. It's important that you take your time. You don't need to furiously masturbate to get to a point of climax quickly. If you haven't got the time, then you shouldn't be doing it. Revisit it another time.

As you continue to pleasure yourself, working towards your point of orgasm, it's important to have your focus on your body, get to know yourself through this process and realize that this is not disgusting or degrading, it's OK. In fact, it's more than OK, and there should be zero guilt. Also, don't let your mind/thoughts wander onto another human being. Let this be about you.

Remember your energy goes where your focus goes, so contain it and focus it on the most important human being in the entire universe: you. Do not use pornography to arouse yourself; it's an addiction, like cocaine, alcohol or sugar. You want to bring yourself close to orgasm but then pull back. You will feel the orgasm building and when you are about 5–7 on the scale where full orgasm is 10, stop. As you do, breathe. You may need to squeeze your perineum and sexual organs, depending on how far you have taken it, to stop.

You will find that the sexual energy has risen, and you can then, with your intention, guide it up through your body. At the same time, keep opening your heart. Feel the energy rising, connect with the energy that has been activated. Feel like you are bathing in sexual energy. The field of the heart spreads 360 degrees through your body and space and the sexual energy merges through it. Breathe deep and slow and relax with your eyes closed, completely inside and connected to your body.

Once you have bathed in this energy, you can go again. Follow the same steps, bring yourself to just between a 5 and a 7 and then stop, pull back, let the two energies combine and then bathe in these powerful frequencies. The more you do this, the more comfortable you will get with the process.

You can do this several times but do not go past the point of no return, even the last time. Now, if you do, when you are starting out, don't beat yourself up. It happens and it is tempting to do this. It may take you a few sessions to master it. You may find that you have to stop at about 3–5 on the scale, but eventually you will be able to build it up until you get to a 9 or 10 and then stop and bathe in even more powerful frequencies, as the longer you go for, the more sexual energy is produced; if you go slowly, building the pleasure, you can go to incredible heights of ecstasy. Remember, do not rush to get to the point of climax. Each time you pull back and let the energy rise and merge with the golden heart frequency, it will get more potent. Take your time between each round. Connect and feel, breathe, and flow. There is no hurry.

Now comes the important part. It's great bathing in this energy but why not utilize it to fuel your body? It can be used to heal your internal organs, which, once functioning at full capacity, will elevate you even further. I want you to aim for six orgasms and at the end of each one, as you are bathing in those powerful sexual energies and heart frequencies, direct this energy to different parts of your body. I have created six sets of codes. Each code sends the energy to different parts of the body. They are as follows:

1. Orgasm 1: Heart and Small Intestines – **XC1**

2. Orgasm 2: Spleen, Pancreas and Stomach – **XC2**

3. Orgasm 3: Lungs and Large Intestine – **XC3**

4. Orgasm 4: Kidneys, Adrenal Glands and Bladder – **XC4**

5. Orgasm 5: Liver and Gall Bladder – **XC5**

6. Orgasm 6: The Brain – **XC6**

These codes have been created to direct the energy from each orgasm to the specific area of the body. To use the code, all you have to do, just after you stop and are combining the heart frequency with the sexual energy, is visualize the code inside a platinum cube. Place it in your heart with your intention. The cube will naturally dissolve, very quickly, and the code(data/program) will communicate with the data/information (sexual energy and heart frequency) and send it where it needs to go. It's all light and information.

Each code has a series of geometries entangled within it.

Practise this. Use it and watch your world change, because when you change your energy, you shift your consciousness and then your subatomic self naturally expands, and with that the physical self will elevate too. I know some people will find it hard to make a regular masturbation practice and others will dive straight in. If you find it hard to take the time to pleasure yourself, with a sacred means to elevate your consciousness, nourish your soul and fuel your human body, you need to look inwards and ask why. Why? Why? Why? Deal with that stuff. Let it go. Heal it. Then start harnessing the most powerful energy source available to you.

Harnessing Sexual Energy in a Partnership

Let's talk about partnerships. Whether you are heterosexual, gay, lesbian, or bisexual, it really doesn't matter. And I know there are so many other sexual orientations and genders than this out there now; but you are a Super-Human, you're not in a box. Whatever your attraction is to another human is perfect. Remember, we are attracted to the energy, the soul, the underlying essence.

Find a quiet, relaxed and private space for you and your partner. You can be naked or fully clothed. It can be nice to start fully clothed and get naked as you progress. You can both stimulate each other to start with but what I have found, from personal experience, is that it's awesome, once you are both fully aroused, for one partner to receive and go through the process of getting to the point just before orgasm and then pull back. The next time you do it you can swap over. This way you can give unconditionally to your partner and, in that simple act itself, massive energy is released. When you give to purely give with no expectation of what you'll receive back, you become so present

and engaged and your partner will feel this, and so will you.

Sit opposite your partner and stare at each other. Good communication is crucial to start with until you really connect and form a deep bond. As you communicate more and more, building trust and a deeper bond, these sessions will get better and better. The more you practise, fully devoting yourself to your partner and remaining fully present, the more you will start to feel everything they feel and be so connected that you feel every sensation and in a way, become them, and know exactly when they are about to reach that point of no return. Until you reach that stage, communicate. It can seem a little daunting at first, but I can assure you, it will become the most magical experience once you surrender.

So, you are sitting opposite each other, maybe in silence or maybe you have some music on. You can light candles, have dim lighting, whatever creates the mood (you can also set the scene like this if it's just you too). Remember, make sure you can see each other's bodies properly. In this situation, it's about being open, letting go. No hiding under the covers or being in the dark because you don't like your bottom or your feet. Embrace your sexuality and know that this is something magical and beautiful. As you stare into each other's eyes, get lost in the light beyond the physical form. Open your heart and feel the love you have for each other. You can smile at each other and touch each other's knees, stroke their arms and legs and caress their face. You can take it in turns or touch each other simultaneously, or if one is receiving and one is giving, let that be. Go with the flow, be guided by the energy in the moment.

As you touch each other, ever so slowly and softly, feel the love flowing through your fingertips and out from your heart. Do this for as long as feels right, don't be in a hurry. You could spend twenty minutes or longer in this space.

You can touch the inside of your partner's legs, go near their genitals, but don't touch them. When the time is right, you can get closer and then your partner can straddle you. You can hug each other, stroke each other's chests and arms and faces. As you do this, you are releasing massive amounts of oxytocin, the trust hormone. This chemical release in the body amplifies the whole experience as nitric oxide is released and the arteries swell, increasing blood flow to the heart. This also strengthens your bond.

When it feels right you can start to undress each other (if you started dressed), continuing to stroke and caress each other as you do so. You can gently kiss each other's hands and necks, shoulders and legs, backs and feet. Again, submerge into the moment and let the energy guide you. No thoughts, just feel, play, flow, enjoy and be.

The one who is receiving may want to lie back and be comfortable. If you are receiving just be and allow your partner to stroke you, kiss you, pleasure you. Remember, you must communicate. So, if you get to that point, say stop. Say it gently and softly. If you are giving, then continue to touch your partner gently. You will feel them getting aroused. Maybe you don't have to touch their genitals for this to happen and maybe you do. Work your way around the body, stroking, touching, kissing, wherever you need to be, bringing them slowly, closer and closer to orgasm. All the time you are pleasuring your partner, keep your heart wide open. Cultivate more and more love and bliss with your feelings and intention. With practice, you will get really good at cultivating this blissful, love frequency almost instantly. A man has an etheric/ energetic penis, and a woman has etheric breasts. They can be used to stimulate your partner too. A man can visualize his etheric penis inside his partner and the woman can visualize her etheric breasts moving around her partner's body. This is potent and the more you play with this the more magic happens. Let go and play.

Keep going until your partner says stop. Once they do, stop completely. Don't touch them at all as once they get to that point, until you have mastered it, one more touch, stroke, kiss may send them over the edge. So, once they say stop, be still, open your heart and feel the love and deep connection with your partner. If you are receiving, lie there, heart wide open, allowing the energy from the orgasm to flow up and merge with your heart frequency. Allow your partner to be for two minutes. You may need to leave them longer; and as you go again and again, and get to orgasm four and five, they will get more and more aroused and the internal orgasms will become deeper and deeper and so more time may be needed before you continue. If you are receiving, once you say stop, you can use the codes to direct the energy or you can bathe in it. Sometimes, when working with your partner, you may want to just be in the energy you have cultivated together instead of sending it to the organs or you may want to. It's your choice. If you are working on a project, you can send this energy into the project to fuel it. That works amazingly.

Use this extremely powerful, creative energy to manifest. When both of you have the same intention in regard to manifestation, it's so much more powerful. When you enhance your intention to manifest/create using sexual energy, boy, it amplifies the creation a hundred-fold.

Once you have settled down a little, your partner can start again, kissing, stroking, caressing and repeating the process. If you are giving, ask your partner, are you ready? Or, if you are receiving, say to your partner, I'm ready! And off you go again, feeling, playing, enjoying, basking in the bliss as you give and your partner receives. You will repeat this two, three, four, five, six times. Maybe you will go eight or nine times and be there for a couple of hours or more. The more time you can give yourselves in this space, the better it will be.

At the end of your lovemaking session, you do not need to ejaculate. Having the orgasms releases the energy from inside but instead of sending out into the ether, like a bullet from a gun, you are using it to feed your body, your soul, your relationship, your life. Sperm is there to create offspring. Animals only have sex when they are mating to reproduce. They don't go and have a wild one-night stand because they are gagging for sex. Making love like this is an amazing way to spend time together, exploring each other, enhancing your energy instead of depleting it.

You may decide that once a month or every two weeks you will have a full-blown orgasm and ejaculate; if you do, still go through the process. Go through the six orgasms, take your time, build it up and on the seventh, let it go. If you do this, you might ask yourself afterwards, why? It's over in a flash and all of that life force has gone. Remember, this is not a means to an end (unless you are trying for a baby); it's a continuation of energy, a circulation of chi. It's a chance for you and your partner to experience each other and fully give or fully receive. It's an opportunity to strengthen your bond and unify as one being.

When you go through this process it's only through touch. For example, a man will not enter the woman with his penis. That is the next stage. Use your hands, your tongue and your energy, that's it. So, you can stop after six orgasms for example, or you may at this stage want to connect and for the man to enter the woman. You may find that the fully engaging part happens faster. Play with this. There are zero rules and regulations. If you do fully engage, take your time, make love and feel each other deeply and continue to communicate. You do not want to ejaculate. If you feel like you are getting to the point, stop. You may need to pull apart from each other for a minute or you maybe be able to just be still, pull back and control your ejaculation with your muscles, by pulling, squeezing, and holding.

Speaking to different women about this topic, I have been told different things in regard to ejaculation. Some women can control it with their mind and others with their muscles. Men tend to need to pull the penis out from the vagina and pull back those muscles but not always.

This is going to take some practice and you must encourage and support each other through this process. Insecurities can arise and it's important you hold space for each other and nurture each other through the process. Your sexual energy can be created and harnessed as little or as often as you like. It will nourish you. It's an infinite storehouse of magic.

I encourage you to masturbate if you are single or, if you are in a relationship, engage with your partner in this way. If you are in a relationship, you may still want to masturbate and practise feeding your organs with the codes also. Talk with each other. Allow each other the space to do so. Don't sneak. Don't hide. Be open and honest.

This will expand you, elevate you, and you will be different. I have many photos of clients who took selfies of their faces and then again after zero ejaculation for forty days. They look younger, energized and totally transformed. When I see couples who have been working together on their sexual energy, building it and directing it, after just two weeks the difference is massive. When I look at a human being it's easy to see, by reading their energy, if they ejaculate often or not. Start using these ways to enhance your life and let your natural life force conjure magic within the cells of your body.

If you are making love and the penis is inside the vagina, something else you can try is this: you can get to the point of orgasm and ejaculate. I recommend doing this after several times of getting to the point of orgasm and pulling back because it will make the final orgasm deeper. When you do ejaculate, you want to time it to orgasm together, and to control the flow of energy.

So, the energy of the man can go up through his body and he will push it/direct it, from his third eye, through the forehead of the woman (through her pineal gland) and it then flows back down through her body and keeps circulating through both of you. The woman's energy goes up through her body and she does the same: she guides it out of her pineal gland, through her forehead and into the man's pineal gland and then down through his body. The energies then move back through the sexual organs and continue to circulate. Both energies are circling in opposite directions and stay within the body. They are never lost. At the same times both hearts are wide open, and an extremely powerful energy field is created in the space. As a divine couple, you reach such a deepened state of connectedness 24/7 and your relationship flourishes. You can place your foreheads gently together, eyes closed, synching deeper into the space.

If you are masturbating and want to try this, you can. Once the energy is released, as you orgasm and ejaculate, the energy flows up your central column. You have two choices. You can stop it in your heart (with your focus and intention) and push it back down to your vital organs, or you can push it out from your heart forwards, see it flow into a natural energy channel that flows over your head and in through the back of your heart. It takes practice and you have to slow time down with your mind to be able to catch the energy in the heart or direct it forwards and over your head and in through the back.

If you are catching it in your heart and pushing it back down you must use your intention, squeeze your chest area and then guide it back down. When you push it out from your heart and it enters the natural energy channel, it's what the Egyptians call Ankhing your energy. The Egyptian Ankh (also used for levitating objects) is the sign for harnessing sexual energy.

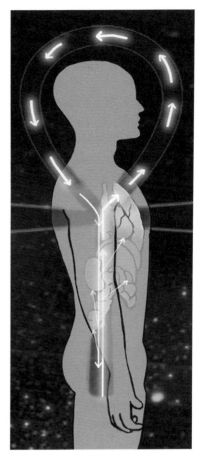

21. The flow of energy coming up from your sexual organs and into the heart where it is guided into the energy channel of the Ankh

The above illustration shows the flow of sexual energy and it being harnessed. Once the energy is harnessed it flows around in that cycle. It's important to note that you should aim to breathe into your belly and fill up your belly and lungs with air to around 75 per cent just before you ejaculate and orgasm. When you orgasm and ejaculate you push the energy out forwards and as it flows out, over the top of the head and in through the back, when the cyclical motion starts, you breathe in the remaining 25 per cent of air. And continue to breathe deep and long and slow. You can then direct the energy into your vital organs afterwards.

Throughout any of these processes, always breathe deeply, especially when you are pulling back from ejaculation. This will take practice but the more you do it the better you will become. Your health and vitality will increase and you will be more energized. Your relationship will thrive. You will have more focus and be calmer. You will see and feel it. You will know but only through experience, beautiful soul!

There are many ways to direct the energy from different bodily positions. Experiment. If you want to know, you will discover them. Use oral sex but try refraining from using plastic sex toys. If you want to use dildos, for example, get ones made from high-vibrational crystals. Treat your bodies with the respect they deserve. Plastic, toxic material is no good. Have fun, don't be too serious. Get out of your comfort zone and start playing around with this. Be adventurous. Be creative. Nurture yourself and your partner and access this storehouse of Super-Human Potential.

Recalibration

Another element of being a Super-Human is rest. We have not reached the stage yet where we can live without sleep and to be honest with you, I don't think we ever will as biological beings. If we succumb to the potential disastrous future that artificial intelligence (AI) has in store for us, (where the crazy cats in Silicon Valley are taking the necessary steps to railroad our species into merging with AI and having it inside of us, where it thinks and learns for us, and eventually dissolves human thinking into an obsolete state of affairs because it can't keep up with the AI software that rewrites itself, renews itself and writes automatically, takes over us and we as humans become digital instead of biological), then it's a possibility that we may not require sleep any more (and becoming AI is a non-starter for me, how about you?). But right now we do and sleep is mission critical to maintaining a high-frequency dynamically functioning you. To be honest, I truly feel that our human brain is the most powerful computer there is. We just have not reached the point in our evolution where we can access its full capacity.

If we find ourselves, in the future, merging with artificial intelligence (AI), I believe that it will take us over and we will forget who we are. It is a dangerous path; the real path to follow is that of the Super-Human, a woman or man who has tapped the full potential of the body, brain and mind, through twelve-strand DNA activation.

It is not only sleep that is very important, but rest and grounding too. Now, there are times when we may need to go without sleep – when we are working on a project or travelling; and some souls need more than others – but on the whole, maintaining discipline around sleep and rest is a mission-critical ingredient of being Super-Human. We must put our bodies into a constant state of recalibration. Meditation is one way of doing this and along with meditation (which we have already discussed) it's important to rest, sleep and ground. How much rest time, sleep time and grounding time really depends on the individual because we are all unique and this you are going to have to experiment with.

I was in this awesome place called Therme. I go there every time I visit Romania. I was with my son Josh and good friend and Star Magic chef, Jay. We had just finished a five-day Training up in the mountains of Transylvania. Therme is a huge complex with baths, swimming pools, saunas, Jacuzzis, infra-red sunbeds, and much more. It's the perfect place to unwind and recalibrate after holding space on a five-dayer, delivering non-stop from early morning until late at night.

I was lying in the lithium pool, looking up at the sky, but my mind was still too active. I was about to suggest to Jay that we get out of the pool and go back to the sauna but just as I was about to, this geometric Greek god appeared in the empty space in front of me. This being said, 'Relax Jerry, you are here to relax.' He (because it resembled a male-looking figure even though it was pure light/code/frequency) reached out, placed his hand over my head (after I checked him out of course and made sure this energy was not corrupted, a natural course of action for anyone who "innerstands" energy) and a stream of intense light entered my head, and boom, I was gone, drifting through a field of colour and light. It seemed to last for ever as I bounced across clouds of energy and then I was somewhere, but I don't know where, and then my eyes opened. I felt amazing, like I had been asleep for a million years. I was so relaxed I didn't want to move, and we stayed there until Jay suggested we go, quite a long time later.

When you are connected, aware, conscious of your entire environment, physical and non-physical, the universe is always communicating with you, guiding you on your path, and it will always help you rest and rejuvenate when you require it. So, listen and accept the advice from the cosmos.

Firstly, we must define sleep, rest and grounding because to some, rest may be going and lying down for an hour in the afternoon, while to others it may be having an early night, and to another human being it may be having a long weekend away, while still checking your emails every thirty minutes because your business and your phone rule your life.

It's imperative that each one of us removes as much stimulus from our environment as often as we can. The more we do this the easier it is for us to recalibrate. We are electrical beings and the natural electromagnetic and magnetic frequencies, available in our environment, coming from the Earth and from the stars and other celestial beings, are sufficient to recalibrate us, sustain us, expand us and elevate us. The issue is there are many other electrical streams at

work and these man-made, artificial versions of electrical energy are not so friendly on the human body. So, it's important we take a break from it, which is becoming more and more difficult to do, especially with 5G rolling out (by the time this book is published, it may well be in towns and cities around the globe in a massive way).

Electricity has been known for a long time to cause an imbalance in our system, which, in turn, stops the body functioning at full capacity. Our brain, liver, kidneys, along with other physical components of our human body, are starved of oxygen and we get ill. This, along with poor nutrition and emotional trauma, creates illness. Food consumption, we can take control of, and also our emotional responses or non-responses. Electrical energy is something that will always be there, though, a constant stimulus, and there are two ways in which we can help ourselves. One is to remove yourself from it and the other we will discuss in the next chapter.

I would like to share with you the way in which our food is broken down and how and where electrons are disrupted within the chain of events, that create problems for us as humans. Our food contains three main types of nutrition – proteins, fats, and carbohydrate – that are broken down into simpler substances before being absorbed into our blood. Proteins become amino acids, fats become triglycerides and free fatty acids and carbohydrate becomes glucose. A portion of these is used for growth and repair and becomes a part of the body and the rest is burned by our cells for energy.

Within our cells, we have mitochondria and within these tiny bodies, amino acids, fatty acids and glucose are all transformed further into even simpler chemicals and are fed into a common cellular laboratory called the Krebs cycle, which breaks them down the rest of the way so that they can combine with the oxygen we breathe to produce carbon dioxide, water and energy. The last component in this process of combustion, the electron transport chain (which is a cluster of proteins that transfer electrons through a membrane to form a gradient of protons that drives the creation of ATP (adenosine triphosphate), which is used by the cell as energy for metabolic processes for cellular functions), receives electrons from the Krebs cycle and delivers them one at a time, to molecules of oxygen. If the speed of these electrons is modified by external electromagnetic fields through the crazy amounts of electricity flying around our environment from laptops, smartphones, TVs, electrical pylons and now with fridges, kettles and every other electrical gadget on the planet being hooked up through Bluetooth to the Smart Grid (or not so smart grid) to a proposed centralized grid with 5G powering it, or if the functioning of the electron transport chain is altered in any way, the final combustion of our food is impaired. Proteins, fats and carbohydrates start competing with each other and back up into our bloodstream and fats are deposited in arteries. This is the start of a series of potential health issues. Glucose is excreted in the urine and the brain, heart, muscles and organs become oxygen-deprived and life slows down.

In the past, doctors and scientists examining humans and animals and exposing them to radio waves (centimetre waves that operate between 3 and 30 GHz) found that there was also seriously disturbed carbohydrate metabolism in animals. They found that the activity of enzymes in the electron transport chain was always inhibited. This in turn interferes with the oxidation of proteins, fats and sugars. To compensate, anaerobic (non-oxygen using) metabolism increases, lactic acid builds up in the tissues and the liver becomes depleted of its energy-rich stores of glycogen, oxygen consumption declines, the blood sugar curve is affected, and fasting glucose levels rise, the organism (animal or human) craves carbohydrate and the cells become oxygen-starved.

Now, all of the above is happening with centimetre waves, which operate between 3 and 30 GHz. It's called a centimetre wave because the wavelengths range from one to ten centimetres. The 5G waves are a whole new playing field of wave forms. 5G will operate on a millimetre wave spectrum, ranging from 30 GHz to 300 GHz. If centimetre waves can affect our bodies and make us sick, what do you think is the potential of millimetre (30G Hz to 300 GHz) waves? I am not saying this to put fear into you. I am sharing this so you can take control of your own consciousness and make the best decisions so you can thrive in this world and not simply survive, living longer but unhealthier. I say living longer because it's been proven, over and over, that electricity can add time onto our lives and at the same time make us sick. Who on Earth would want their fellow sisters and brothers to be sick for longer? It's an interesting question and that we will discuss later.

Rest

When it comes to rest, I am talking about a complete shutdown from everyone and everything, as often as possible. On a daily basis you can turn the Wi-Fi off in your home, turn your laptop and smartphone OFF, not to silent or aeroplane mode, but OFF. And just be. You can read a book, go for a walk, spend time in the garden or a nearby wood or forest or go to the park or beach. In our home we turn the Wi-Fi off at 9 p.m. every day and back on the next day.

Investigate orgonite, a unique material made up of organic and inorganic materials layered together. Orgone means prana, life force or chi. You can place orgonite objects (usually inside a geometric shape such as a pyramid) around your home, such as by your laptop or Wi-Fi box and the frequencies from them will keep your space clear. Shungite is another incredible crystal that is used to dissolve harmful frequencies. There are also EMF stickers (small, encoded stickers that dismantle the negative waves), which you can place on devices to do the same. Do some research.

Obviously when you turn off your phone and laptop no one can contact you (unless you are already at the telepathic stage). I know, that sounds scary, doesn't it? What if my mother needs me? What if my children need me? What if my boss needs me on my day off? A lot of us have these thoughts. You know, I have two children and am a single father. My children's mother lives in a different country. If I am away or they are away, my phone still goes off at night. When I was growing up, I couldn't contact my parents from my mobile phone, because I didn't have one. They couldn't reach me 24/7. I survived and so will my children. Step out of fear and into TRUST. If you live in fear, then expect things to enter your reality that you really don't want. Remember you are the co-creator of your own universe. And if your boss thinks he or she should be able to contact you in the evening, days off or at the weekend, get a different job or go and speak your truth and straighten them out – with love of course.

On a weekly basis, you must have a whole 24-hour period where all of your gadgets go off, your Wi-Fi is unplugged at the wall, and you become unreachable for EVERYONE. On a monthly basis, you must be out of the loop for one 48-hour period, where NO ONE can reach you. Every six months a two-week period where you are on holiday, away from ALL THINGS, ALL INFLUENCES – totally engaging in pure ME time. You may feel you want more and if you do, create that space. I am not telling you what to do. These are simply my suggestions for the minimum, based on practice, that work.

Rest also means resting the mind. So, when you go into your quiet space and the distractions go off, be still or go into pure observation mode. By the way, I forgot to mention the television. Make sure that TV is no longer a distraction. It's called a television because it tells you a vision. What you should eat, drink and buy in every area of your life. If you have a TV, throw it away but before you do, smash it up and make sure it's so broken that no other poor souls can retrieve it from the trash and get it working again. Life should be a constant meditation, and with zero possible distractions this is a golden opportunity for you to be the observer, create space inside your mind and see what incredible flowers blossom from the weed-free garden inside your head.

You could use this time to try something new. What about painting? Drawing? Writing? Yes, get some paper and a pen . . . Oh no, not a paper and pen! How could you possibly go back to the Stone Age? Try it. See what happens. You never know, if the electrical frequencies dissolve into the background from time to time, you may just reignite your creativity, or kick-start it for the first time.

It's so important that you step away from everything; in doing so, the natural frequencies of your body will recalibrate. Your inner geometry will recalibrate and that will connect you with the original universal geometry/code once again, and you will synch back in with the God Worlds at large, instead of feeling like a frazzled atom, separate from all of the other atoms. You will feel the energy in your body connected with the energy of the space around you and you will feel like the whole puzzle, instead of a tiny piece of a gigantic puzzle that actually doesn't fit together any more. Living in an electrically stimulated environment, we are "fried" by the electricity and then placed into a world of energy, our planet, our home, the cosmos, which no longer recognizes us (or us it) and the natural processes our body was designed for are hindered.

Sleep

I have no contact with screens for an hour before bed. The frequencies coming out from your laptop or smartphone stimulate you, and relinquishing them in this way allows your brain waves to slow down. Before bed I have dim lights around me and then always sit in the dark and go into silence for twenty minutes, with my eyes closed, becoming my breath and then going beyond. Sometimes I will end up on a deep and intense journey and then fall asleep, and other times I will slowly cross into a deep sleep. Either way my brain waves slow down, from alpha, to beta, to theta and then delta.

I always aim for an early night. For me that is 10 p.m. at the latest, but I love it when I hit the sack at 9 p.m. I know that extra hour means more potential the next day. It excites me. I remember when I was younger, I used to laugh at the idea of an early night, doing my very best to stay up as late as possible. During my drug-fuelled benders, throughout my teens and twenties, I wouldn't sleep for five or six days. "*Eating is cheating and so is sleeping*", was my motto at the time. Now, I LOVE my sleep! The hours between 9 p.m. and 1 a.m. are the best for me personally, and in total 7 hours a night.

People say it's best to sleep in 90-minute cycles as this is how long a sleep cycle lasts, during which we go through five stages of sleep. The first four stages make up our non-rapid eye movement (NREM) sleep, and the fifth stage is when rapid eye movement (REM) sleep occurs. The first four stages are when our brain waves get slower and slower as we move from light to deep sleep. REM is when we are said to be in the dream state. In my opinion, we are all different beings and whether ninety minutes is the best is down to the individual. I often sleep for two hours and feel fully charged, or meditate for thirty-five minutes and feel like I have come out of a deep sleep, fully revived. The more you can master your heart rate and brain waves, the better you become at resting and sleeping well and maximizing your time. If you go to bed with a fully activated mind, worrying about your problems, you may take an hour or more to fall asleep properly, and still be thinking about your problems during the night. You are creating a stressed-out inner environment and wasting valuable recovery and rest time. This is why taking away all stimulation before bed – including your thoughts – is important.

I can be fully charged, but if I decide to rest, I can fall asleep in minutes. I can be on a park bench, a busy airport, anywhere. I switch myself off like a light switch. Breathing correctly, being in your heart and having an observational mind are crucial to be able to do this.

It's also important to know that when it gets dark, melatonin levels rise in your brain. When it gets light, serotonin levels rise. So, sleep in a dark room. No LED or laptop lights, phone lights, alarm clock lights. Sleep with your gadgets out of the room. If you go to bed early you will train your body to wake, like clockwork, without an alarm clock. With practice, as you fall asleep you can control the journey into dream time, a little like meditation, and get good at recall from your dreams. If you go to bed so completely shattered that as soon as your head hits the pillow you are gone, you are not getting enough rest or sleep. Start making different choices and change the game. If you wake up in the night to go to the toilet, keep your eyes closed and go in the dark. Don't let your eyes see light; it will activate serotonin, and the mind will start to activate.

Grounding

Grounding is the next piece of the recalibration puzzle. As we know, Mother Earth is magnetic, and our energy comes from this incredible celestial being, hovering in space, constantly spinning. And so connecting with her energetically and physically is a must.

Mother Earth has a field of energy moving through her and around her, called a toroidal field. She also has a rod and a staff, two spinning vortices (you have those two and other components). She also has a merkaba field in her core and around her celestial body. (We looked at this in the qigong section.) These fields can be tapped into, along with her strong magnetic nature. Remember, our energy comes from the ground and our knowledge from the stars. Mother Earth is a source of formidable strength. She is, by the very nature of being she, feminine. When we talk about masculine and feminine, we are not talking about men and women. Energetically it is positive (masculine/ male) and negative (feminine/female). She carries the spark of divinity to ignite the divine feminine inside you.

Many people think that power and strength come from masculine forces. In truth, real strength comes from harnessing both masculine and feminine forces and bringing them into perfect balance. It's the deep Mother Energy that gives the fearless masculine its depth and the deep masculine energy that protects and serves with intensity, the divine feminine. They say behind every man is a strong woman. This is true. Also, behind every powerful woman is a devoted, fearless man. Together they create an unstoppable force. Neither is better than the other. Both are integral and essential. With this being said, both feminine and masculine energy can be found in every woman and every man.

I highly recommend that you spend twenty minutes every day with your shoes and socks off, walking on the Earth. When you take off your shoes and socks and connect to the Earth, you heal and energize. The magnetic fields merge with the electromagnetic fields of your physical and esoteric body and naturally harmonize. You are after all a part of your environment; but often, through the electrical fields, our physical disconnection with the Earth, through the clunky fashion statements on our feet and the heavy concrete on our roads, we have lost our connection. When you connect physically with the Earth, energy starts to flow.

If I have a client with cancer, I have a certain protocol that I suggest to them. It involves a number of elements and one of them is walking on the Earth. Another is tree-hugging. Trees also have a merkaba. When you hug a tree, it responds. You can also talk to trees and extract massive amounts of wisdom but that's another story. If you stand with your feet on the Earth and hug a tree, open your heart and allow the field from your heart to submerge into the field of the tree, magic starts to happen. An energy circuit starts to flow. Your merkaba fields and other energetic components interact with the fields of the tree and the Earth. Energy starts to flow through all three of you and your physical body goes into healing, a massive extraction of physical and emotional toxicity occurs, and you recalibrate. It's amazing. I highly recommend you do this every day.

If you live near the sea, go and stand in the sea and ground your feet into the sand. Stay there for twenty minutes or more. If you live in a sunny climate, try to combine your grounding with sun-gazing. Go out and stare at the sun (in the first and last hour of sunlight, when the light is softer). Those photons from the sun will nourish you and feed you and assist with your recalibration. If you've never done this before, start with five to ten seconds a day and build up, don't go out and stare at the sun at midday, although, once you are accustomed to the sun, walking around without sunglasses is important, even in high sun. The photons activate your pineal gland and feed the body and also charge your DNA.

If you are starting sun-gazing and grounding together, you could have your eyes open for ten seconds and then closed for a minute, and then open your eyes again for another ten seconds. You could also ground on the Earth and sun-gaze. Both options are there for you. This is like plugging you into the power supply. While you are doing this your mind is empty, so zero energy is leaking away. Remember, large amounts of energy are wasted on the incessant stream of repetitive thoughts. Once they slow down (and eventually cease to trouble you) and you are plugged into the Earth and the Sun at the same time . . . **WOW! Now, add deep conscious breathing to the mix and you are switched on, BIG TIME!**

You can buy grounding mats and other grounding devices. I have a device that wraps around my ankle. It's a strap with a metal face on the inside, connected to a wire that can be earthed through a plug into the wall or into another attachment with a metal rod that can hang out of your window and run directly into the ground. Grounding mats go on your bed. You lie on them and again, they plug into the wall. You will be surprised how good a night's sleep you'll have. Add a Wi-Fi-free zone into the mix and your time in the pit will be maximized.

You are a Super-Human in the making and these three suggestions will accelerate your potential. The more you do these things, combining all of these high-performance ingredients together, the higher your frequency will go and the easier it will be to stay in the space of strength, focus, clarity and zen with a bombproof consciousness that cannot be affected by the outside world. Nothing should ever alter your state, unless you decide.

Electromagnetic Heart Transducer Shield

I mentioned in the last chapter that there are two ways to deal with some of these harmful electrical waves hammering their way through our environment. I suggested stepping away from them, which isn't always easy. As I mentioned you can turn off your Wi-Fi and get into nature and do the things already outlined, but there is another piece to this puzzle.

As humans we tend to go into fear when people spread the news about 5G. We certainly should not go into fear; we should always remain in love as fear is the biggest killer on Earth. The mm waves of 5G are kicking out a serious force and can truly affect the human body but what if we could shift our frequency and alter these waves? What if we had the power to change or shift the potency? What if we could change the way these waves interacted with our body and our body's electromagnetic field?

I was in Madeira with my son, and we were taken up this incredible mountain by two friends of ours. The views from the top of this mountain, stretching out over the diverse landscapes, carving their way through the valleys below, in and among the sunshine and clouds, was utterly breathtaking. As we walked further up the last part of the road, before we had to hit the dusty pathways, my head was feeling strange, and I could hear massive amounts of noise as well. Like a buzzing sound. Up in front of me was a café and shop at the end of the road and the magical scenery was off to the left and right. I got closer and closer to the shop and then stepped onto the pathway, walked around to the left and then behind the shop was what looked like a gigantic white and silver golf ball. It was huge. It was surrounded by barbed wire fencing and a ton of security cameras.

I asked the lads what it was, and they told me it was a huge radar from the Portuguese Air Force. It detected anything moving in the air space within a 500-mile radius. Now, the ultra-high-frequency (UHF) region from 300 to 3000 MHz is extensively populated with radars, although part of it is used for television broadcasting and for mobile communications with aircraft and surface vehicles. The radars in this region of the spectrum are normally used for aircraft detection and tracking. We discussed the potential of millimetre waves (30 GHz to 300 GHz) in the last chapter. If military radars are kicking out 300 to 3000 MHz then you can imagine how much my head was buzzing, or should I say frying (Wi-Fi/We Fry) in this environment.

Underneath this radar tower was a small office and a car parked outside. I can only imagine that whoever that car belonged to must have had a short lifespan working in that job – or maybe even being on this Earth. Radar waves are emitted in pulses, so they are not constant, like a TV antenna or a 5G tower, but due to the sheer size of this golf ball-looking radar, the pulses were strong enough.

I climbed to the tallest point on the rock and on top of this rock was a stone marker. It was about 1.5 metres tall with a square flat surface, just big enough to stand on. I climbed on top, which required focus and pure present moment awareness, because as soon as you looked down you had rocks, and valleys hundreds of metres deep. I went to the top because this was the highest point and it was directly in front of the golf ball radar, right in the middle of it in fact. I stood there and felt the energy. I closed my eyes and then tuned my third eyesight into the pulses of these waves being emitted. I could see them. There were literally giant vortexes of energy. The pulses of these vortexes had gaps in between but still energetically, they were linked. They seemed to pulse, stretch and explode as they travelled. That is how I interpreted them with my mind's eye.

I decided to stand in this space, relax and try to alter the frequency of these energetic pulses, and allow them to flow into my body but in a harmonious fashion and not a harmful one. It took me a minute or so to truly focus. There was a gentle breeze, and I could feel my body sway slightly. The fall would not be a pretty one so overcoming this first challenge was key. I thought back to Philippe Petit, the guy who walked across the metal tightrope between the Twin Towers in the 1970s. He was interviewed after and said he was able to do it because he became his environment and in doing so was supported by

it. He said when he felt he was falling forwards, the sky would gently pull him back. I thought about this and smiled. I said to myself, stop being a pussy Jerry. This guy was on a tightrope, two kilometres above the concrete. You are stood on a solid square. Get a grip, sunshine. I then took some deep breaths and boom, I was in my heart and present.

I opened my heart and saw an inverted crystal-blue tetrahedron inside a sphere, in the centre of my heart. I connected with this geometry and felt it. Then I asked if it could assist me in changing the frequency of these radar vortexes. It asked me to pick one cell inside my body and then to choose one proton from that cell. I brought my awareness into my body, down into my stomach, which is where I felt drawn to. I saw a cell, expanded it and then took my awareness inside. I connected with one proton. The tetrahedron in my heart told me that this proton contained more energy than I could ever imagine. I connected with this proton, and it grew and expanded into a black hole, like a vacuum. I saw lights with codes stream from it up through my body, into my heart and then into the tetrahedron. The tetrahedron and the sphere started to expand.

They expanded out past the boundaries of my physical body and the tetrahedron started spinning clockwise. I was given a code. The code was a series of geometries, all floating within this orange and pinky, bluey green fractal pattern that expanded and contracted and grew back into itself and then reappeared from the other side, becoming even more glorious in its nature. By this time, I was feeling nothing, not actually knowing if I was on the square surface or not, balancing 1,800 metres above sea level. I was just observing this code and this mesmerizing pattern. I then heard a voice. It whispered to me, a voice I have heard many times on my journey. You could call it the universe and we will for now. The universe told me that this code is **RT14009** (it had taken the underlying geometrical code and created something simple). It told me to place this code inside of my heart. I connected to the code and did so with my intention. I focused on my heart and thought "**RT14009**" in my head.

This code just exploded in my heart and then I was feeling my body. My legs, arms, everything. I was stood on the flat surface, eyes closed, watching this tetrahedron spin inside the sphere and as the radar vortexes moved towards the sphere, they got lighter and brighter, and the length of each vortex/pulse grew. As the energy entered the sphere it continued but got brighter again. As it encountered the tetrahedron, it shifted from a vortex into a tetrahedron. Suddenly there were lots of radar vortexes/pulses, transforming into lots of tetrahedrons. These tetrahedrons flowed into my body and danced around, flowing through my body, getting smaller, turning into spirals of light, and then they dissolved and disappeared into my cells. I stayed in this space for what seemed like a few minutes.

I then opened my eyes and stared at the giant golf ball. The noise, the static sound, the pressure in my head, it was not there. It had all gone. The entire environment, in my reality, was different. I stayed there for a bit and felt great. I then got down off the piece of stone and walked down to the café. I sat in the café for an hour eating the best mangoes I have ever tasted. Afterwards I went back up and stood back in front of the radar. The pressure was back but not as strong. So, I closed my eyes and placed the code **RT14009** into my heart. Immediately the tetrahedron and circle were outside my body. I connected with my third eyesight again and watched the same things happen to the vortexes of energy coming from the radar. I felt awesome within several seconds. I decided to hold this space for ten minutes. I then got down off the stone marker and walked back to the café. I sat

there for forty-five minutes. I then stood up and placed the code back into my heart. I then walked back up close to the radar, and I had no pressure, no noise, static, nothing. I closed my eyes and could see the vortexes of energy/frequency, transmuting into tetrahedrons and then into spirals of light and then they dissolved. I've since tried this in other situations with frequencies, including 5G. It works. What I have realized is that it needs to be re-enforced and the more you use it the more potent it becomes.

EXERCISE *Electromagnetic Heart Transducer Shield*

I still recommend shutting yourself off from Wi-Fi and other electrical frequencies as often as possible but when you are around them, make doing this a habit.

It's very simple. These are the steps you must take:

1. Close your eyes.

2. Breathe deeply.

3. Connect with your heart and feel love.

4. See the inverted crystal-blue tetrahedron inside the sphere in your heart.

5. Bring your awareness into one cell, connect with one proton and see it open like a mini black hole and infinite energy flow from it, into your heart.

6. Connect with the code **RT14009**.

7. Place it with your intention, into your heart, inside the tetrahedron.

8. THAT'S IT! Just observe the rest.

It will then just happen. The tetrahedron and sphere will grow out from your heart, the tetrahedron will spin and you just have to watch and feel. I have given this code to more electrically sensitive people and with consistent use, it starts to take effect. It's the same as anything. Use it or lose it. If you are not electrically sensitive, use it also. I install it every morning. I re-enforce it if I go into a town or city, on a plane, shopping centres, pretty much everywhere. I have found that I can go a few days and I don't have to do it. But I did that just for a test to see. It will get more and more potent as more of us human beings use it.

So, let's work together as a human family and use this code. Let's transition from 5G to 5D and use the electromagnetic power that we are, to change the man-made pulses/vortexes/data streams in our environment, into frequencies that make our bodies thrive and expand. You are in control. Remember this! Step up and be your beautiful, authentic, powerful soul self. You must know that you have the power to create change, to influence change at will. You have the capacity to tap a whole world of internal chemical potential. Experiencing is knowing!

6

Resilience and Gratitude

Resilience is a beautiful thing, and it stems from our inner foundation, built upon layers of geometry, which has been infused by energy from compounded positive chemicals released in our body and brain, time and time again. This compounded growth, activated by our psycho-chemistry, is the basis of everything. As humans we get to make choices, powerful choices, every given second. They can grow us to extreme heights or plummet us to the depths of despair.

Resilience is a by-product of your inner growth, self-love and your dedication to be sovereign. It's also a by-product of discipline. When you keep moving forward, attacking life, and things don't go to plan and you get back up and go again, resilience is woven into the tapestry of your human fabric on a mental, physical, emotional, and spiritual level.

People often say to me, "Jerry, why do you attack life? Why do you see it as a battle? With that attitude, don't you think you create that?" But life is a test. Life is harsh. Those that are happy sitting in the background, getting by, being average, can go about life, working a 9–5, kidding themselves that this is it. That is OK. That is their choice. Life will never be too tough for people like that because they fit into the mould. The second you want to break the mould, raise the bar, amplify your frequency, stretch and raise your head above the parapet, life is going to come on strong and beat you a little, maybe a lot, to test you, to see if you really want it; and also to make you stronger, fitter, more able and to furnish you with new skill sets and abilities for the next level of the game. So, the battle can be both positive and negative, a double-edged sword. It beats you to try to keep you from breaking the mould but also beats you to sharpen you and strengthen your will.

One thing I do not tolerate is excuses. When you make an excuse, you are destined to head nowhere. I was going to do this but . . . I was about to, but . . . I was so close, but . . . Eliminate the word "but" and realize that you either do it or you don't. It's OK to fall down, but just don't quit. Failure is only failure if you decide to stop. Get back up and go again. My own brain has a whole encyclopaedia of excuses, ready to be brought to the forefront of my mind at any given moment. Here is a small extract:

1. Horrific birth process.

2. Raped as a baby.

3 Beaten by my adoptive mother with a wooden ruler regularly.

4. Embarrassed and beaten by my first schoolteacher.

5. Picked on as a kid for having big ears and dark skin.

6. Being a drug addict and an alcoholic at a young age.

7. Losing every bit of money I had made when I was nineteen.

8. Losing everything I had made at twenty-seven and being hundreds of thousands in debt.

9. Being ripped off by my best mate and my daughter's godfather, at twenty-nine, to the tune of 1.4 million pounds, after clambering out of debt and getting back in front.

10. Being in a crazy car crash eight weeks before Star Magic started. Attempt on my life by the darker forces.

11. My wife leaving the children and me just after Star Magic started. I had to home-school them and get Star Magic off the ground.

12. Being arrested for healing people with cancer, one year after Star Magic had started.

This is just a small snippet of the excuses I could use to give up or pull back or take it easy or quit. If you knew everything I had ever been through you would wonder how the fuck is this fella still going? I use everything to grow, as fuel for life. I use every opportunity to extract knowledge and wisdom. You should do the same. Going through life's challenges builds resilience.

Resilience allows us to be in control, emotionally, and harnessing our emotions, in a world that tries to manipulate them, is a skill, a mastering of one's mind, body, and soul. By following the suggestions I make in this book, you will develop a way of being in this world that is absolute, energized and courageous. You will rarely stray from your path and if you do, you will find your way back ever so fast, using the derailment as an incredible opportunity to see through the eyes of a human being, being in a space that you don't wish to be, just for a few minutes or possibly hours (because when you are firing on all cylinders as your Super-Human 5D self, you will not allow your external reality to drag you into the dark for long); and then boom, you are back on track, in full flow, grateful for the experience, buzzing once again on this magical ride.

To change the world and our human species is a simple act of changing one's emotions and internal experiences and detaching from the external focal points of our ever-changing, ever-constant disruption from this radiance we call life.

We often let life and its model of reality shake and shape us, instead of us, the powerful, uplifting, galactic beings that we are, shaking and moulding our inner worlds to collide with the light and information of the quantum field, to blend the inner and the outer into one, to bring nature and humanity into a coherent harmonic field, where the vibrational resin, the rich empty space (which is far from empty), glues us together with infinite flexibility. But, and this is a huge but; we not only want to bring nature and humanity into a coherent field, we want to change our own mathematics and through that change the mathematics of nature. Nature itself has been corrupted and we must bring it back into alignment. Nature is an extension of us as are we an extension of nature. The problem is that nature has followed the Fibonacci mathematics and so the mould of reality has taken nature (and human beings) into it and shaped it. So, it's down to us to change our inner geometry, in turn change our mathematics, and then the extended elements of us (nature itself) will blend into the Krystal Spiral New Earth Mathematics. We will discuss this in detail soon.

Back to resilience and gratitude. Super-Humans prepare for and adapt fluently in the face of adversity by managing emotions and regulating energy, by returning to the heart and keeping the heart–mind connection in perfect equilibrium.

Having this balance within one's soul allows a woman or man to ride the storms of life from an observational standpoint. Just like an eagle, flying high above the storms, watching, gliding, not affected by the commotion below, waiting patiently to return to the blue skies, to re-engage with life, not disturbed by the noise.

It's imperative to be able to facilitate this much self-control. It gives you massive clarity and a sure-fire focus and enables you to bounce back from any and every situation with a smiling force. Life is short. A Super-Human doesn't have the time to be wallowing in pity or disturbed by others' actions, reactions, judgements or external situations within the local or global environment.

Our inner world is the key to all things. Great sages throughout history have guided us in, to the stillness and peacefulness that we create through practice, through repetition, harnessing the thoughts that flow in unfathomable, incessant streams. We create effectively when our heart and mind is coherent and we are on the frequency of love, compassion, gratitude. Observation and acceptance are key triggers as they lead to the state of surrender and freedom; no attachment to the external and pure trust in the internal world, where we get to create, as quantum architects, the grand structure of our infinitely divine lives.

When we feel gratitude, we send out positive signals from the heart. Even if there is chaos in the environment, you change that potential field of destruction into the paradigm you are living within. You become bombproof – and you also become the alchemist for rapid frequency change. In other words, you can transmute any energies, from any situations, into harmonious frequencies, because in your reality nothing outside of you exists unless it exists in harmony with the reality you are creating within. Remain present and you stay powerful.

Resilience and the Autonomic Nervous System

When a human being lives in constant stress, our heart centre becomes incoherent, and this hinders our ability to create fluently and effectively. The brain also becomes disintegrated and incoherent in response to chaotic or disrupted heart rhythms, which is reflected through the autonomic nervous system (ANS), a control system that acts largely unconsciously and regulates bodily functions such as heart rate, digestion, respiratory rate, pupillary response and sexual arousal.

The ANS has two main components, the sympathetic nervous system and the parasympathetic nervous system, which act in completely opposing roles. The sympathetic nervous system prepares the body for intense physical activity and is often referred to as the flight-fight response. The parasympathetic nervous system does the exact opposite: it relaxes the body and inhibits or slows down many high-energy functions.

When the heart and brain are incoherent, it triggers dysfunctional patterns and the sympathetic nervous system, which is like an accelerator, and the parasympathetic nervous system, which is like a brake, both try to perform their roles. So, one is preparing for battle while the other is putting its feet up on the couch. One is running the hundred metres and the other is in dreamland. Take the analogy of a car. If you slam your foot down on the accelerator (sympathetic) and press the brake (parasympathetic) at the same time, you are going to stress the drive chain and wear down the brakes, waste energy/fuel and the car will eventually need repairing. You are the same. When you de-balance your system, throw out the electromagnetic workings, the body gets tired, the stress wears the body down and in the end it eliminates our ability to repair, maintain health and vitality and depletes our resilient nature. So, it's mission critical for you to stay balanced and coherent and live from your heart space, on the frequency of love, in an accepting fashion, with zero judgement, being compassionate and vibrating within the vortex of joy.

Gratitude and Heart Coherence

I highly recommend that you spend twenty minutes a day being in your body, opening your heart and feeling love and deep gratitude for all things. Focus on everything you are and everything in your reality and love the people, the business, the health, the body, the material things you have at your disposal. Love everything and everyone and your entire life. Cultivate the strongest feelings of love and deep gratitude that you can possibly muster and sit in this energy. Your heart will overflow with joy the more you practise, and you will shed tears of joy as you go deeper and deeper. Eventually this conscious twenty minutes will become unconscious, constant and always.

Studies have shown that elevating your emotional state through daily gratitude signals the immune cell genes to make a protein called immunoglobin A (IgA), a powerful antibody that strengthens the immune system. The massive increase in IgA is an incredible example of just one of the many benefits of focused heart coherence. Make gratitude a daily habit and synchronize your mind, body and soul and the electromagnetic fields of charged energy that connect it all and you will become the most resilient Super-Human on the planet! This doesn't have to take lots of time. You can incorporate it into your meditation, qigong, sun-gazing or grounding. You can combine all of these. Many of our Super-Human exercises can be stacked on top of each other.

Live in joy, love, peace, gratitude and compassion and fill your cells with the nectar of pulsating magnetic and electromagnetic vortexes of inspiration from the Earth and the Stars. Life is magical. Let your soul see the world in wonder. Allow your heart to guide you.

Be Deliberate

By following these principles, ways of being in this body, in this world, you start to live life extremely deliberately, like every other Super-Human that has been before you and every other Super-Human that will emerge in this supposedly physical space, after you. Life is a creation. Many people are like pinballs in a pinball machine, bouncing around the inside of the game, being dictated to by the fear of falling down the black hole, after bumping into every conceivable object in a chaotic fashion. This is how many people live their lives, being pulled from pillar to post, pushed and bounced by the actions, reactions, judgements and moods of others, along with the false information streams, fed systematically through our screens to alter our emotions and manipulate us to take some kind of action, that serves an elusive spectrum of women and men who have their own sole interests at heart. Power and control.

When you act deliberately, you take charge of your emotions, your reactions, you live as an observer, with high energy, smooth octaves of light running cohesively and coherently through your field, ensuring the operating system, your physical body, the biological computer that you are, living in a holographic universe, is in harmony with its environment, thus being its environment, connected to the Source, the primary light and sound fields of Source energy, the centre of our magnificent universe. When you don't act deliberately, the complete opposite takes place. You relinquish yourself to the depths of despair, begging for mercy as a slave, encapsulated in a fear-fuelled pinball machine world.

Many humans are scared to be who they truly are, but when you follow the suggestions in this book, you will completely alter your frequency and in turn your perspective. Remember, this world can be viewed in so many ways. Every single situation has a myriad of perspectives, none of them right or wrong, they are simply different observational standpoints. When you take control, as an observer of life, you liberate yourself to choose your perspective freely. Those not-so-incredible souls that do their very best to control our world and programme our biological computers know that perspective and perception can be massively influenced, and so do their best to warp our minds at every opportunity.

There are believers and seekers in this world. Believers think and seekers know. At school we are taught to believe in many things, to regurgitate useless facts, figures and information. Believing can be the pathway to death. Death of the heart and death of the soul because you are closed, governed, told what to think and then critical thinking dissolves and then a warped world view becomes your associated death sentence. Once you believe in something you tend to go deeper into the indoctrination. You think you have found what you were looking for, where you belong, and once you belong you settle.

When you settle you enter dangerous territory! Whether you settle with a religion, a church, a group of people, even the rules or values of a family, handed down, it's terrifying to think that this idea, concept, in whatever manner it presents itself, is all there is to life, to the universe. Once you belong you obey the rules and become a good little indoctrinated human slave. You have handed your power over and then to stray away from the rules of your religion, church, family (quite often one of the most dangerous places on Earth) or group instils fear. What if they reject me? What if I lose them? What if I leave and don't like it and they won't let me back in? What if, what if, what if . . . ?

When you engage in a system, your potential, if shown, is a shock to the system the human being entrusted and most of the time stamped out because free, critical thinkers, with open hearts, do not help the system. These kind of people (like you and I), Super-Humans, tear down

the system and create their own path and blaze a new and empowering trail (with no hierarchy), inspiring others to do the same. Soon, the system crumbles because the system can only exist if the people allow it to.

It's intrinsic to human intelligence to want to seek. It's natural. You don't need to teach it, it's within us all as sovereign, free, kind and compassionate beings, to want to evolve and expand and seek out the very best in ourselves, and others. Deep down, real deep down for some, no one wants to see anyone else less off than them. Poorer, unhealthier, in low-vibrational circumstances in any way, shape or form, whether it be relationships, business or health matters. We all want to flourish and see others succeed too.

We teach belief systems. Inside a belief system people lose the true spark to seek. Instead, they seek inside of the rulebook, the structure, the belief system itself, which is controlling and limited. It's like tying a boat to the pier and then rowing. You won't go very far. Seekers take the perpendicular approach, like Christopher Columbus. They row straight out to sea, away from the land, knowing there is something else out there and also that if they stay near to the land they are leaving, keeping it in sight for safety, they will never discover anything new because fortune favours the brave and the magic lies within the unknown world. An inward step (into the heart) of a perpendicular nature is the only way to know the truth.

That is why seekers, on the other hand, work alone, diving deeper into their own consciousness, knowing that there is more to life, more to the world, more potential to harness. Seekers are hungry for knowledge, information and know that they must take full responsibility for everything. Seekers discover many wonders, so much beauty, they see life in a different way and live to expand and flourish, wishing the same for others. Believers on the other hand are like crabs in a bucket. They will pull each other back in, to hold the system in place. Seekers smile when others make new discoveries, excel, change, transform and become more. Seekers, once they discover their conscious power, tend to vibrate towards other seekers, hanging around and enjoying each other's company, sometimes forming communities but never becoming attached like a believer. A seeker will move on easily, pack up camp overnight, like a gypsy on their travels with zero attachment.

When you start putting yourself first and focus inwards, loving unconditionally, realizing you are a kaleidoscope of infinite universes, flowing through each other, you step into a new paradigm of conscious power. I say conscious because we all have power, it's just that some of us use it to serve and others use it to control. When you connect with your conscious power source, your mind and heart, balanced in perfect equilibrium, you become unpredictable and start not giving a fuck. When you are still in sheep mode, unaware that you are in a holographic game, thinking that your job, your house, your mortgage and earning a living is your sum total of life, you are totally predictable and with data being the number one commodity on the planet right now, enslaving you into predictability is the number one priority for a minority. It begs the question; how did a minority take control of a majority?

When you live from the heart, you are a loose cannon, but a conscious loose cannon. You choose when to fire and in what direction and no one will ever light your fuse because no one can find it. Why? Because it doesn't exist in a Super-Human's psyche – and if it still does with you, it will get shorter and shorter as you practise these ways of being, doing and acting. Eventually your fuse will disappear, and you will become totally non-reactive and, in that moment, truly liberated, free to sing and shine. You slowly move into a new arena where you harness formidable conscious power. This new arena is called the "NOT GIVING A FUCK" arena. And why would you give a fuck? You are a walking, talking, undefinable kaleidoscope of magic, spiralized geometry and code, a vibrating instrument of truth. How could something as powerful as you give a fuck about anything? You created it all anyway. You created the sun, the moon and the stars. The animals, oceans and rainforest, jungles, rivers and streams and nine other billion potential Super-Humans to interact with and show you your own wonder. After you created it, elements of it got a little lost and started manipulating the entire playing field but that is the game, the beauty of exploration. Consciousness itself got a little bored too and created duality. Look where it took us. But it's cool. Now we can play the finding our way back home again game, which we are doing right now. A little like Hansel and Gretel, but we are not trusting the breadcrumbs we sprinkled, we are using our life compass, our heart.

We must be Unfuckwithable Beings. Unfuckwithable beings do not give a fuck. Here is the definition of Unfuckwithable: When you're truly at peace and in touch with yourself, and nothing anyone says or does bothers you, and no negativity or drama can touch you.

Your soul is infinite. Your beauty is extraordinary, and your talent is breathtaking. You should see the angelic and extra-terrestrial beings you created, watching you from above and all around, beyond that ever-thinning veil, rooting for and supporting your brilliance. They are awe-struck.

Let go, surrender to this human experience and allow the universe to play your human vessel like an instrument from an orchestra. There is a frequency, an intelligence, that is talking to you right now, guiding you back home. Let go and dance, shine, play, run, skip, smile and explore. Be the glowing beacon of love that you know deep inside you are. Be you and let your soul shine through every cell, drawing exuberant energy from the infinite vacuum inside every proton, and light the world in bliss.

Do not give a fuck about how others behave and are in life. Do not put anyone else on a pedestal. Everyone on this planet is a little or a lot fucked up in their own unique way. Some people just hide it well. You cannot live on this planet and not have experienced your share of trauma in some way, shape or form. So, forget about the other nine billion fucked-up humans on this planet. Those that thrive are those that embrace their vulnerability, realizing that is the foundation for ultimate power. They take their pain and alchemize it. It becomes pure energy and that kind of energy is unstoppable when harnessed and applied correctly.

Start not giving a fuck and feel how liberated you become. Whatever happens and unfolds, let it happen, with zero judgement. If you feel like doing it, do it. If you feel like saying it, say it. If you feel like dancing dance, crying cry, laughing laugh, jumping up and screaming the world is pink from the tallest rooftop, then do it. Don't give a fuck about what others think. If you want to quit your job, quit it. If you want to leave your marriage, leave it. If you are sick of the rules and regulations in your religion or church, exit. Do it now. Smile as you change, shift, transform, move on – and remember, don't give a fuck as you do it!

BE FREE!!!

7

Going Quantum

Follow the Signs

Taking control requires a lot of effort and sometimes to be in full control, you have to be comfortable out of control, moving with the tides and the natural flow of the river of life. Everything is a double-edged sword. I've told you how I came into this world. The birth process my birth mother endured. I was split/fractured mentally as a kid, through this process, and then raped as a baby. I remember when I was a boy and into my teens, all I wanted to do was go into the army. I wanted to be a soldier. I hated being told what to do as a kid, by anyone in authority but I loved the thought of going to war and following orders to kill people/enemies.

In my last several incarnations on Earth, I have killed others. This is the first one I haven't killed another human being in, so I am primed to kill. Or was anyway, until I did the inner work. I am still primed for war and will always be ready if war breaks out. I fight this spiritual war every day, as so many others. It's why we are here.

I actually booked an interview at the army recruiting office in Gloucester, where I grew up. I was walking down there for my appointment and went past my local pub. I looked through the window and saw my old mate, Lewis. He was stood at the bar on his own. I popped in. Three pints later, I thought, shit, I better go. Anyway, I turned up to the army recruitment office stinking of beer and they told me to get out. That day I was rescued, guided by some force that put Lewis in that place to entice me for a beer. If I had gone into the Army, the dark side would have got

me right where they wanted. I am pretty sure I would have gone all the way into the Parachute Regiment and the SAS and been involved in some kind of special ops team at a high level, killing and murdering. It's crazy because there is this part of me that loves the thought of war and battle. It's why I do everything to the maximum every time. There are never any half-measures with me. It's all or nothing and I love pain and suffering, mentally and physically to push myself and to see how far I can go.

The malevolent forces wanted me executing on their behalf and had trained my psychology since birth to become a soldier. The benevolent forces had another plan and that was Star Magic. My major test came a year after this experience and this test lasted approximately six years.

I got a job at Walls Ice Cream, a large factory near me. I packed ice cream and sold drugs and my plan was to save some money, buy an old camper van and go travelling around Europe with my girlfriend at the time. We brought the camper van. The plan was to get away from the crazy influences in my life, get off the booze and drugs and sort myself out. The night before we left, we were in the pub drinking and a man walked in. We had never met him or seen him before. He walked up to us and said, "I hear you are going travelling. Don't do that. Take this name and number," and he handed us a piece of paper. It said "Chris" and had a Spanish mobile number on it. The man said, "Go to Tenerife, call this guy and he will give you a job. You will get free accommodation and earn at least £300 a week." We looked on the map. I'd never heard of Tenerife. It's one of the Canary Islands, off the coast of Africa but a part of Spain. We sold the van the next day and brought two one-way tickets.

We ended up working for a guy by the name of John Palmer. John was allegedly involved in the Brinks Matt Gold Bullion Robbery at Heathrow Airport in the early 1980s but was never convicted. He earned the name John "Goldfinger" Palmer because of it. He was actually shot dead a few years back in the UK, in his garden. Working for this organization taught me so much about life. It also took me into a real deep dark hole. I was earning lots of money, by ripping off tourists. Being in this environment I was exposed to criminals from all walks of life. I got involved in the selling and trafficking of drugs and other commodities.

I also met my now ex-wife Laura in Spain. Our daughter Aalayah was born in Tenerife. Aalayah is a real blessing to this world. She is nineteen now but has the intelligence and wisdom of a million people who have walked the universal planes for millennia. I am so blessed to have her in my life and will be forever grateful.

The universe guided me to Tenerife through this man we'd never met or seen. We didn't question him at all. We just went with it. We had been preparing for a year for our trip in a camper van and it all changed in three minutes flat. My local boozer was the space where both of these guides, Lewis and the unknown man, got me back on track.

When Aalayah was born the situation on the streets of Tenerife was getting pretty crazy. Two different mafia groups were having a turf warfare. Aalayah had just been born and so we thought let's go somewhere else. Laura had left Romania illegally and so didn't have a passport. That meant we couldn't get Aalayah one, so I had to smuggle her and Laura back into the UK, so Laura and I could get married.

In Tenerife I also met a fella who became my best mate for about ten years. He also became Aalayah's godfather, once he had come out of prison. He came back to the UK just before me and had to do some time in the nick. He ended up stealing a lot of money from me in a business deal, which ended our friendship, and he also introduced me to my first spiritual teacher/ Earthly guide. From this guide I remembered so much, and my inner journey went into overdrive. You see, everything is a double-edged sword: lessons, magic, love, pain and suffering, it's embedded within every situation. You choose to take from each event what you will. It can haunt you for the rest of your life or the knowledge can fuel parts of the rest of your life.

You have the Devil on one shoulder and God on the other. It doesn't matter who you are, both aspects reside within you. Who you choose to listen to, is on you. Both have their pluses and minuses. Balancing both is key, as discussed in the "Master of Dark and Light" chapter. There is a battle for the right passage of your soul. Certain forces believe they own your soul. It's up to you to fight for it and know that no one owns you and you can make the choices, which will lead to your ultimate destiny. The universe will guide you back on track, but you have to listen.

Something made me choose to go for a beer with Lewis and something made me sell the old camper and go to Tenerife. It was not plain sailing. I went through darkness, which I actually enjoyed. Being in my late teens and early twenties, having lots of money, living in the sun, not having a care in the world. All I had to think about was how much cocaine I would sniff and smoke at the weekend, where we would party and what new clothes I would buy to go out in. It was one of the best times of my life. At the same time, the dark side was getting its claws deeper into me. I was governed by dark entities and my ego and trauma were driving my behaviour. The spiritual war is ongoing. It's invisible to the unaware. It's why so many people never break through the mould.

Following the signs was the best thing that ever happened to me. Most importantly, Aalayah came out from this journey and then Josh, my son, two years after. I met my first spiritual guide and that was priceless.

There are other times you have to follow the signs. These adventures are all a part of the spiritual war we are in. In August 2020, I was in Transylvania at a house I have there. A friend phoned me up and told me that there was something I needed to collect from an old casino, in a place called Constanta, which is by the seaside, eight hours by train from where I was. I was due to fly back to the UK three days later. I connected and tuned into the situation and saw a golden cloak. I know, this sounds bonkers right?

I was with my girlfriend. We brought two overnight tickets and jumped on a train two hours later. It was about 9 p.m. The train left at 11 p.m. By the time we arrived in Constanta it was about 7 a.m. the next day. We booked into a hotel, got changed and went down to this casino. The casino was run down and being repaired. It had scaffolding and security in cabins guarding the site as it was the weekend. The casino is on the beach. We walked around the front and there was no way in without being seen.

We then walked around the left side, jumped the fence down to the beach and started walking around the back. The building was not in a good state in places. I climbed up the back wall, through a hole to get a better look but on the other side of the hole was a 20-metre drop. I turned to go back and the piece of iron I was holding onto, that was sticking out from the wall, broke. I fell but managed to grab a piece of jagged rock to stop the fall.

I climbed back down, and we continued walking around the back. At the far side was a hole. A big hole, maybe one metre deep, two metres tall and one metre wide. There were some things carved into the stone. Now what I am about to tell you is pretty crazy.

We saw the letters Culote. The number 8. The number 9:

- The number 8 is my girlfriend's life path number.
- The number 9 is my life path number.
- Cu = Control Unit.
- Lote = With hidden meaning and it also means lesser of two evils and lives of the elite.
- The numerology of Culote breaks down to nine, which is my life path number and also symbolizes spiritual advancement.

We are sat there deciphering these encoded messages. Could we have smoked too much Cosmic Crack? Could we be totally off our fucking heads, and all this is just a massive coincidence?

I stood in front of this hole and this massive wave of energy comes around me. It sits me down. I literally could not stand up. This being comes behind me and puts a golden cloak around my back. I am downloading these codes and it feels amazing. My girlfriend is next to me downloading information too. The next thing I hear is "go now". I get up, scale the wall behind me, jump the metal fence, run to the right, across the open space between the wall and the casino and towards a door about fifteen metres away. It's an entrance into the casino. I go though the door, down a staircase and into the basement.

The place is run down but with incredible architecture. I go down as far as I can and into this huge basement. There is scaffolding holding the ceiling up in places and it's dark as dark can be. Other areas were lit up. I am guided to this back part and the energy is crazy. I knew I was not alone. I was told to turn and be still. I started uploading this energy from the ground. I looked forward and saw two lizard-looking beings come into the space. They zigzagged left to right and came towards me. I put up this real strong force of energy around me and they couldn't get through. I stayed in this space for about four to five minutes. To be honest I could not wait to get the fuck out of there, but I knew I had to wait until the upload was complete. I then left the basement, walked back up the stairs, back out of the door, ran back across the open space, passed the security and jumped the fence.

I scaled the wall and sat back down. My girlfriend was still in her space. I sat back down and went freezing cold. I was there and then the being that gave me the golden cloak told me to look in the left pocket. I did and there is a golden masonic book, with a compass on it. There was also a crystal inside the pocket. I started looking through the book. What was in it, and still is, is a whole world of knowledge.

I went back into the casino later and underneath the basement was a chamber. It was used for sacrifice, and I had to let some souls out. In 2009 when I was remembering how to meditate, Jesus appeared in front of me, my feet turned to balls of fire and he told me I could walk anywhere and not to be fearful. He then took me into the Last Supper, where I was Matthew.

What I realized during the experience in Romania was that I was retrieving a masonic book I, as Matthew, had given to the dark forces, many years ago. I had sold out and gone dark and now I was making up for it, righting a wrong as such.

I know this sounds bonkers. I am sure some souls reading this have had their own similar experiences and other souls will think I am a "roll and butter". But you know what, I don't give a flying you know what. The wisdom in this book has been split into parts and is being kept safe. I am dissecting it in parts, as and when I am being guided.

The truth is often hidden in plain sight, but we only see what we are conditioned to see. It

takes trust to follow your heart and the signs the universe leaves in your path. When you do, you will get more and more, and your life will open up like a cosmic portal that leads you into a labyrinth of beauty and magic.

This next experience is something that most would have not ventured forwards into, because it took a lot of trust, faith and commitment. It also would seem to many like something out of a Harry Potter movie and too far-fetched to even contemplate. I have a different character. Ever since I was a kid, I have given anything a go. I always throw caution to the wind and just do it. Sometimes it has landed me in beautiful places and other times it's got me in trouble. One thing I know for sure, however, is that I learned more from the trouble and strife. There are no good or bad decisions and there are no positive and negative experiences. It's just a game. So, play it, beautiful soul.

I woke up one morning, having had an intense dream about a small blue, Greek artefact. It had the picture of the sun on one side and the other side was worn away. In my dream, I had taken this artefact to Ireland, to a castle there called Cashel Castle. In my dream, I was also aware that I had been/was the King of Cashel in a parallel reality (known as a past life to some – I use the term parallel reality as there is no past or future in the quantum field). The Queen of England was also in my dream, and I had been shown her playing a part in constructing a grid. But it made no sense when I woke.

I opened my laptop that morning and Amazon popped up on Google. The screen clicked itself (as it does when you are being guided) and there on Amazon was this blue artefact from my dream. I bought it immediately and it arrived a few days later. The vibration in this was crazy powerful. My heart expanded and my pineal gland vibrated as soon as I held it. I knew I had to take this artefact to Ireland (just like in my dream), so I dropped everything I was doing (this felt very important – even though I didn't have a clue why), bought a plane ticket and flew to Waterford in Ireland a few days later. Waterford was approximately an hour-and-twenty-minute drive from Cashel Castle if I remember rightly.

I plotted up in my hotel that night after hiring a car at the airport and the next day drove up to Cashel with my little blue Greek artefact, not knowing what to expect. I parked in a car park at the bottom of the hill, had a quick look around the museum and then headed up the road to the castle.

It was actually a bright sunny day and with Ireland being such a beautiful space, the views from the top of the hill, where the castle lay, were awesome. I paid my entry fee and one of the first things I noticed was a picture of the Queen and that she had visited this castle two years earlier. I then started to walk around. At first, everything seemed pretty normal. Looking at the displays, the old kitchen, chapel and various other rooms that you'd expect to see in an eleventh century castle. I love looking around old buildings as when I am in the space, I can see exactly what it was like, what the people dressed like, how they behaved, and what the energy was like back in that other reality or further back on the timeline. The veil between the physical and non-physical worlds are thinning so much on Earth right now. Maybe you too, are getting glimpses into the quantum, but very real world as dimensions bleed through?

I then headed to a different part of the castle, which was more run down, and I was walking through a corridor. I looked up and saw a being coming towards me. I won't say man or woman because this was like a zombie. This being had a hood up, was well built. It looked completely out of place in this space, among a load of human tourists sightseeing for the day. We walked towards each other, and it looked straight through me. I knew that this being was there to

try to disrupt whatever it was that I was supposed to do energetically. I've been face to face with negative Reptilians (and there are some lovely ones too) and their comrades in the physical on several occasions, so these things don't faze me. It's only when you are fearful that they can manipulate you. Love is the key.

So, I walked past this being into a part of the castle that was a dead end. I just stayed there contemplating, feeling, just for a few seconds, what to do next and then a smooth soft voice asked me to go back down the corridor and out onto the grass, in front of the building. I did this and, once I was there, just stood admiring the views. Next, a powerful wave of energy surged through me and lifted me off my feet and I ended up lying face up on my back. I couldn't move but was very aware of everything that was happening. A white stream of light flooded out from my being, straight down into the Earth and I saw a heavy black energy line that went from the Vatican to Cashel Castle.

Just as I was there in this space, as a spiritual tool, so was the Queen there two years previous as a spiritual tool. We were being used by opposing forces of nature, however. Dark and light. Quite often physical beings are needed to do certain things (insert codes into the grids for example) as we live in this heavier third-/fourth-dimensional reality. Most energetic work can be done at distance but there are exceptions.

The white light that surged down through the Earth penetrated this black tunnel of energy and smashed it in half. Bright light exploded in the most exquisite way and the connection between the Vatican and this space was broken. Within the explosion of white light were angels, unicorns and other mythical beings I do not even have names for. When I eventually opened my eyes, I looked up and there was a spacecraft hovering in the midst of the air. The support for this mission to Cashel Castle was immense. It was far more important than I could have imagined. I was completely aware through the whole thing, however, what seemed like minutes was almost an hour. No time. No space. A friend of mine back in England knew where I was going and held space for me throughout the process. She experienced everything just as I did when we spoke on the phone later that evening.

I still had this blue Greek artefact in my pocket and was wondering what I should do with it. I stood up after several minutes feeling a little dazed and I was staring out over the castle wall, down the hill and into a field. I saw a calf. I looked around and there were no other cows to be seen. It felt a little odd to see a calf with no mum, dad, brother, or sister and so I decided to make my way over to the field. I climbed over the castle wall, down a massive drop, over a few barbed wire fences and then looked up into the field to see this calf running off along the hedgeline. I ran after it. I must have looked like a fruit cake chasing a calf through a field. It's caring what other people think about you that holds you back. The calf went around a corner, and I couldn't see it any longer. I ran and chased it until I turned the corner also.

I was expecting the calf to be with a load of other cows when I got there, or maybe it would have slipped through a fence and back into another field, with the other cows. But no! Once I reached the end of the hedgeline and turned the corner, the cow was looking at me. Its hoof was on a rock. Again, the rock looked so out of place. I walked over towards the calf, it removed its hoof from on top of the rock and I lifted it up. There was a hole in the ground just the right size for this blue Greek artefact. I took it from my pocket, kissed it and placed it in the hole, put soil and grass over the top and threw the rock into the hedge. The smooth soft voice then said to me, "You can go home now, thank you." This soft voice is my inner self. Some people call it your

higher self. I don't consider anything higher or lower than me, so inner fits the bill.

So, I left the field and walked back around the castle to where I'd parked the car. Got in and took a slow drive back to Waterford, wondering to myself "what the fuck just happened?"

This world is not what it seems. There is a spiritual war being fought behind the scenes for the right passage of your soul. The solution to this war is love. We must love all beings, even the ones that are misguided or malevolent. We must live with zero fear, on an elevated vibration, playing this game by our own rules. The only rule that is a must is love. It's the driving force that will unite our global family and create heaven on Earth. You get to choose always, but when you don't know there is a game being played and your consciousness is being corrupted continually, how can you make the best choices? Some people do know bits and pieces of the truth but they only know some of the rules and truths that hold illusory structures in place. If you are fully aware of the game, you already know how to handle business, mentally, physically, emotionally, and spiritually. If you are not, keep on reading and dive deeper into your heart. Eventually you will alchemize a deep knowing, carved from your own experiences and then you too will know. Once you know, you know, and there is no turning back.

The Queen of England had been (maybe unknowingly) used to run lower vibrational energies, through Mother Earth's ley lines, across the planet from Rome to Cashel, from the Vatican to the castle. Once this grid had been set up, which is a part of a much larger grid, being used for dark and light, it needed another human being, in this case me, to facilitate the undoing of this dark and devious deed. I say dark and devious but that is judgemental. We must look at this in terms of vibration. High and low-vibrational frequencies.

There is no good or bad. It's just a game. As you read on you will understand the rules and become a master in this Earthly realm. Also, to put your mind at rest, the Planetary Grids that were once majorly hijacked by darker forces are now moving back into the control of the forces of light, the positive, the benevolent. There is still a little work to do but we are getting there as a Global and Galactic Family.

Having a dream, waking up, seeing elements of the dream on the laptop, going to another country, following a calf, listening to a soft voice in your head, transmuting negative energy lines, seeing unicorns and other mythical beings, sounds far-fetched and quite possibly like a script from a movie or maybe the thoughts of a crazy man who just escaped from a psychiatric hospital. For me, this is normal. My life has been like this since a car crash and a trip in a spacecraft. But that's a whole other story. These missions we go on as souls are important. They are an integral part of us winning this spiritual war. Follow your heart. Follow your intuition. Have the composure and the courage to follow the signs. Remember, some are tricks but even within the tricks there are opportunities to grow, beautiful soul.

Love or Fear

We have talked about the spectrum of emotions from love to fear, and how any other emotion is just a diluted version of one of these or a slightly varied vibrational version.

This kind of love, like we've looked at, is the type of love where there is no turning back.

Meditation, breathwork and the pineal gland work I am going to share with you later is your ticket to this beyond-human-words love. The first time I experienced it was on Alpha Centauri, when I met the Lyrans there. I had never felt so peaceful, so at home, so loved. It was a love, so pure and untainted, by thought forms. When the Lyrans hugged me, I melted into an ocean of nothingness. I will never truly be able to describe what happened in that moment. The next time I experienced this magnitude of love, was when my ex-wife and I were discussing our relationship. It was the first time we split up and the only time before we ended our sixteen-year marriage three years later.

I was not living at the house but went over to have dinner with the children. After Aalayah and Josh went to bed we were talking. I was sat there on the edge of the sofa, and I had this massive realization that I had never loved myself. It hit me like a steam train. A wave of energy pushed me back onto the sofa and I was looking up towards the ceiling. I popped out of my body and was floating in the space above. I felt so much love. I felt loved beyond this human world. I also felt like I was the love that was loving me and everything everywhere, throughout all space, and this love, this energy was connected to me, a part of me and it loved me, and I loved it. In this moment there really was no separation. It was like I could be everywhere, and I was. I was so expanded and had no boundaries.

The next thing I knew I was outside the house, taking my clothes off because I was so hot. My body was on fire. It was late at night, and I was stripping in the street. I have no recollection of getting from the sofa to the street. Laura told me that I walked into the kitchen, was crying intensely, sat down and then made my way to the front door. I remember nothing. My body was soaking wet, I was still crying as I was coming back into this reality, and they felt like the happiest tears I have ever shed. It was years of not crying and bottling up my emotion flooding from my soul in one gigantic gush, like a dam that burst through, and the water was racing to the other side. In this moment I had the realization that I had never loved myself. I had never truly been held and loved properly by anyone, including me. When I floated above my body on the sofa, I felt like I was being held in an infinite blanket of magic and love, and, at the same time, this infinite blanket or magic and love, was me. It was such a life-altering moment. When the Lyrans hugged me, it was like coming home. The love was immense. The love I felt with them was beyond, just like when I floated above my body in the living room. The difference was, in one experience I was being loved and the other I was the love that was loving me, but the magnitude of both experiences was the same.

You can't teach this stuff to people, but you can help them remember. Everything I am sharing with you in this book is to help you remember. I am not a teacher giving you new information. I am a guide, offering you the opportunity to step back into your own ancient wisdom, to remember your truth. To be your divine sovereign self and activate yourself.

In every situation love is the only choice for a Super-Human. I remember one day, Josh coming into my bedroom in the night. A heavy, green and brown-looking being with a shadowy exterior had come into Josh's bedroom and started to strangle him. Josh was suffocating and he tried to call my name but couldn't. He then remembered what I told him. Be in love and stay calm. Josh then stopped struggling and fighting and opened his heart. As soon as this being felt Josh's love and the total lack of fear, Josh was able to push it off of him. The being then disappeared.

Remember, we create our own reality. If you stay in fear, you fuel the enemy, and everything is a co-creation, so your own fear is fuelling you to create this situation.

Now, I am not saying that this being didn't exist. It most certainly did but on some level, Josh would have co-created this. His energy would have

had to feed into this situation to make it possible. This being was also a great opportunity for Josh to practise his skills. This being that came into his room, in my opinion, was a holographic insert. Reality can be layered over reality and made to look very real and if you play into the reality that has been inserted, it becomes very real.

I was lying in bed a few years ago and I opened my eyes to see this orange and black electromagnetic spider in my room. Some people may have gotten scared and gone into fear, but I smiled, chuckled, told it to piss off (in a gentle loving way, of course), closed my eyes and pretended to sleep. I opened them ten seconds later and it was gone.

Love is always the question and the answer, the solution to every circumstance. I won't say problem but there are situations and circumstances and all of them require a sprinkling of love. From a crying baby to a homeless sister or brother to an electromagnetic spider, love is the way!

If you want to irradicate a disease or stop a war, you do not give that war or that disease any attention. The observer affects the observed in every situation, so it's important to move your energy in the right direction. Always remember, your energy follows your focus and attention. If you want to stop war, focus on peace and if you want to irradicate disease, focus on perfect health. When people come to me for healing and tell me they have this or that disease, it doesn't show up in my reality. I create a whole new reality, with no disease and quantum-entangle the two. We must, as a collective, choose love in every situation. We must cultivate a love culture but not just any love culture. It must be a fiercely, loving love culture where we accept each other in our totality, with zero judgement, and be kind and compassionate towards the world and its inhabitants: humans, animals, insects, Mother Nature in her entirety.

Love of a fierce nature is the order of the day. I cannot stress this word "fierce" enough. If you do not love fiercely, a constant barrage of negative potentials will eventually break you. You will crumble, react to another person or event and your vibration will dip. You must love fiercely to stay on track, continue to elevate and be your Super-Human self. Fierce Love is the geometric universal code, it's the fuel of our universe.

The Quantum World and Healing

For a long time I resisted coming out into the public eye and starting a "healing business", which has now developed into a passion and a mission, which I will move heaven and Earth to fulfil. It was a radical U-turn. I came from a life full of criminals, mixing in what some would deem unsavoury circles, living with a "get there fast and never mind everyone else in my way" approach to life, striving for more money and material possessions because I thought it was cool – and then moved into a world full of love and compassion, living with a purpose each day to be a better human being, a Super-Human, and create the space to transform the lives of as many of my fellow sisters and brothers as possible. At school I couldn't stand physics, biology or chemistry. I didn't like maths even though I was good at it and if someone mentioned an atom or a molecule it would be like the sound of long nails scratching a blackboard. I would be headed to the gardens at the back of the school to smoke a spliff.

Now I live every day fascinated by a world that once made me sick. I grew up a total non-believer and still am a total non-believer, but I am a hardcore "knower".

I have witnessed some incredible healings, when clients have gone back for scans showing no cysts or tumours, or suddenly been able to see or hear, or move a limb that had been disabled for twenty years. When it happens over and over you just know that these things are not miracles. You simply have to create the right environment for healing to take place. Every single human being was designed to self-heal; once a healer sets up the environment so the woman, man or child can self-heal, the healer must get out of their own way and let nature take its course. Even though I have a healing business, I am not a healer. I have never healed anyone in my life Yes, thousands of people's lives have been transformed by the work I have instigated. Many who were told they were going to die, are still alive. People who were "disabled" are now fully functional. I say instigated because all I do is create the environment, set up the space, connect with the right frequency through my heart and bring in data streams or light streams, unplug the human being I am working on from a data stream that is causing illness or disease and plug them into a new data stream that is pure, clean, full of life force and harmonious energy.

Our body is an amazing instrument. And it is just that: an instrument. It plays tunes, melodies, songs. Sometimes those songs are full of joy and bliss and other times the sounds emitted are just that: noise, horrible sounds that are incoherent and scrape and prod your consciousness. When the body is out of synch it communicates with you and lets you know something needs a little attention. When our car breaks down, we take it to a mechanic and when our body breaks down, we head for the doctor. Your own physical body is a gigantic pharmacy, and you have access to all of the chemicals you require. Just a simple example: if you ever get a mosquito bite and it is itchy, close your eyes, talk to your body and ask it to release its natural antihistamine stores. You will see, it works.

The space around us is rich and full of information. There are unfathomable amounts of energy everywhere. The empty space is not empty. I am able to see code in the empty space. I have done since 2013. It just appeared and that is when my healing journey went into overdrive.

I see zero separation between objects, people, trees, plants, buildings; just code. Streams of moving geometries, spirals of information and this other type of code that carries this moving formation. These codes are the codes I use to heal with Star Magic.

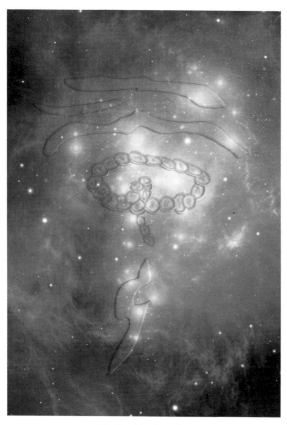

22. Star Magic codes

You will notice they have horizontal lines at the top, then some code and then vertical lines underneath. The number of horizontal and vertical lines varies but there is always more horizontal than vertical. The entire universe is code and it's the code, which is fully accessible to each of us, that creates the healing. The quantum world is everywhere. What I mean is that time, distance and measurement do not exist in the world beyond form. If I have a client in New York, I can be sat at home and hold out my left hand. I can then imagine a miniature version of my client

hovering over my hand, and can tune in to her or his body and connect with it. I decide that this image in my hand, this visualization, is her or him and I quantum-entangle the two realities. That means whatever I do to the body in my hand will happen to the body in New York.

This is a mathematical equation in the form of geometrical code. The codes are balanced numerically and are fractal in nature, unfolding from within themselves and unfolding infinitely, geometrically in a spiralized fashion and quantumly. When you connect with these codes, the underlying architecture of our physical reality, you can see which light-encoded data streams are creating an illness or injury and remove them. There are two primary ways.

The first is to work with the actual light codes themselves and the second is to tap into or connect with the reality or realities that are creating these data streams.

In healing someone who has a cyst, for example, I can see the light codes feeding into that cyst to create it or I can go past that and into the reality that created the data stream. Now, in actuality, the data stream and the reality that created the data stream could not exist without each other, they are one and the same, so one does not come before the other. The data stream is the light codes/data and the reality is the experience that is creating the cyst and the data stream. So, if a woman has a cyst in the ovaries, it could be that in this earlier life she had a father who left her and her mother; so her masculine and feminine are out of balance and there is also deep anger, a lack of trust in the masculine, and huge resentment issues. This has resulted in a physical ailment. Which is really just the body's way of communicating to the individual. So, if I go into that reality, I can change it, recreate it or collapse the timeline. Once I choose what to do and take action, the data stream, the light-encoded frequency running into the human being's biological computer is now different. This changes the human being at a cellular level and the cyst will often disappear. If it shrinks and is still partly there, I may need to connect again and access a second reality and change that too. If the experience no longer exists within the universal field, it cannot feed into the human being's consciousness. Delete the programme and you delete the dis-ease. It also works in reverse: if we want to bring something to life, we must first create it quantumly. The quantum world contains the building blocks of all physical life.

Data is always being fed back to the universal field and from the field into us. We are one and the same. Inside every human there are between 50 and 100 trillion cells and inside every cell there are approximately 100 trillion protons. Each one of these protons is like a mini universe, sharing and collecting data. Wherever there is an action there is an equal reaction somewhere, and in some cases multiple reactions. There are two polar opposites feeding back into a singular point, a singularity, what some would call the zero-point, which has no start, middle, or end. It's infinite and from within this infinite space, all things occur or are.

We can control the data to some extent but not in its entirety because we are all connected. So, we have access to multiple streams of data at all times. We can control the data surrounding our cells and then feed this data into our cells. Remember, the cells are affected by their environment. If I go into the quantum space, the place where nothing or no-thing exists, I can visualize, imagine, and create any reality I want. I can tap into a past life where a person was murdered and rewind that timeline until the point before it happened. I then create a different outcome. I can hold this data in the quantum field, entangle it with one of the cells in the person's body that I am working on and feed that data into the cell. I can then entangle every cell in the human body with this reality and the programme disappears.

Nothing in the physical world is real. Nothing is unchangeable because in this reality, it doesn't exist. Everything that you do and see was born out of the quantum field, from the womb of space, the dark, infinite labyrinth of magic that exists in our universe and inside every proton in our body. This space is so richly energized that anything can be created and moulded, recreated and remoulded from it. Energy never dies, it simply moves through form, into form, back out of form and into form again, therefore with the right technology (a human being who knows how to manipulate the quantum field), all things can be changed. Why? Because when you change consciousness, you trigger a change in energy. I see people regularly in our trainings and workshops, going into deeper states of meditation, where they go beyond their bodies, into the world of spiralized geometry, fractal patterns of light. Their brain waves and heart rates are slowing, they're altering their consciousness and there are explosions of energy in the brain, people leave their bodies, they see indescribable colourful sights/visions, access parallel realities, meet beings from other dimensional spaces and take the mind completely out of the way. In this space the body naturally does what it's supposed to do. Neurons fire, nerve fibres light up, the central nervous system and the entire nervous system start to transport huge amounts of light/data and the body naturally self-heals. For some it's easy to get there, others need to work harder, but everyone eventually will go to that space. Discipline and surrender are crucial.

I want to share rewinding timelines with you. We can collapse/change many realities on one or multiple timelines, in one go, by altering the deepest experience. Anything thereafter, in linear time, in this human's field, will dissolve also. My mission is to absorb all of this human being's soul experiences back into the now space so they can be whole, unfragmented. This is real healing! We have a very specific technique or way of doing this, which I will share with you later.

"After" may not be the best word, because there is no before or after in the quantum field. Everything is now. However, when I am searching for a trigger, a reality, a past life (which are all one and the same) in the field of information, I am looking for the deepest wound. I want to hit that wound wherever it lies in the field. Sometimes I may hit a wound that is deep, but not the deepest, but which is all the human being I am working on can handle right now, emotionally for example. So, they will partially heal, get some relief, feel the shift (maybe an arm that was totally dysfunctional will get some feeling back into it), but there is still more work to do. I would go back in and repeat the process, or maybe I will be shown something completely different that needs working on that wasn't available the first time, and that will heal the human being.

If a human being is willing to do the work and completely surrender, information is restructured, energy is reorganized, and miracles take place. Every human on the planet has the ability to tap into these subatomic fields, through practice and discipline. Unfortunately, not everyone is willing or able to put in the effort; for some people there is self-pity, low self-esteem, blame and judgement. Some need a kick up the bum, while others require a more loving touch and soft guidance. We are all different and unique.

You are reading this book, so I know you don't require any persuasion. It's time for you to go to work. It's time for you to play, have fun. Journey deeper and maintain the discipline even once you feel healed, elevated, expanded, and keep going. You must keep going, because there are always deeper levels.

It's a bit like an alcoholic. They stop drinking for a week and feel a little better. After three weeks, better still, and after eight weeks totally transformed. The thing is this, the reformed alcoholic doesn't know what it's like to not drink for three, six, nine or twelve months. Those milestones will see them operating on a completely different frequency. Then you have exercise and clean eating to add into the equation. The sister or brother becomes clearer and clearer, moving fully online with more health and vitality.

Two years down the line they are master meditators. You cannot compare the journey from teetotal for seven days to two years, combining eating clean and exercising or even just teetotal for two years without the other components; they are worlds apart! The same goes for you on this journey. Even when you feel that life cannot get any better, and you feel this is the pinnacle, keep going. I guarantee there is always uncharted territory to explore and when it comes to the quantum world and healing you will be fascinated, over and over again.

Real-Life Transformation

I want to share with you some experiences that I have had with clients. I want to give you an insight into the kind of transformation that can take place, how it happens, and to show you that the people who come for healing or to a workshop or training are not highly spiritual people, for want of a better phrase. They are not monks, religious believers or worshippers of some archetypal figure. They don't go around dressed in robes thinking they are the next Jesus Christ or Mary Magdalene. These sisters and brothers are just everyday folk, like you and me, who made a choice, to step up, change and surrender to the experience.

It is important to "innerstand" that my approach is not always the same. Sometimes I work with the code directly and other times I work with the data streams/past lives/parallel realities. These stories will give you an insight into what is possible and how it works, in case you want to try it yourself, which I am trusting you will, of course.

Facial Paralysis

A young woman, Agata, who came to our Facilitator Level 1 Training Experience in the UK, had a stuck face. Its right-hand side, from the cheekbone down, was paralyzed. When I asked her how long she'd had it for, she said as long as she could remember. Agata had tried different medications, alternative medicines, herbal doctors, massage therapy and a whole list of other things. The paralysis in her face was very painful at times and she was receiving regular Botox treatments, as recommended by her doctor. It gave temporary relief, but the pain and paralysis always came back. After a while it became too expensive, so she stopped, and the pain and paralysis returned. No one could tell Agata what the condition was, and no one had any answers on how to solve it.

I asked her to stand in front of me and I asked the same question I ask at the start of every healing session. "Please show me something I don't know, to help me facilitate the healing of this incredible human being." A soon as I asked, I dropped into the space of the heart and felt the situation. To drop into the space of the heart, you simply have to bring your attention and awareness into the space of the heart, consciously, and feel. Feel and see it open. Feel love for all things. The more you practise being in this space, the easier it is to access. Eventually the access will be 24/7.

As soon as I did this, I immediately saw the geometry in Agata's face and how one side was different from the other. With my hand I moved the geometry on the right-hand side of her face into alignment with the geometry on the left-hand side. As soon as I did this the pain and paralysis was gone. She felt her face and couldn't believe it. It took me twenty seconds. That night she went to bed and when she woke up, she reached for her face, expecting it be the same as before the healing. But she could move her mouth and there was no more pain. Each morning of the training she woke up expecting it to be back, but it was still

the same, pain-free and paralysis-free. Eighteen months after the training, at the time of writing this, Agata's face is still perfectly OK. A lifetime of pain gone in twenty seconds and all I did was change the code.

It took about twenty seconds from the time I asked the question to the time I realigned the geometric code in her face. Is this a miracle? No. It's just energy/light/frequency/code. It's what we are and it's how we access the truth and create massive change.

No More Wheelchair

This is quite possibly one of the best stories, because it totally shows how one human being can empower themselves with a simple shift in perspective. I was giving a talk on Star Magic one day and there was a lady, Sarah, in the audience who was in a wheelchair, paralyzed from the neck down. She asked if I could help her and so I asked her a question. Remember, in every situation I never know what is going to happen and I don't always know why I say what I say, but I am intuitive, feel and listen and go with what always feels right. The head is your worst nightmare in a healing scenario, so stay away from your thoughts.

The question I asked Sarah was this. "Have you accepted, fully, that you are in a wheelchair?" Her response was: "How can I accept I am in a fucking wheelchair? Look at me!" So I said to her, "Once you have accepted you are in a wheelchair come and talk to me." I told her I loved her and then continued talking. She was seething. Really unhappy.

At the end of my talk, Sarah blocked my path and asked me again for help. Again, I told her that she needed to accept that she was in a wheelchair and then come and talk to me.

Sarah called me a couple of times, and we had the same conversation.

Three months went past during which I heard nothing, and then she called out of the blue. Sarah sounded so happy. I asked how she was, and she told me she was walking.

Eventually, she told me, she had had no other option but to try what I was suggesting. So, one day, she sat there in her wheelchair and surrendered. She had watched my YouTube videos about dropping into your heart, so breathed, opened her heart, felt gratitude for life, that she was alive, and said to herself, "I am in a wheelchair and I totally accept this. I will make my life the best it can possibly be in this situation and accept, in its entirety, everything that happens on my journey." Within a few days of her acceptance, Sarah started to feel her fingers and small pulses of electricity in her arms. She then started to wiggle her fingers, slowly at first but then things built. Within a few weeks she stood from her wheelchair. Another week or so later she had balance and took her first step. More and more love, more and more gratitude poured through her body and out from her heart with every small improvement, from the first feeling in the fingers to the first time Sarah wiggled them, all the way to her first step.

As soon as Sarah surrendered, her thoughts, her head was out of the way. Her pain disappeared. She was in total acceptance, with no judgements, and her body was able to do what it was designed to do: self-heal. The body always knows what it must do and when we get out of the way, it will heal, Mother Nature will step in. In fact we are Mother Nature and our body will take care of itself just like the environment around us does. We don't have to tell the sun to shine, the rivers to flow, the flowers to bloom, the clouds to rain. Mother Nature does it all by herself. Our bodies work in the same way, when the thoughts and body are not working against it. Remember the body becomes addicted to the chemicals produced by pain, so it searches for more chemicals, more drugs, to feed it. When you take control of your own consciousness, it will do magical things and all that means is total surrender to the situation.

Once you do this, you create a platform and nature will take its course.

In this situation I did nothing, apart from give this lady the best piece of advice I could. It seemed a little harsh at the time (in her eyes and the eyes of everyone in the audience listening to my talk), but in the end the healing took place. This goes to show the power that we possess. Sarah changed her consciousness and in doing so, her energy. She went from being a wheelchair user, full of despair and misery, to being a Super-Human, and self-healed. I did nothing. She did it all.

Ten Years of Pain

A lady called June at our Facilitator Level 1 Training Experience in the USA suffered from chronic hip, leg and shoulder pain in the left-hand side of her body. It was excruciating and her mobility was limited. As usual, I said, "Please show me something I don't know to help me facilitate the healing of this incredible human being." I saw that June had suffered a deep trauma to do with a child. I felt huge guilt and the word "hurt" was ringing around my consciousness. I asked her what happened with one of her children. June's son had died and she felt responsible. Within weeks of his death the pain had started in her leg and hip, and spread to her shoulder. June also had strong mediumship skills, but they were currently stifled.

I saw two men, brothers, in a battle, in a previous life or parallel reality. One was an aspect of the soul of June's son and the other was an aspect of her own soul. They were fighting and then June's brother was killed. In that reality June's soul (the man) again felt guilty for not helping her brother (her son's soul) in that life and saving him. In this present-day reality, she was playing out a similar scenario: her son had overdosed on drugs, and she wasn't there to save him. Same emotions, guilt and hurt. I rewound the timeline to a few days before the battle took place and saw the two brothers in military quarters. I advised them that if they were to escape this war, and live, they would have to leave now. I watched them pack their bags and leave, then turned this new reality into code and downloaded it into June's biological computer, her brain, which downloaded the information into her cells and in turn every proton in her body, each and every mini universe.

To do this I dissolved the reality into light (which is code). I asked her how she was feeling now and she told me she felt full of joy and huge relief. She moved her hip, leg and shoulder around, a great big smile came over her face and she said, "It's gone. I can move. I feel no pain. Oh my God, this is amazing."

Saving the life of the soul aspect of her brother then, and son now, completely removed the underlying, core trigger point that was creating the guilt, hurt and loss, and so the pain (the symptom and communication from the universe letting her know where she needed to look) vanished.

Chronic Adrenal Fatigue

Ben had been in bed for six months. After losing a very successful business and being involved in some very heavy personal relationships, his life deteriorated. He had been to some of the best coaches, healers, alternative therapists on the planet and gained slight relief, but kept falling back to where he was.

When I asked the crucial question, "Please show me something I don't know, to help me facilitate the healing of this incredible human being," I saw the right side of Ben's body was heavy and weighing him down. The energy I was observing was running right down through his body and into his right foot. I could see heavy energy in his kidneys and adrenal glands and his heart was like an old mine that had been covered over with wood and nails and boards: zero access.

I knew that his sexuality was at play. Again, I left it and went deeper. I then asked the questions

again: "Please show me something I don't know, to help me facilitate the healing of this incredible human being." I saw a black box and started drilling into it with a pneumatic drill. When I got to the middle there was an older man inside. As I connected with the man, I saw him on a ship in a storm. The ship capsized and the man lost his crew. He survived and he felt extremely guilty. I spoke with him and he understood that he didn't need to carry this burden any more. I brought this aspect of Ben's soul into healing by opening Ben's heart and the heart of his soul aspect (the captain of the ship), dissolving the soul fragment into light and then bringing the light/code from his dissolved soul aspect back into the now space and into Ben's body.

Then, in another reality, I saw a man and a woman walking down a road. I knew that Ben was the man. A car came past, and the lady stepped out in front of it. She died in the arms of the aspect of Ben's soul. He was angry, upset, felt guilty: the same emotions he was experiencing as the captain of the ship.

I decided to rewind the timeline. I saw the man and woman walking, before the car came down the road. I tapped the man on the shoulder and told him a car was coming. He turned and as the car came past, he pulled his partner away from the road and the reality changed. I collapsed that reality, turned it into code and downloaded the new reality into Ben's brain in this current reality.

All of this healing was done at distance, so I sent Ben the report by email and we spoke a few days later. Ben told me that his father had disowned him because he had come out as gay. He also fell in love with an older man but that relationship fell apart. Ben felt abandoned and rejected, hurt and guilty for sharing the truth. He was angry at his dad and his ex-lover. Then his business fell apart. Within weeks he was laid up in bed, and had been for six months when we connected. The guilt he was experiencing was the guilt of not saving his crew members and his female partner in those other realities. The events in this present-day reality were simply beautiful opportunities to deal with this deeper traumatic experience. After this healing session Ben was out of bed within a matter of days, full of energy.

Lose the Colostomy Bag

I had a call one Boxing Day from a gentleman named Mark. He had been in hospital for the last forty-eight hours fighting for his life. His blood tests showed E. coli and peritonitis. Scans showed three cysts in his intestine and a large growth.

The doctors told him if he made it through the next forty-eight hours, they would refer him to a surgeon to have ten feet of his large intestine removed, and that he would have to have a colostomy bag for the rest of his life.

Mark did make it through the next forty-eight hours, found me on YouTube as he was searching for a healer, contacted me, and explained the situation. I asked him to lie on the bed and relax. I centred myself in my meditation/healing space and I then went to work and entered Mark's room. He was in Coventry, England, and I was in Cheltenham, more than fifty miles away. I gave Mark a healing on this day and then another one a week later.

In the first healing, Mark said, he had been in a room full of people who looked like surgeons, in a tall, ancient-looking stone building that he felt was Egypt.

In the second healing I worked on his stomach again and also on his spine, where he'd had some major problems – he was an ex-jockey and had fallen in a race and been trampled on by several horses.

When Mark went to the doctor he was amazed. Mark no longer had any swelling in his stomach, he was eating, had no diarrhoea and zero pain. Mark's doctor told him he didn't need

the operation after all. His blood tests came back with no trace of E. coli or peritonitis and scans showed that the cysts and large growth had totally vanished.

People would refer to this as psychic surgery. For me I see all healing as the same. Healing is healing. I am simply changing frequencies at a level of light and information, rearranging code and shifting data streams. In each case I am just a vessel for the energy or light. I am "The Facilitator". This for me is no more serious than a headache. It's no less serious than a life-threatening road traffic accident. I treat everything the same, with zero judgement.

Something else I did with Mark was to change his nutrition. I always take a full holistic approach and recommend exercise and nutritional changes when necessary. Remember, your body is a natural organism, and it requires nature to thrive. Putting man-made so-called food into your belly is not going to aid you on your journey, to unlock your greatness and release your full human potential, out into the YOU-Niverse.

It is possible to bring in 5th density + light rays, codes, information streams from other worlds or spaces, and your body can metabolize this light as energy. After all, we are light. Our human body is an illusion. I eat less food now and feed off light more. If you ask anyone who has been to one of our workshops, they will tell you that their nutritional needs completely change afterwards. This is because I take them so deep in the deep frequency-encoded meditations, and bring so much light and code through their bodily hologram, that it activates something within them. It activates dormant genetic encodements within their human DNA.

As the observer of Mark's situation, I simply created a different reality. He was told there were cysts, growths, E. coli and peritonitis . . . and I simply chose to see it differently – a body containing none of this. The power of alchemy! What is important to note is this. Mark said he felt a hand going into his belly where the major pain was. He said it was mine. It wasn't mine. It was one of the Egyptian surgeons I was working with during this healing. I simply observed and oversaw the surgery. I did nothing apart from create the environment so all of this could take place. You can watch the video on the Star Magic website of Mark telling the story and showing his scar that was left across his stomach during the healing. It's fascinating.

Energetic Kidneys

A lady, Kara, on one of our trainings was yellow. She had zero confidence, her face was full of big scabs. She was using dialysis every day. She was not in a good space.

This story will stretch you a little or maybe a lot. Stay in your heart, listen and internalize the information. Don't let your head jump in the way.

I used a healing way/technique on Kara to install some specific codes into her biological computer. As soon as Kara downloaded this code, she fell backwards to the floor and I caught her and lowered her gently down. What happened next, as she downloaded the code, was phenomenal: she writhed around and screamed for maybe fifteen to twenty minutes, then shook and vibrated uncontrollably for another twenty minutes. She stopped and became freezing cold. We wrapped her in a blanket and left her resting, for maybe one and a half hours. When someone goes very cold or hot it's a sign of deep healing.

I programmed the code to remove all of Kara's trauma, apart from the deepest trigger point. I didn't know at this point what the deepest trigger was, but I knew it was heavy and she wasn't ready for this. What she went through in this space was traumatic enough. Two days later I went in to see what the deepest trigger was and I saw Kara as a

being, an extra-terrestrial, flying a craft through space. She was being chased. I let her know what I was seeing. She was having vivid recall. Crystal-clear memories. She burst into tears as she re-experienced this reality.

It was during the galactic wars, hundreds of millions of years ago. Kara in this reality was chased through space and eventually captured by some dark green beings who took her and her family and tortured them all, killed her family and locked her up for a long time. The level of fear that was created, on a soul and a cellular level, was extreme.

We changed the timeline; we superimposed these time-space coordinates onto another reality (one that was full of peace, health and happiness) and quantum-entangled the two. Kara's whole energy changed, big-time. An electromagnetic green light poured from her heart centre. Her light body went violet and the geometry spinning in the space was extraordinary.

Once this was done, I took Kara's light body onto a Pleiadean spacecraft owned by a being I work with called Rianar, who helped me create two new kidneys, quantumly. The kidneys store massive amounts of fear, and they also communicate fear and flow issues/blocks/trauma with their host.

Rianar removed the old kidneys and then we entangled Kara's light body and holographic body together and brought her back down into the physical space. When she was able to sit up, she was glowing.

Kara didn't use her dialysis that evening, or the next day. In fact, she went weeks without it. But then one day felt she was deteriorating, so she used her dialysis and then called me. I did two more healings and since that day (almost two years ago) her dialysis has never been used.

Energetic Gall Bladder

I was in Los Angeles at the Conscious Life Expo and was approached by a lady, Heather, and her mother, Claudia. They explained Heather's situation. She'd had to have her gall bladder removed and she was experiencing uncomfortable symptoms such as diarrhoea and large bile dumps. They asked if there was anything I could do.

I said yes. I always say yes, even if I haven't got a scooby doo how I will help/assist or what will happen. I have no expectation and carry zero judgement. I said, "Let's go to work and see what happens." I have worked with many people who I had to help across to the other side, to transition back to spirit, energy, frequency and go on their merry way. So, I never judge a situation and never know what will happen.

I had a chair in the Star Magic booth and Heather sat down. I attend this expo regularly, give talks and workshops and do one-on-one healings the rest of the time. It's very rare that I get to work on a human being, one-on-one close up, unless it's at a training, so it's something I enjoy.

I approached this healing session the same way as I always do, but I had an agenda at the same time. Firstly, I wanted to shift the deep emotional triggers, from this reality and any others. So, I asked the question, "Please show me something I don't know to help me facilitate the healing of this incredible human being." I went to work with the information I was shown, cleared the trauma/triggers, recoded the timelines and changed the data stream and then I created a quantum gall bladder.

When I started facilitating healing, I didn't have a clue how the body was/looked internally, but after working with so many people, you get an idea of where things lie within this interesting avatar. And even if you don't know anything about the body, the bone structure, the lymphatic system, vital organs and other components, it

doesn't matter. I have developed a way of training anyone to heal, simply using code and patterns. Even Noddy or your teddy bear can use Star Magic to transform relationships, businesses, health and even save lives.

So, back to Heather. I created/visualized an operating table on a spaceship. Well, actually I just saw an operating table on a spaceship, that actually exists. One I use regularly with some benevolent E.T. friends of mine. Whether you are comfortable with creating it, visualizing it or knowing it's actually there, it really doesn't matter. When you have seen as many incredible feats of healing as I have, you practically live on these crafts. So, as Heather was sat in the chair, floating through the field somewhere because of two frequencies that I brought in at the start of the healing, to put her into a deep state, with hundreds or people walking past, loads of noise all around, I took Heather's light body onto this healing/operating table. I started to create a gall bladder from code. I asked to be shown the perfect codes to create a gall bladder, that also carried the right frequency for Heather's physical body, and then I went to work and created this quantum gall bladder from spiralized code. I assembled the codes and put it together, a bit like a complicated, 3D jigsaw puzzle that looked exactly like a gall bladder.

Once the quantum gall bladder was created, I placed it into Heather's light body, which looked exactly like her physical body, but light, transparent, translucent, with extended streams of light flowing out from it, full of tetrahedrons, merkabas and octahedrons and spirals of light. As soon as I placed it inside her quantum body, electromagnetic streams of light started to connect to it. Connections were made between this organ and the rest of the body on a quantum level. I waited and watched and held space. It took maybe three to five minutes.

Once it was over, I brought this quantum body off the operating table and back into the space we were in. I entangled it with Heather's physical body, and she jolted. A quick point to mention. I have found that taking the light body from the physical body, in a situation where you are creating organs, is best – and not entangling it with the physical aspect until the work is done brings the best results, rather than bringing up a hologram and entangling it from the start or working on the physical body directly. When Heather came round, which took a little while, we talked and then she went on her way.

I received an email from Heather's mother two months later. It said this:

Dearest Jerry,
I wanted to let you know that the energetic
gall bladder that you placed into Heather
is working great. No more diarrhoea or bile
dumps, everything is working normally.
Thank you so much for helping Heather, she
is continuing to heal and is moving forward
in her life. AWESOME I say!

If this isn't awesome, just like Claudia, Heather's mother, expressed, I don't know what is. If we can create an energetic organ that works, it proves, way beyond any doubt, that we are not physical beings, limited to what we have been conditioned to believe. We have some serious potential locked inside of us. Super-Human potential

There are some people who you do quantum operations on, and they are not successful. There are people who have real transplants too, that are unsuccessful. Work with zero expectation, with love and commitment and you will get awesome results the majority of the time – and remember, some people are not supposed to be on this planet any more. Your job while facilitating their healing is to assist their transition. Other times, people get too much secondary gain from their illness and so choose to hold onto it.

Mary's Lung Transplant

Mary came to our Facilitator Training Experience Online and told me that she has never been able to breathe properly. Breathing was painful. Mary had been to every specialist you could imagine. No one could help her. Mary's SP02 levels were around 86/87. There was no known cause. Mary could not run more than five metres. What must it be like to run five metres and run out of oxygen? Can you imagine how much that would hinder your life?

During the training I gave Mary a new lung, a little like Heather's gall bladder and Kara's kidneys. Her SPO2 levels are now up around 98. Mary went from five metres to running a kilometre very quickly and doing hill walks. Mary was experiencing zero pain and she could stand tall and felt incredible. Before, she was hunched over.

I found a past life experience where a man, Mary's soul fragment, was experiencing trauma. We brought this piece of Mary into healing and did the lung transplant. Within two months Mary was walking and slow-jogging ten kilometres. After fifty-seven years of pain, Mary now has her life back. We have agreed to do a marathon together as a celebratory goal. Mary is in training right now. If this isn't a mind-blowing transformation, I don't know what is. We are Super-Humans and we are creating a new way in this world by going back to what we all know deep down is possible.

Interface

We are souls inhabiting a vessel and that vessel is the human body. When consciousness wants to communicate with consciousness, in human form, in other words when a soul wants to speak to a soul, it does so by speaking and listening or touching and feeling. The human body is the interface in which consciousness communicates with consciousness.

We are walking, talking, biological computers and consciousness is the underlying force that controls this interface. There are other components, such as the electromagnetic frequencies that move through the empty space, coming down from the stars, powering our internal batteries, the heart and our mesentery, as well as the energy from the Earth, fuelling our lives. We are a mixture of chemicals and electrical currents, inside a physical vessel, the body, the interface, full of bones, blood, muscles, tissue, ligaments and organs. Flowing through all of this is consciousness. The body is literally an interface.

You can follow these suggestions and train your interface to tune in and perceive a more expanded bandwidth of information. In other words, I'm giving you the keys to higher frequency bands or bands of frequency. You are like those blue beings in the movie, Avatar. When the character Jake goes into the laboratory and is rigged up to his avatar, through electrical wires that tapped his brain's frequency patterns, he is able to be the blue being. His consciousness interacts with other blue beings on their planetary home, through an interface. Just like Jake, your body is your avatar.

As a consciously aware stream of data, vibrating in an infinite field, it's important that you fall in love with and nurture this avatar and, at the same time, keep degrees of separation as to not get lost in the game and be a chocolate-loving, junk-food-eating, vodka-drinking space cadet. You must nourish your avatar with clean food, water and exercise. You must meditate, exercise and qigong it and keep it strong and vibrant. If your avatar dies, your consciousness loses its Earthly home, which might not be a bad thing for some, but as a Super-Human, let's be here on Earth and stretch the boundaries of what's possible. Our bodies are amazing!

Your perception is the dominating factor that controls the emotional response of your interface. As an expanded Super-Human, you can control the ebb and flow of the data stream and decide what to pull from it. You can choose what you see, what opportunities you take.

The faster your frequency, the lighter and more potent your energy field. The faster you vibrate and oscillate, the more aware you are and the better access you are granted to higher frequency bands and light/data streams. If you want to heal others, you must remember to be in control of your avatar.

As a quantum being living inside a human vessel, it's important to know that your vibrational code, your frequency is always transmitted out, into the universe, through every proton; and seeing as there are trillions of protons in one single cell, that's a lot of data. So, as an aware Super-Human, be consciously aware of your vibration and be sure to send out frequencies, light, data that will elevate your fellow sisters and brothers. If we all consciously choose our reality, less and less low-vibrational information will be communicated with the field and then there will be less and less potential for certain data streams to enter your field and derail you. Do it for you and do it for others.

We must take full responsibility for every transmission, in and out of our interface. If it's carrying negative potentials, i.e., drama, then crush it instantly by changing your focus and directing your energy onto something more positive. That way, what you bring into your field and redistribute will be on a shifted/elevated frequency. A frequency of a higher vibration. If you take in low-vibrational data, stew on it and regurgitate it, it flows back out into the field for others to download. Would you intentionally let a virus harm your friend's or loved one's computer? No way. This is no different. Let's transmute every negative potential and emit loving frequencies that spark divine magic in the souls of our sisters and brothers.

When you are healing another human being (or yourself using your own hologram) you bring up an image of the person's hologram and quantum-entangle this with their physical being and also their quantum being. which are one and the same. It's just that you see them on different levels of information. The physical depth is the superficial depth which shows us the symptom, i.e., the tumour or cyst or damaged nervous system. When you view the quantum being you can see the truth, the patterns and code, that lie beyond the physical nature, the ebb and flow of data that is causing the illness, whether it be a tumour, cyst or damaged nervous system.

You have to communicate with the hologram by opening your heart, being on the frequency of love and then playing the game. Playing the game is what we show you how to do on our Star Magic Training Experiences, but I will give you a glimpse into this playful world of science and spirituality in the next chapter.

Just know that you and your body are not the same, even though the body is an extension on your metaphysical makeup. You are consciousness inhabiting a body and this body, your avatar, is fully at your disposal. You can operate it however you want – but know that it's your method of communication with every other living thing in the physical world, as well as the fuel you pour into it, that determines the state or vibration of your avatar; and know that, like any other technology, it will deplete or malfunction if it's not nurtured.

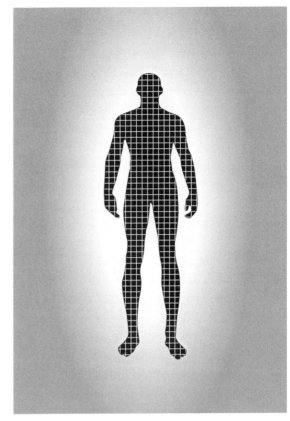

23. A human hologram

Subatomic Healing and Space Memory

Did you know that the densest atom is a diamond atom? If you enlarged a diamond atom to the size of an orange, the next diamond atom would be two football fields away? Space is rich, full, dense, extraordinary. There is enough energy in a cup of space to power the world for thousands and thousands of years. This space is the key to world issues. We can harness this energy for free. I see what is inside the space or should I say, what the space actually is. It's an incredible communication network of vortexes, spiralling and merging, sending information backwards and forwards. I use this communication network to facilitate healing.

It's common now in the spiritual world to talk about the fifth dimension. When we talk about dimension, we are referring to space. Height, width, length. When we refer to density we are talking about frequency. Within a frequency band/density, there are multiple dimensions. In our time-based matrix there are three dimensions in each frequency band. So fifteen dimensions in total. However, there are many more and this topic is huge, so for now we will leave it at this. Densities 1 through to 5 are our total playing field and there are versions of us throughout all frequency bands and dimensions. Information is exchanged, and physical realities are healed by accessing all reality fields. We are playing in all frequency bands at once, on many levels of vibration. Some of us are aware and others are not. One thing I know for sure is that when you do this work, you will start getting glimpses of other realities, densities bleeding and other fields of consciousness presenting themselves.

It's important to "innerstand" that there are multiple dimensions and multiple frequency bands/densities and that we operate out of many at the same time. The structure of the universe is completely mathematical, so I am sure someone or some being/s know/s the entire landscape.

When you operate beyond the physical vessel and in this field of magic regularly, you realize how vast it is and that trying to systemize it is extremely difficult. I am sure, however, that this vast, expansive, kaleidoscopic universe is systemized in some way.

What I do know is that it goes on and on and I have never found an end or a start or a middle. It is just an infinite, expansive, divine space with multiple layers/levels/frequencies, that leave you in a state of complete excitement and wonder. Or fear, if you are that way inclined.

From my own personal experience, one can be in this so-called 3D reality (which we have all truly moved beyond now) and at the same time, be bouncing around in multiple other quantum spaces, or densities or fields of information. We can coexist simultaneously in the same space on different frequencies. As you go deeper on your spiritual journey and discover more of who you are, there are fewer and fewer thoughts in your head and there is more and more feeling in your body. Or maybe you simply become aware of the feeling in your body and also the subtle energies moving through you and all around you. Healing is becoming faster and more efficient and methods and systems don't cut it any more. Healing modalities that follow systems are limiting. "Star Magic is a non-systematical way of knowing": and the more you play and experience it, the more you will "innerstand" this quote. We have trained many healers from different healing backgrounds (quantum healing, reiki, re-connective healing, and many others) and they all say Star Magic goes way beyond what they have previously learned. It's the next level.

The subject of energy healing can seem very mystical. When people use terminology like quantum entanglement, it can shut down others' brains. People tend to switch off at the very mention of quantum physics or technologies as they find it too complicated.

You on the other hand, reading this book, are very different. You may be completely sold on the idea of quantum entanglement and know it to be a very real thing, proven by science. Or you may be like I was (and still am), completely in awe of it. For me, seeing the emails from people who have recovered after one or two healing sessions that my team or I have facilitated still just blows my mind. I have had thousands of these emails and they never get boring. In fact, it inspires me to work harder, try different things and find faster ways of getting the result so I can assist more people. In fact, we have a method/way for healing large groups en masse and the more people there are, the higher the frequency we can achieve as a group. Life-changing events occur regularly. In this world, science and spirituality are kept separate (like most things) and that is because if they merged as one, absolutely everything would make sense, and those that control the game, don't want us figuring it all out and becoming empowered.

Entanglement

If a human being is not in your space so you can work directly on the physical body, you can bring up an energetic, holographic version of them in front of you instead. When you decide that one thing is another thing, they become entangled. Because you have decided/intended that this hologram is that human being, and by working on the hologram, you work on them.

I have used all sorts of objects and entangled them with people. I've used a banana to heal a serious case of fibromyalgia, a light bulb to heal a brain tumour where the doctors said the man would be dead in eight weeks, an iPhone to heal an irregular heartbeat, an empty toilet roll to remove three cysts from a lady's ovaries . . . the list goes on.

I simply have the object in front of me, decide that the object is the human being and go to work. Everything in the universe is connected by empty space and no-thing actually exists inside the empty space because the things that you can see, that we call physical, are 99.99999 per cent space anyway. It's all pretty much space and a little something else. A twisting, bending, ebbing multitude of vortexes, spinning and spiralling through nowhere, connecting all no-things. So, when I take an empty toilet roll (a no-thing) and connect it to a human being (a no-thing) they become entangled. Well, actually they were already entangled; all I had to do was direct the frequency, the energy, the code in that direction specifically, which, if you really look deeply, is no direction at all. Because all things in the quantum world are everywhere all at the same time. Time, distance, measurement – they are all illusory.

Subatomic Healing with Isosceles Triangles

I want to tell you a story about a lady called Lesya who came to our Facilitator Training. She arrived with severe kidney stones and her spine forming a double C-shape, which means the spine is curved not once but twice. Some people call it an S-shape spine. This creates bends in the spine and the body and can be very painful and often make it difficult to sleep or walk. She left with none of these symptoms.

Lesya had been to see numerous surgeons, chiropractors and physios. The latter two could do nothing and the surgeons wanted to remove parts of her spine and fuse it together. Lesya had felt this would be the start of the end and said no.

Something to point out before we really get into this is that spines bend when there is pressure in someone's life. A double-C-shaped spine is some serious build-up of pressure; pretty much guaranteed, it spans more than one reality/lifetime, density or dimensional space, often several.

I got another participant to do the work for Lesya under my guidance. People think *I* can do it but *they* can't, so it's good for them to witness another human creating a so-called miracle. So, I asked the volunteer to drop into their heart and connect with Lesya's spine.

I asked her to ask the universe to see her vertebrae as isosceles triangles.

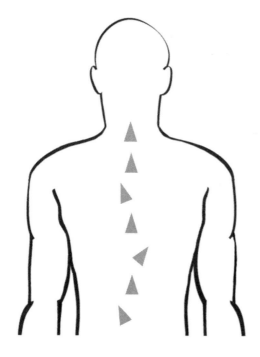

24. Experiencing the spine as Isosceles triangles

When you see the vertebrae as isosceles triangles you can see there is one angle at the top of each triangle that is different from the other two and one side that is shorter from the other two. You may see the spine as in the example above.

You may also see it like this:

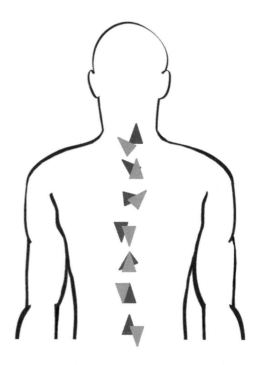

25. Observing two different realities

This means you are observing two different realities, one illustrated by the lighter triangles and one by the darker ones.

You may also see it like this:

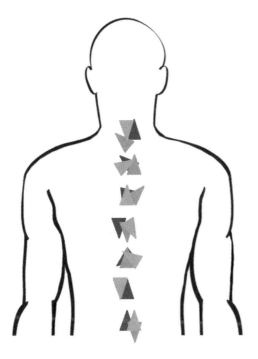

26. Observing three different realities

This means you are observing three different realities, illustrated by the three different colours. Remember these are just examples (for better distinction of the triangles also see the colour insert after page 160).

In Lesya's case she had four sets of triangles, as in the illustration below.

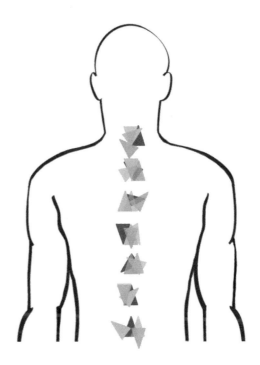

27. Observing four different realties

This means you are observing four different realities. One reality is blue, one is orange, one is pink and one is green, and this is exactly how it showed for Lesya (see the triangles also in colour insert after page 160).

Once you see the triangles, the aim is to turn all of them so they are pointing the same way. The correct way may be pointing down, or pointing up; you won't know until you start playing, but after a while you will get a strong sense of which way is correct. If you start turning the triangles/ vertebrae the wrong way, the human being you are working on might bend and contort even more out of shape. I remember this 6 foot 4 guy whose left shoulder was touching his ear, his right hip dropped, and his spine twisted when his partner in one of our trainings started working on him. We all laughed for a minute (he saw the funny side too!) before putting him back the way he should go.

Sometimes you can have triangles that are bent, or face forward with their base to you. It can be like the child's game where you have to put the square block in the square hole, the circle in the circle hole and so on. As the child is learning, they may try to put the triangle in the square hole and so on. This is just the same; you keep playing until you get it right.

The lady who was working on Lesya followed my instructions and was drawing on the whiteboard exactly what she saw. It took around fifteen minutes and then Lesya's back was straight. I don't think she could believe it, even though she felt the movement and the hot and cold sensations and energy shooting up and down her body. A little while later she went to the toilet with one of our team, who took a photo and showed her. She came back in, beaming, overjoyed. Still a little shocked but very happy. Many years of pain and discomfort had gone.

So, how did we go about correcting Lesya's spine? There are four colours and one spinal column. This means that there are four realities playing out, as there were in Lesya's case. You cannot move the triangles around until you have found them in all the colours/realities. By found I mean, if I saw a spinal column as triangles and there were seven triangles in four different colours, I would have to find seven of each colour before I went to work.

In other words, if we're looking at this illustration, all of the different colours must be in alignment as separate streams of consciousness/realities and must be dealt with separately or you will make a mess of the human being you are facilitating the healing of. They can bend more out of shape.

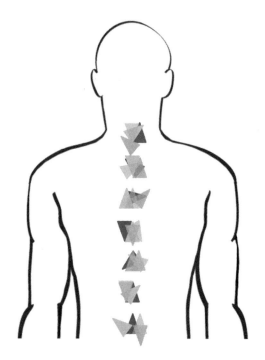

28. Observing four realities as one spinal column. The rest must be found before you can start

29. All four sets/colours/realities of triangles have been found. Now they must be separated

You need to find all the differently coloured triangles and separate them like this.

Once they are separate, you can go to work and straighten them all up so they are facing in the right direction.

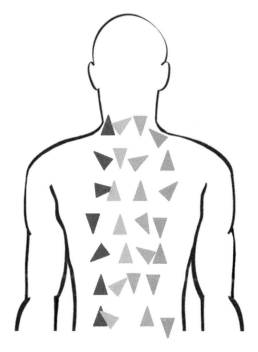

30. All four realities separated for clarity.
Now you can work

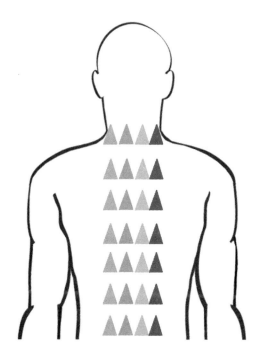

31. All four realities corrected

Let's say, for argument's sake, that they all have to be pointed up, just like in the illustration above.

You then have to bring them all into alignment and superimpose them over each other, just like in the next illustration.

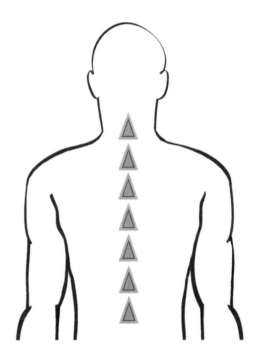

32. All four realities super-imposed over each other

Now you have four realities, all in the same space, brought into healing. What I do next is get an electromagnetic pole and stick it down through the top of the triangles to stop them turning back out. It doesn't always happen but sometimes it does, and if it does the spine can come out of alignment, so I put the poles/rods in to stabilize it. The healing is complete. This is a huge release for the human being having it done.

As I've said, it is mission critical that you separate the triangles and the colours. Anyone can do this. It's just like playing a game. Now, you may say to me, "But Jerry, I don't see yet. My third eyesight isn't functioning very well." So, let's move on to the next story.

Your Favourite Cocktail

I want to share a similar story that was executed in a different way.

I was in India and showing people the isosceles triangle technique/way. A lady came over to me, really annoyed. "Jerry, I can't see anything. This doesn't work for me. It's useless," were the first words that came out of her mouth. I asked her to take a few deep breaths and show me who she was working on.

It was a lady named Pia, who had a bad right knee and back. Her physical pain had taken her to New York, London, Los Angeles, all over India, searching for top doctors to help her. But none of them even knew what the problem was, let alone how to deal with it.

Something I have come to realize is that trauma can be held in our body from many other quantum spaces. It comes down to memory. As our soul has many human experiences, these experiences leave a memory in the field, in space, something I would call Space Memory of the reality still playing out in the field. This is a memory but also very real, as a Soul aspect can be still having that other traumatic experience. To shift a dis-ease, injury, illness you must remove the memory from space, i.e., the Space Memory. Sometimes you can do this at the front end and sometimes at the back end and there are times when it needs to be done at both ends. I would consider the front end to be the physical (so-called) problem which is the symptom and in Pia's case, her knee and back, and the back end is the memory, the experience, the life that the soul lived, in another quantum space. The back end would be the past/future/parallel life experience, the trigger.

We went over and Pia was stood there with her back to us. The lady was getting a little more stressed at the thought of not being able to do this. I asked the lady doing the healing to breathe and tell me what her favourite drink was. She said she didn't drink any alcohol but she liked this particular non-alcoholic cocktail. "But what has that got to do with anything?" she asked, sounding stressed. I asked her to close her eyes and bring her awareness to Pia's knees and to see/imagine a glass of her favourite mocktail in each knee. Then I asked her to describe them. She said the one in the left knee was full and the one in the right knee was half full. I asked her to fill the glass in the right knee up, until it was full. She did so.

Next, I asked her to see glasses of mocktails all the way up the centre of Pia's body where the spinal column is. She did that and told me that there were two empty glasses and one glass that was upside down. The upside-down glass was where the pain was, but at this stage the lady working on Pia didn't know this; nor did she know Pia had a bad right knee. She turned the upside-down glass the right way up and then filled it up along with the other two glasses that were empty.

Literally within seconds Pia turned around with a huge grin on her face. She was moving her body, trying to feel the pain, but couldn't. It was at this point she told us that the issues had been with her back and knee.

I remember the first time we visited Asia for a training and went to Taiwan. A guy had very wonky hips. The man I was guiding to correct them couldn't see much either, just like the lady in India. As soon as I asked him what his favourite beer was, he was able to see very well indeed. He loved Budweiser. He saw the guy's hips who we were working on as two bottles of Bud. One was straight and one was off to the side and facing forward at a 45-degree angle. I asked him to straighten them up. Once he did, the guy whose hips we were working on straightened up. His hips realigned and so did his entire body.

These are some very simple examples of how to create healing that show we live in a world that is connected. A world, galaxy, universe connected by space. Everything is entangled, and we can enhance the entanglement of any situation to change or shift our own or another human being's reality. The space is not empty. It's full of information and we can plug into or unplug from certain data streams, held within the memory of the empty space. When we know how to control or tap the flow of data, we can induce rapid states of healing. We can choose how we interface with another human being's hologram and play like a little child to make changes in the quantum field, to have a massive impact on our physical lives.

I'm a kid from the streets, who spent a lot of his life hustling for a living. No one ever taught me this stuff. I haven't been on one single healing course/workshop or training in my life. If I can do it, so can you. I wanted to share a couple of stories regarding healing with you. Next, we are going to really start activating your body, and after that we are going to come back to healing. The reason being, once your body, brain, third eye and heart are switched on Super-Human style, the healing becomes second nature.

Chapter 7: Going Quantum

The Quantum World and Healing

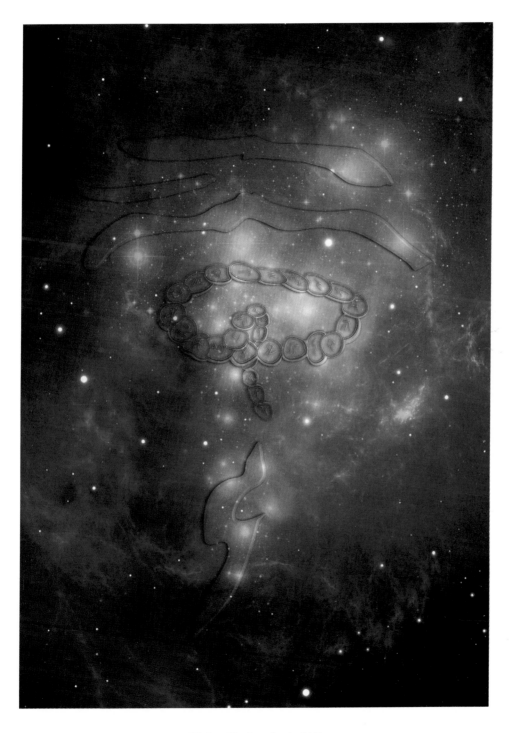

22. Star Magic codes (p. 140)

Subatomic Healing and Space Memory (pp. 154–58)

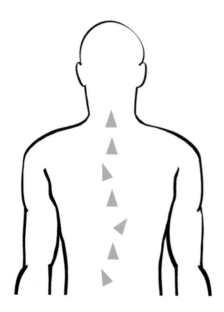

24. Experiencing the spine as Isosceles triangles

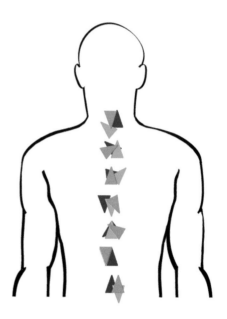

26. Observing three different realities

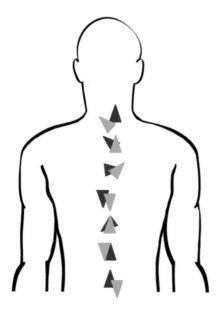

25. Observing two different realities

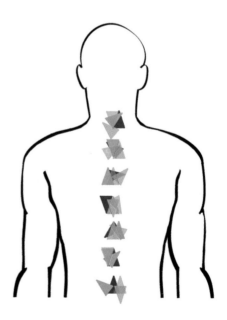

27. Observing four different realties

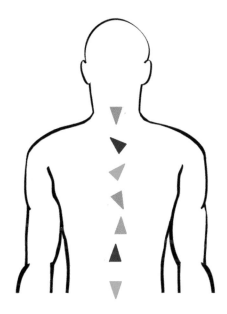

28. Observing four realities as one spinal column.
The rest must be found before you can start

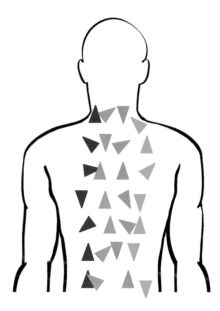

30. All four realities separated for clarity.
Now you can work

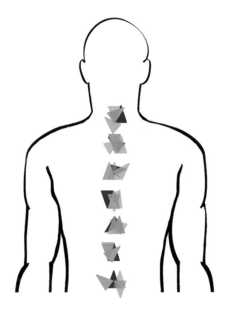

29. All four sets/colours/realities of triangles have
been found. Now they must be separated

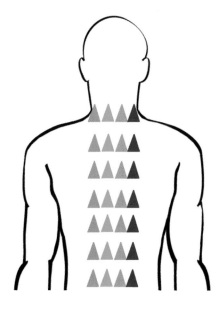

31. All four realities corrected

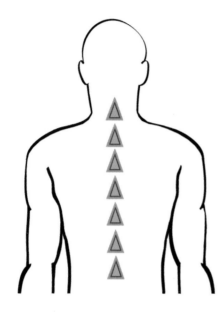

32. All four realities super-imposed over each other

Chapter 8: Switching On

Creating a Unified Heart Field (pp. 169–70)

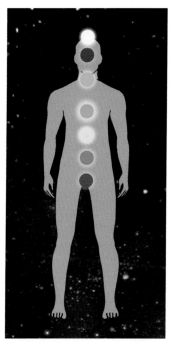

44. Showing the basic 7–chakra system

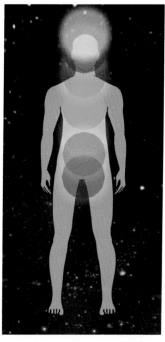

46. Chakras growing larger and dissolving

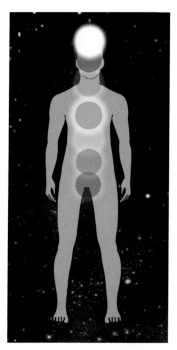

45. Chakras start to grow and merge

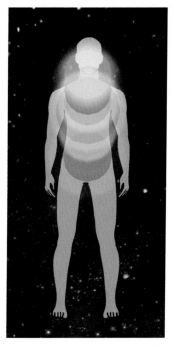

47. Chakras continue to merge and the
heart starts to dominate

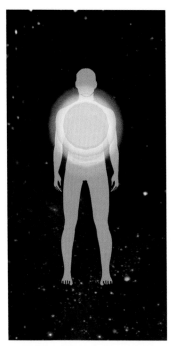

48. Chakras are dissolving into the heart

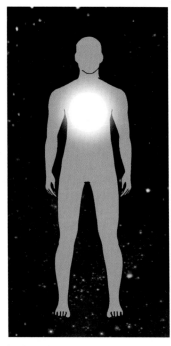

50. The heart becomes a bright diamond light

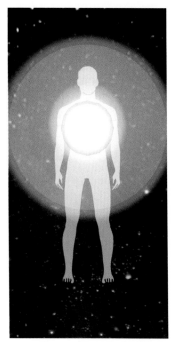

49. The heart grows larger, taking
over the entire field

Third Eye Merkaba Matrix – Pineal Gland Activation (pp. 196–99)

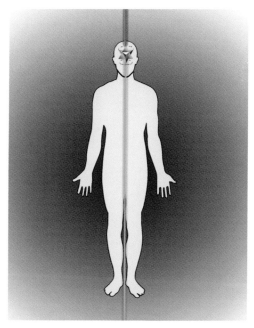

65. Merkaba around the pineal gland and the frequencies of Sirius and Earth flowing into it

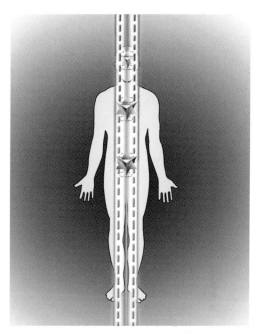

67. Introduction of third merkaba and the continuation of light/energy flowing

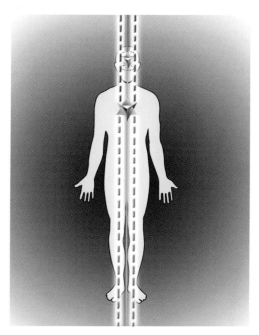

66. Introduction of second merkaba and the flow of pink, green, and platinum light from Sirius and Earth

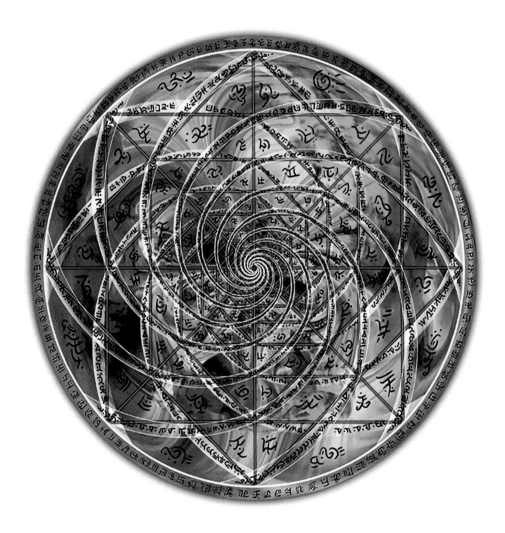

105. Krystal Spiral and the New Earth Mathematics Code (p. 280)

PART 2

Switching to Higher Frequency

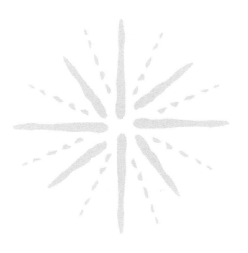

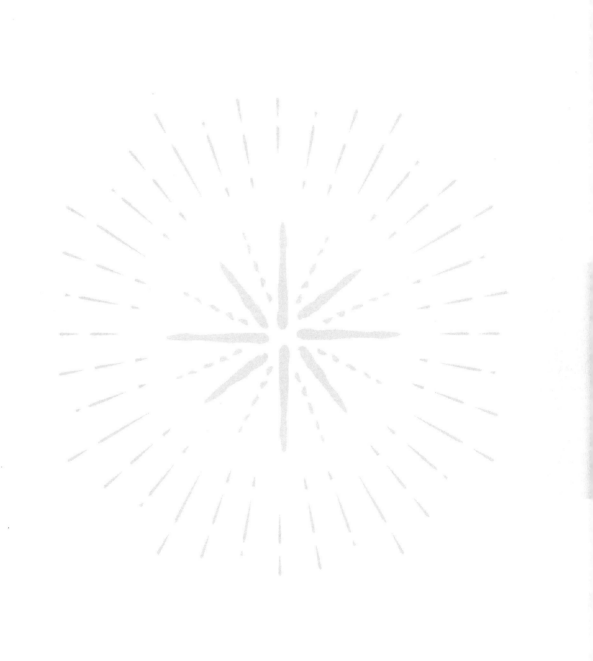

8

Switching ON

The Torus Field

Around every living being there are a number of different mathematical/geometrical structures or fields of energy/light. One of those fields of energy is the torus field. We have a torus field within our heart, around our physical body, and also the planet has her own torus field. It looks a little bit like a doughnut in shape.

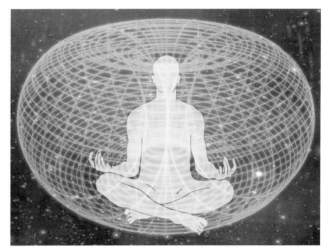

34. Meditating inside your torus field

This illustration above shows a human being in a meditative position, inside the torus field.

To truly get the torus field functioning, our hearts must be clear and open. This is important for many reasons. An activated, open heart can then synchronize with the brain and bring the body and mind into total coherence. When this coherent state occurs, magic happens. The body starts to do what it is supposed to do: and that is heal. In this state you can also heal others. It's also in this coherent state that you truly activate the pineal gland, which we will be doing in the next chapter, so it's important to cleanse your system now, ready for the next step.

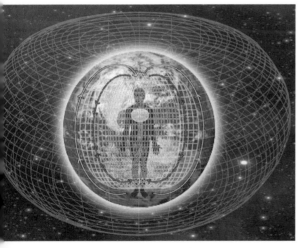

33. Showing the three torus fields.
Remember, it doesn't show the torus created by the activation chambers

The illustration shows the toroidal field in the heart, the toroidal field around the whole human being and the planet's toroidal field. It's not in proportion, as you can see. Or maybe it is, if you know how to expand your energy out through the field/space.

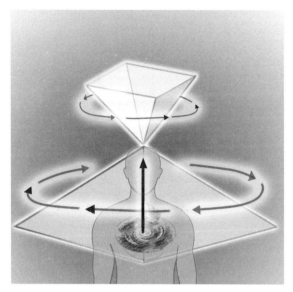

35. Heart space clogged with emotion/toxicity

In illustration 35, you see a heart space that is clogged with stuck emotion. It can look like tar, black energy, rocks, or there are many other ways you can see or feel the blockage. Often people have iron grates over the heart where they have closed it down to avoid being hurt.

EXERCISE Clearing the Heart and Lower Energy Centres

You can do this exercise on yourself or another human being. If you are doing it on yourself then I would bring up a hologram of yourself first, entangle that hologram with your physical body and then go to work. If it's someone else, bring up the hologram in your space and say, "This is the hologram of Jerry Sargeant" or whoever you are working on. If it's you, say your name. Say it three times. That will entangle the two quantum spaces. Remember, once you've finished working, dissolve the hologram. Don't leave it hanging around. Dissolve it into light. Intentionally scrub it out of the space.

You will see a pyramid, over and around your body, the apex over your crown and the base below your heart space. You will see an inverted pyramid above your crown with the apex just

above. The larger pyramid will spin clockwise (pushing/driving stuck energy up and out) and the inverted pyramid will spin anti-clockwise (drawing the stuck energy up and into it to be transmuted). You don't have to use your own hologram. You can of course, just visualize and create this structure around your own physical body. Personally, I use a hologram. I like to treat myself like a third party. I find it makes it easier.

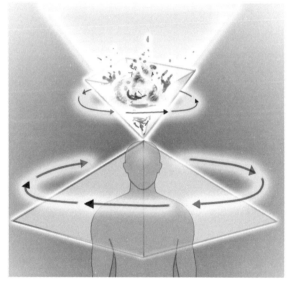

36. Two pyramids spinning and clearing out the heart and then toxicity from lower energy centres

You will spin the two pyramids as in illustration 36 until the heart is completely clear. Once the heart is clear, you will sit there in your space, with your hologram or with your partner, and clear the lower energy centres. You will squeeze your perineum, your genitals and buttocks, pull your abdominal muscles back to your spine and consciously pull energy from your bottom three energy centres, up through your body and into your heart. You will hold the squeeze for ten to fifteen seconds as you pull and visualize the stuck energy rising up, from the space between your perineum and just below your heart, into your heart, and then let go of the squeeze. You can repeat this several times. Any toxicity that is blocking and hindering your flow will be drawn into the heart space, collected by the spinning pyramid and sent up into the inverted pyramid to be transmuted and sent back into the cosmic fabric as clean, positive energy. If you are working on another human being, you can squeeze for them within your own body, and see the energy movement with your mind. Remember, imagination is reality. They can also squeeze themselves.

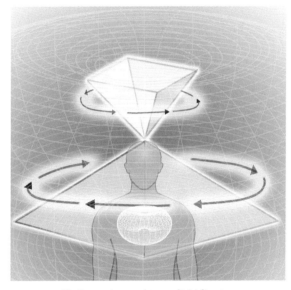

37. Heart clear and torus field flowing

Once you have cleared the heart, you will become aware of a torus field flowing inside of the heart centre, as shown above. As you squeeze and clear the lower energy centres the old toxic emotion/energy from them will flow into the heart. Once they are clear, the heart will stay clear.

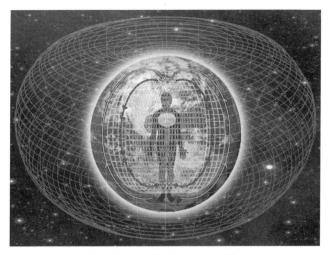

38. Heart's torus field connects with the planet's torus field

The torus field in your heart connects with the planet's torus field, as in the illustration above. Once we activate the pineal gland another torus field will come into operation, flowing out from your crown, running around to your perineum, creating a two-way flow of information, as in the illustration below.

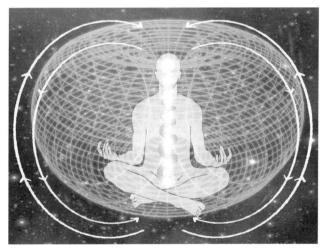

39. Two-way flow of data/light/information

I recommend that you do this exercise regularly until your heart is completely expanded and you feel like you are in bliss always. You should wake up and go to bed with joy and bliss as your natural default state. If you feel your vibration has shifted, check your heart and revisit this exercise. If you find there are iron grids or coverings over your heart, take them off. Sometimes you may have to unscrew them.

You want your energy centres (even though we will be removing them soon) from base to heart completely clear. It is also important to mention your throat: through this process the bottom pyramid will also naturally clear and cleanse the energy centre in your throat. You are creating a clear channel for energy to flow up through your body and into your brain.

Dissolving Your Chakras and Creating One Unified Heart Field

Now, the last exercise will have enabled you to clear a lot of toxicity from your energy centres and that will make the next part of the process much simpler. I am going to refer to our lower energy centres as "chakras" for this explanation, as that's how they are commonly known. In fact, they have been created quantumly for thousands of years and we have played an active role in creating them and in how they're thought of.

People say, for example, that one chakra relates to a certain type of trauma. But remember, reality can be created in any way we like. I just always come back to this question: Why would we create a system to trap energy? Is it not supposed to flow naturally? The truth is our lower energy centres are a control mechanism. They are part of the indoctrination, like religion, like the information taught at school and our false history. Chakras are only real because we have been indoctrinated to believe they are a part of our system.

We higher-vibrational beings have a heart. A great big cosmic heart. That is all you require to be a multidimensional being. Your so-called chakras hold trauma and keep you stuck.

EXERCISE *Opening and Clearing the Chakras*

For most people, the lower energy centres are like ice cream cones: large at one end and smaller at the other. We can imagine the two small points meeting in the middle of the body, with the larger end of the ice cream cone on the outside.

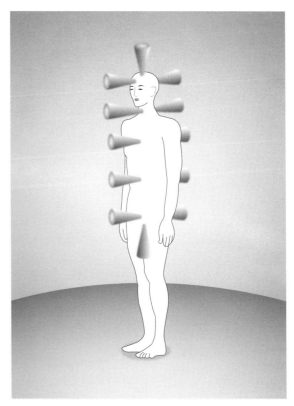

40. The common form of chakras in the body

Now when your chakras are like this, much emotion is carried/stuck in the smaller end. Stuff gets blocked. What Star Magic enables you to do is open those chakras fully so that they become free-flowing cylinders, straight through the body. This releases you from the game of duality. Step one is to open each chakra to its full capacity and step two is to clean the inside of each chakra. Following on from there we can merge these chakras into one unified heart field.

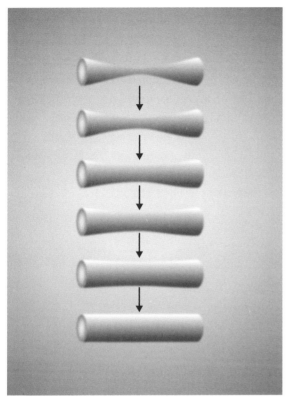

41. Chakra transitioning into cylinder
through clearing

Step 1

To open the chakras you will need mental strength, as you may come up against resistance. Opening the chakras can also bring up deep-seated emotions that have been clogged inside the energy centres for a long time. To open these chakras, you simply visualize the smaller end of the cone becoming larger, until it's the same width as the wide end. Do that on both sides of the body until you have created a cylinder. You are going to need your third eye for this or to feel the process taking place.

Creating the cylinder cannot be forced; however, a little gentle persuasion is sometimes necessary. Remember, we are Super-Humans and Super-Humans are quantum architects. We can create and recreate reality exactly as we wish to. If scholars and sages can condition us to create a system that keeps emotional trauma stuck in

our body and energy field, then we can un-create that system and recreate a unified heart field where love is the driving force and there is no requirement for low-vibrational energy/emotion to be stuck in our field as a hindrance.

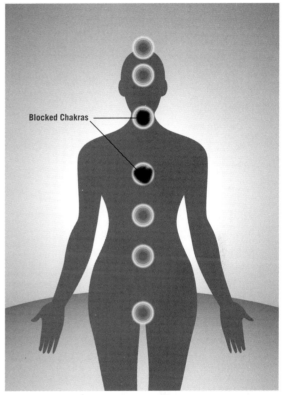

Blocked Chakras

42. Blocked chakras

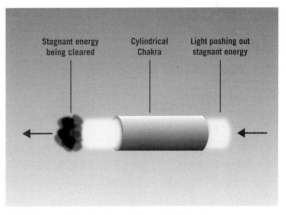

Stagnant energy being cleared Cylindrical Chakra Light pushing out stagnant energy

43. Clearing the chakra with light/energy

Step 2

Once the cylinder has been created and there is a channel from one side of the body to the other, any stuck energy can be moved in a much easier fashion. You will sometimes notice energy inside; this is stuck energy that doesn't need to be there, old toxic residue that has been there for many years.

Three ways to move this energy on are as follows.

1. Shine light through from one end to the other and watch it filter through. It's not always as easy as this because the old stuff doesn't want to shift.

2. Imagine the cylinder is like a straw. A large one at that; but you could shrink it in your mind if it helps. Put your mouth around the end of the cylinder and blow extremely hard and see this stuck energy moving on until the pathway is clear for you, and the clean energy can flow freely.

3. Sometimes I see big chunks of energy, like in illustration 43 on the previous page. They may look like clumps of coal or rock. They are very heavy and don't want to budge. If this is the case, I will take an imaginary rod of light and push it through the chakra. Sometimes it takes a lot of mental strength, but I will not stop until I have pushed that rod of light all the way through and have seen the clump fly out the other side. Remember to see that stuck, blocked-up energy turn to white light upon its release. The size of the rod that you will use is just small enough to fit inside the chakra, so no stuck energy escapes when it's being pushed out.

EXERCISE *Creating a Unified Heart Field*

Once the chakras are open, then you must make them bigger. You must grow and expand them with your intention and imagination until they all merge into one unified heart field. As the heart opens and becomes stronger, it will create a huge field of love all around you. It will merge with your toroidal field, your platinum light body (we will discuss this in detail later) and those old structures we call chakras will become obsolete.

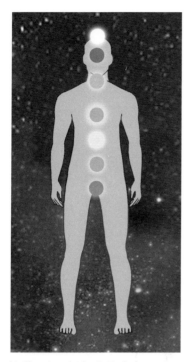

44. Showing the basic 7–chakra system

As you expand them they start to merge.

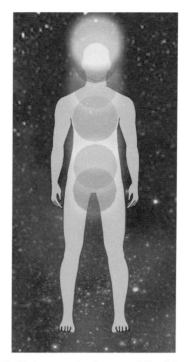

46. Chakras growing larger and dissolving

They continue to grow and start to dissolve.

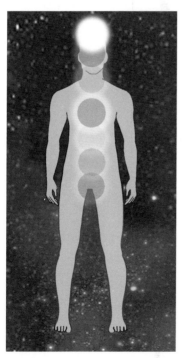

45. Chakras start to grow and merge

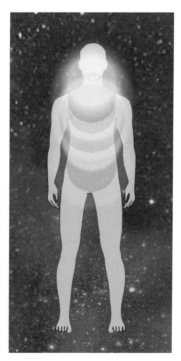

47. Chakras continue to merge and the
heart starts to dominate

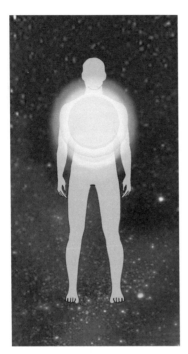

48. Chakras are dissolving into the heart

You see the field of the heart growing larger than the rest.

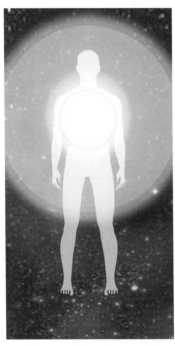

49. The heart grows larger, taking over the entire field

You continue to expand them, they dissolve, the colour fades and the light gets brighter.

Eventually the heart takes over the entire field and your true nature, love, rules your world.

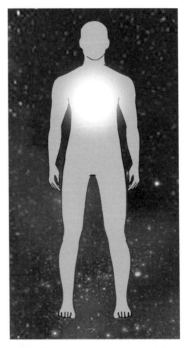

50. The heart becomes a bright diamond light

Your heart becomes a bright diamond light that you can expand and contract at will.

You are a walking, talking beacon of love. Stop buying into these chakras/energy centres that lock you in a space. You are quantum. You are magical. You are divine. You don't need anything in your field that keeps energy from flowing. It's old-school, old-hat, primordial low-level energy work. We are on the Super-Sonic Shuttle, baby!

Star Systems

Now I want to talk to you about transmission centres and star systems. Some people call them multidimensional chakras, but let's just forget about this word chakra altogether. It's time to move on from it.

When we are moving from a 3D/4D reality or consciousness to a higher frequency reality or level of consciousness, we activate a different system within our light body. Before we talk about this system, I want to introduce you to the stars and how they can heal your body, as this will set us up to move into the area of transmission centres and how they control the flow of light/data through your body.

Something that we share on our trainings is how to heal the body using star systems. There are really thirteen zodiac signs in our charts, not twelve. There are supposed to be thirteen months (each of twenty-eight days) in our calendar year to represent this; however, with our modern system one month (one zodiac sign/star constellation) is missing. This is Ophiuchus, the Snake Bearer.

All of the zodiac constellations link to different body parts; Ophiuchus is linked to the nervous system. Interesting how the zodiac sign that links to the most important element of our human anatomy is missing.

The illustration 51 shows the thirteen zodiac signs and the body parts they are linked to. For example, if you wanted to heal a left arm you would communicate with the constellation of Gemini, the twins, and intend that star frequency into the field of your client's hologram. When you set up the link and entangle the two spaces, the human being you are working on will heal.

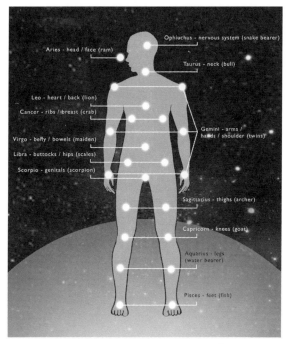

51. 13 Zodiac signs and the body parts they link to

Here is the full list of the body parts each star constellation links to:

- OPHIUCHUS
  The entire nervous system.

- ARIES
  Head and face. Rules the skull, the brain, the upper teeth and everything in the head except the lower jaw.

- TAURUS
  Neck and throat. Rules the lower jaw and the throat region, including the larynx (voice box), the tonsils, upper cervical vertebrae, tongue, mouth and thyroid gland.

- GEMINI
  Rules the respiratory tree (lungs, thoracic cavity and diaphragm), the trachea (windpipe), the arms from fingers to

171

shoulder blades and the upper thoracic vertebrae.

- CANCER
Rules the upper abdomen/chest and upper portions of the liver. Also rules all of the body's containers – breasts, stomach, womb, peritoneum (the membrane encompassing the abdominal cavity), the pleural sac surrounding the thoracic cavity, the pericardium surrounding the heart, and the meninges (the sac surrounding the brain and spinal canal).

- LEO
Rules the heart and spinal vertebrae directly behind the heart.

- VIRGO
Rules the lower abdominal cavity, which includes the lower liver, pancreas, gall bladder and small intestine.

- LIBRA
Rules the "belt" area (along with Sagittarius) and buttocks at the level of the navel, which includes the kidneys, the adrenal glands and the lumbar and sacral vertebrae.

- SCORPIO
Rules the organs of reproduction, the large intestine, the rectum and in men the prostate gland.

- SAGITTARIUS
Rules the hips and upper legs down to the knees, as well as the very important sciatic nerve.

- CAPRICORN
Rules the knees as well as the skeleton and the skin.

- AQUARIUS
Rules the lower legs and ankles.

- PISCES
Rules the lymphatic system (including the white blood cells used in defence) and the feet.

There is another system that is a part of our light body and must come online, fully functioning, if we are to raise our vibration into a 5D state of being. It's a part of the structure that controls the flow of light once it moves through the alpha transmission centre and out through the omega and down into the Earth's grids. It happens naturally for some people and for others it is a struggle. Some don't even know about it and others are aware to a certain extent but don't fully "innerstand" the importance of what, essentially, is a massive part of the reason they are here on Earth.

We have looked at the platinum light body, and the fact that we are planetary guardians, here on Earth to bring high-vibrational light streams/codes/information and act as a conduit to send/ground those codes down into the Earth. Transmission centres control the ebb and flow of light and information. They are actually a two-way channel, allowing electromagnetic frequencies/ information to flow from the stars down through our bodies (upgrading us on the way) and into the ground, and magnetic frequencies to flow from the Earth up through our bodies to the crown and back up to the stars, to energize us and maintain this total cosmic connection to our celestial sisters and brothers. Remember, information comes from above (the stars) and energy comes from the ground (the Earth).

EXERCISE Activate the 13 Transmission Centres

To switch on these transmission centres (which run throughout our body), we must enter a meditative experience and connect body parts to stars and constellations. Unlike the body and star connection for healing (where one body part links to one constellation), when we are using star frequencies to bring our thirteen transmission centres online for 5D activation, we sometimes connect one body part to one constellation and sometimes one body to two or three stars and constellations combined or simply two constellations.

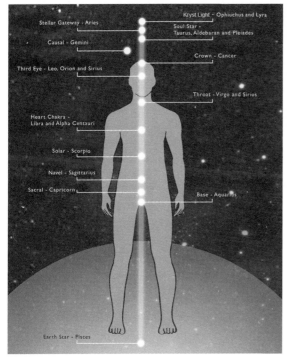

Stellar Gateway - Aries

Kryst Light - Ophiuchus and Lyra

Soul Star - Taurus, Aldebaran and Pleiades

Causal - Gemini

Crown - Cancer

Third Eye - Leo, Orion and Sirius

Throat - Virgo and Sirius

Heart Chakra - Libra and Alpha Centauri

Solar - Scorpio

Navel - Sagittarius

Sacral - Capricorn

Base - Aquarius

Earth Star - Pisces

52. Transmission centres and the stars and constellations they link to

In the illustration above you can see the thirteen transmission centres and the star and constellations they link to. Again, open your heart and connect, communicate and set your intention. The stars are intelligent, and you are stardust, so kick back and let the codes within the streams of light go to work. I recommend connecting every day for five minutes for a thirty-day period – but it can happen much much faster, and we are all unique, so feel it. With the rest of the work you are doing, they may switch on very fast indeed. All you need to do is sit with the information in front of you and one by one go through them, set up the connection and then close your eyes and feel and observe the experience. You can use your hologram to set up the link, or your physical body. It's up to you. Personally, I always like to use a hologram when working on myself. Even though the transmission centres are in the same places as you would see what people call chakras, do not get confused: your chakras are obsolete, or soon will be, and these transmission centres are there instead to assist your growth, safely and efficiently. In actuality, there are many more transmission centres than this in our light body's architecture; you have them in and among the ones depicted, and they also flow through other energy channels within your light body's architecture, and they will all automatically start to switch on fully as you move through this process. This is a natural part of our esoteric structure.

After your thirty-day period (or maybe much sooner), your light body will start to reach out and communicate with the stars of its own accord and your whole energy will shift. You will feel it before the thirty days but continue anyway. I want to share with you a code. It's a cheat really, so please honour this work and do the process manually for the first seven days, but then you can use the code for the remaining twenty-three days.

The code is an orange octahedron with **CZ13K7** vibrating in the centre. Visualize this and then place it inside your heart, close your eyes, be, and enjoy the experience. The octahedron will spin clockwise and start distributing geometries into your cells and the bio-photons within your light body. This will signal a communication link between your light body and the stars and constellations. After the thirty days you can forget about this. Your light body will be upgraded, reprogrammed and your transmission centres will come fully online.

If you want to be a perfect conduit and fulfil this part of your human mission as a planetary guardian, do this work. It will shift you into a new and expanded vibrational space that has no ceiling. Enjoy, beautiful soul.

Powerhouse 6

Before we hit the pineal gland for activation, I want to give you some more tools for your ascension toolbox. The first of them is called Powerhouse 6. We have an incredible body and there are certain components that, when switched on, truly work magic in your body, as though a wizard has waved his wand.

We must turn our attention to the following components; they are mission critical in the body's ability to recalibrate, heal, elevate, move into higher states of consciousness and access more information from the quantum field. The pineal gland, pituitary gland, hypothalamus, medulla oblongata, spleen and the substantia nigra are areas of the body that we must turn our attention too. Remember, wherever your focus goes, your energy follows.

Pineal Gland

Firstly, the pineal gland. Later I am going to dedicate an entire chapter to this incredible little pine cone, located in the centre of your brain and back slightly, as it is so vitally important and there is so much to it. For now, let's just say that it is a receiver and transducer of information. There is so much information available in the empty space, within the fabric of the cosmos, beyond matter and beyond the speed of light. When the pineal gland is activated (through certain techniques I will share with you), it picks up these frequencies, which contain codes. They are information streams that don't make much sense to the logical, left, male brain. They do make sense to the right brain, however. What the pineal gland does is take this information and transduce it for us. It's a form of translation, literally. It will present to us the information it picks up in the form of spiralized geometry, fractal patterns,

images, knowings or thoughts or feelings. When you feel this information, it translates into real communication. "Innerstanding" the communication is a skill in itself and that requires practice. This we have touched upon but will cover further later on.

Pituitary Gland

The pituitary gland is another powerhouse piece of this extraordinary puzzle. When the pineal gland is activated, it stimulates the pituitary gland and two very important chemicals are released: oxytocin and vasopressin. Oxytocin is known as the trust hormone. Studies have shown that you cannot be mad at someone or hold a grudge against them when this chemical is released in the body. It produces elevated emotions, the heart opens, and deep love is felt, along with states of bliss and joy. As oxytocin levels rise, nitric oxide levels increase also and the arteries open, causing a higher blood flow to the heart, in turn opening it and amplifying the love frequency.

When vasopressin levels go up the body naturally retains more fluids, causing the body to become more water-based. This is vitally important because as you bring more frequency into your body, a greater spectrum of information, you need more water to carry this frequency around the body so the information can communicate with the cells and deliver the messages. These messages embedded within the vibrational coding are what is unlocking the knowledge and wisdom inside our DNA. With more water in the body the information will naturally reach its destination easier as it's a beautiful conductor. Elevated vasopressin levels create a more stable thyroid gland, which affects the thymus (critical to the immune system) and the heart, which affects the adrenal glands, which in turn affects the pancreas, which produces a knock-on effect of a positive nature all the way down to our sexual organs.

The pituitary gland looks like a pear and sits behind the bridge of the upper nose, right in the middle of the brain. The front part of the pear is responsible for making the majority of the chemicals that influence the glands and hormones in our body, and it's the back part of the pear that produces oxytocin and vasopressin.

Hypothalamus

Next up we have the hypothalamus, which is responsible for the regulation of certain metabolic processes and other activities of the autonomic nervous system. The autonomic nervous system is itself a piece of the powerhouse puzzle, as when we enter that space of no-thing, the emptiness in deep meditation, beyond the physical form, and we switch off the mind from repetitive thoughts and switch on in a turbo-charged fashion with high-frequency, multicoloured data streams (a bit like a fluid cosmic firework display of kaleidoscopic proportions), the autonomic nervous system goes into full flight and starts recalibrating the body. Most of the pieces of the Powerhouse 6 Puzzle link into the autonomic nervous system, so it's important that we focus on them and distribute our energy there. The hypothalamus controls body temperature, hunger, important aspects of parenting and attachment behaviours, thirst, fatigue, sleep and circadian rhythms.

The hypothalamus also contains several types of neurons responsible for secreting different hormones.

- Thyrotropin-releasing hormone (TRH)
- Gonadotropin-releasing hormone (GnRH)
- Growth hormone-releasing hormone (GHRH)
- Corticotropin-releasing hormone (CRH)
- Somatostatin
- Dopamine

The hypothalamus is a deep region of the brain and while it's also responsible for basic impulses like hunger and thirst, it even triggers lust. Lust can be misread but when you drill down into it, it's an element that triggers/fuels love. Or maybe love triggers/fuels lust. Who really knows? What we do know is how important the heart and the energy it produces is to everything we are aiming to achieve as a Super-Human. The hypothalamus, when stimulated through frequency, also enables us to connect into the future and past, accessing timelines with mission-critical information from our soul's experiences. With this information we can retrieve knowledge and also create healing.

Medulla Oblongata

The medulla oblongata (or medulla) is a long stem-like structure located in the brainstem, where the spinal cord meets the foramen magnum of the skull. It is a cone-shaped neuronal mass responsible for autonomic functions ranging from vomiting to sneezing. The medulla oblongata helps heart and blood vessel function, digestion, sneezing and swallowing. This part of the brain is a centre for respiration and circulation. Sensory and motor neurons (nerve cells) from the forebrain and midbrain travel through the medulla, a powerful passageway. The medulla oblongata monitors the body's respiratory system using chemoreceptors. These receptors are able to detect changes in blood chemistry. For example, if the blood is too acidic, the medulla oblongata will increase the respiratory rate, allowing for more oxygen to reach the blood. It will also regulate blood pressure, pulse and cardiac contractions based on the body's needs.

This area at the base of the brain (top of the spinal cord) is the principal point of entry of life force/chi into the body. Cosmic energy is received and flows down through the body. The energy is stored in a reservoir in the top of the brain, and in the mesentery, a "battery" also known as the second brain and a focal point when doing your qigong routines. This energy also flows down into the area of your perineum and triggers a reaction within your eight genesis cells. These cells come into existence forty-nine (13 Divine Goddess Energy) days after conception and are the only cells in the human body that never change. There is a flow of information/energy from this area, back up through your body and into your brain. In essence, the medulla is the main switch that controls the entrance, storage and distribution of life force, qi or prana.

The medulla also secretes a liquid, like honey, that communicates with the Divine Father (the pineal gland) and the Divine Mother (the pituitary gland). The Divine Father and Divine Mother then communicate with the Divine Child, the hypothalamus, creating the Trinity, and the liquid flows down though the claustrum, down the spinal column, and into the perineum. This activates the kundalini, and the energy rises, travelling back up towards the pineal gland, through the ventricles and into the third house of Solomon, the right brain. The claustrum is Santa Claus coming down the chimney and the resurrection of Jesus Christ (Kryst) is the activation of your pineal gland and right brain. We will talk more about this later.

Spleen and the Spleen Vortex

We are more focused on the vortex of the spleen than the spleen itself. The centre of the bottom rib on your left is where your spleen vortex is located. The location of this vortex thus corresponds to the actual location of the spleen.

Unlike the actual spleen in the human body, which is not believed to be of crucial importance, the spleen vortex serves greatly. The vital functions are not merely physiological, but spiritual and psychological as well.

The spleen vortex is a focal point for life force or chi once it enters the body and is the source of power needed for success and victory. Interesting to note is that in the Lord's Prayer, the phrase "Give us this day our daily bread" refers to the spleen vortex, the bread being symbolic of the energy needed for sustenance and growth.

This vortex may manifest as depression due to low energy levels. When healthy and energized it leads to a feeling of strength and general well-being. Several years ago, pre-Star Magic, I was discovering healing and a healer told me my spleen needed cleaning. He blew through my skin over my right collarbone, down towards the middle of my body, and the strangest thing happened: I felt his breath move around what felt like channels within me and then my spleen area made a "whoosh" sound, as though lots of air or energy was trying to get through a hole that was too small. This made me even more curious as to what is possible with healing.

The physical spleen is the largest organ of the lymphatic system and is related to the process of blood purification, as it tackles dis-ease-causing germs and cleanses old and worn-out blood cells, along with producing antibodies. The spleen vortex energizes the physical spleen and causes the body to be victorious over dis-eases and illness. Air/prana is also absorbed, digested and distributed through the spleen vortex. And it controls the quality of blood and the immune system.

Health conditions of the spleen vortex reflect conditions of the physical spleen like lack of vitality, weak immune system, arthritis and rheumatism. Rheumatoid arthritis patients are usually found to have dirty spleen vortexes. A malfunctioning or depleted spleen vortex is also often observed among individuals with chronic fatigue syndrome. In other words, if this vortex of energy is thriving, we are booming with energy. As mentioned previously, we want the field of our heart to run through our entire physical and non-physical bodies; once it does, every energy vortex, including this one and the ones you have in your vital organs (yes, there are many) will thrive and be fuelled by love, the only fuel we need as humans.

Substantia Nigra

The main job of mitochondria is to perform cellular respiration. This means it takes in nutrients from the cells, breaks them down and turns them into energy. This energy is then in turn used by the cell to carry out various functions.

Mitochondrial diseases occur in the body when mitochondria fail to produce enough energy for the body to function properly. Deletions in mitochondrial DNA (mtDNA) are an important cause of human disease and their accumulation has been implicated in the ageing process. As we get older, so does our substantia nigra, and it contains very high levels of mtDNA deletions. These may be directly responsible for impaired cellular respiration. This in turn creates less energy and in turn our bodies slow down, and we age.

The substantia nigra is also responsible for molecular change and when it's not functioning, this becomes impaired. If we have impaired cellular respiration and impaired molecular change, we get older faster and have much less energy. So, it's vital that we concentrate and focus our energy on this particular part of our body. By focusing on it we draw energy into it and stimulate it, which has a positive knock-on effect throughout the entire body.

There is a specific exercise that I want you to practise. I recommend you follow this process every day for forty-nine days and then do it once a week at least, or as often as you feel necessary. If you want to, continue with it as a daily practice. For me, I link this in with meditation. It's like anything: once you have done it enough times, with a little focus, your multidimensional nature takes over and you do it automatically. This is one of those GOOD habits! You will realize as you start working with this information that you can combine things together, they are not all stand-alone exercises. You will naturally find your way.

EXERCISE *Powerhouse 6 – the Process*

1. Please be standing. Close your eyes and take some nice long slow deep breaths.

2. Breathe into your body and bring your awareness into your heart.

3. Hold your awareness in your heart space and keep breathing. Breathe, through your nose. In and out 9 times.

4. Squeeze your perineum, genitals and buttocks. Pull your abdominals back towards your spine.

5. Bring your awareness from your heart into your perineum (while squeezing). You will see a platinum light. Concentrate on this area, breathe out all of your oxygen, then breathe in slowly and as you do, pull the platinum light up into your heart and see the light collect inside your heart. Feel your heart expand.

6. After 6 seconds, breathe out fully, let go of the squeeze and bring all of your awareness and focus back into your perineum. Repeat step 5, two more times. On the third turn, hold your breath and awareness inside your heart as long as you can and see the platinum light radiate out through your entire body, filling it up and getting brighter as it expands out into the space. Then release the breath and squeeze when you need to and breathe out slowly.

7. Next you will repeat step 5 again. This time, as the platinum light is pulled into your heart, you will see/feel/know a stream of electromagnetic energy flow from your heart and into your spleen vortex (same area as the spleen). You will bring all of your focus and awareness to your spleen and hold your focus there (as you hold your in-breath at the top) and the light flows from your heart into your spleen. When ready, let go of the squeeze and breathe out. Repeat these three more times on the spleen.

8. Repeat step 7 for your pineal gland.

9. Repeat step 7 for your pituitary gland.

10. Repeat step 7 for your medulla oblongata.

11. Repeat step 7 for your substantia nigra.

12. Repeat step 7 for your hypothalamus.

PLEASE NOTE: when you hold each breath at the top, don't get to the point where you start turning blue. Just hold it for as long as is comfortable. I recommend you do this exercise every day for forty-nine days and then continue with it once a week. Feel your body. Always do this exercise standing or lying down, and never sitting.

The following illustration shows you where these components lie within the brain and body. Remember, if you intend/command the light into one of these areas, that is where it will go. You are in control, so exercise your dominance over the control of energy in your body.

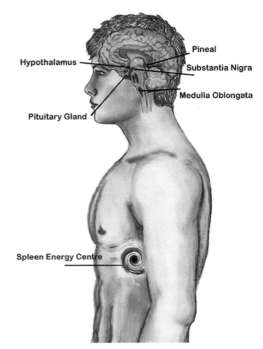

53. Location of the components of Powerhouse 6

The Truth about the Pineal Gland

When there is a change in energy, there is a change in consciousness and when you increase the energy in the brain, and do this in a specific way, magic happens. When we change the energy in our brain (regularly) it stimulates and brings our pineal gland/third eye online, and opens us up to information streams beyond our third-/fourth-dimensional reality. When you increase energy in the brain, it changes your levels of awareness and you are able to tap into vast amounts of data/information, held in the space all around you and inside you. When you change energy, you change consciousness and when you change your frequency, you change the levels and the information streams available to you, similar to a radio station. Most of us are plugged into the familiar channels of our external environment but there is so much more we can access beyond what we see, hear, feel, smell, taste with our five senses. Our five senses are actually extremely limited.

When a human being connects with the fabric of the cosmos and dives into the multiple layers of beauty and wonder, the brain itself is activated by a greater energy that carries information in the form of flowing, spiralized geometric and fractal imagery, thoughts, feelings, knowings, pictures. This information often doesn't make sense to the logical mind, but the pineal gland starts to decode it, and with practice you can "innerstand" it.

One thing that will happen is this: The brain will track and capture these information streams, however they are presented, and the human being will have a profound internal event or experience. It will be vivid and 100 per cent more real than any past event or potential future scenario and in that moment the mind is submerged totally within that experience and the body and brain receive a biological upgrade. They shift at an extremely deep level. I've seen miracles take place in our workshops in hours, sometimes even just minutes or seconds. Once that download of information comes, boom, electromagnetic energy changes the woman, man or child from the inside out, at a cellular, subatomic level.

If someone (no different from you or I) can have such a profound internal sensory experience and move a limb that was paralyzed or dissolve a cancerous tumour, or hear again or see again or shift so much that their IBS (Irritable Bowel Syndrome) disappears after sixteen years, or becomes confident in a body that was ruled by anxiety or depression, in hours, minutes or seconds, what is taking place internally? What chemical or biological processes are happening? How does the body communicate or interact with the quantum/universal field (which is like a database of information) and create such mind-blowingly epic, Super-Human experiences?

The human body is an amazing biological machine. It knows how to self-heal, self-regulate and become coherent in every way – under the right conditions, the primary condition being a state of oneness. When thoughts and emotions, concepts and reactions are eliminated from the equation, the body does what it's supposed to do. When stressors are removed the body can recalibrate. We create this environment by using Star Magic Healing Techniques/Ways or by the human being going into meditation, into the void, beyond body and thought so the body's latent systems can switch on and do what they do best, HEAL AND TRANSFORM!

If we can interface with the cosmic fabric, a field that is naturally coherent and instigate such incredible inner events there must be a biological, neurological and chemical chain of events to shed light on these Super-Human feats of healing and transformation that people experience. What physiological components are lying dormant inside the body, waiting to create such profound change? What organs, tissues, glands, cells and neurotransmitters get involved in our inner process to catalyze such profound changes mentally, physically, emotionally and spiritually?

There are four states of consciousness that we will discuss. The first is wakefulness, the second is sleep, the third is dream state and the fourth is the magic of the fractal/transcendental/inner spiralized geometric experience brought on through meditation, light codes, high-frequency downloads and high-vibrational light/data streams.

Wakefulness is simply when you are awake and fully conscious. Sleep is when we are unconscious, and the body is restoring and repairing. The dream state is when our body is catatonic, and we are in an altered state of consciousness. In this state the mind is engaging with visual imagery, symbolism, quantum data/geometry and is actually often travelling in other dimensional spaces, working and creating as the multidimensional being that we are. This is one reason why you may feel tired in the morning – it's understandable if you are out and about doing grid work, laying new architecture on other planets, battling lower-vibrational forces in other realities!

The fractal/transcendental/inner spiralized geometric experiences are often beyond our logical understanding, based on the reality of the five senses. When you have one of these otherworldly, hallucinogenic experiences, which are vividly real, there is no turning back. You can't unsee what you have seen or dis-experience what you have experienced first-hand. Let's talk about the chemistry, neuroscience and biology of these extraordinary experiences and how I perceive them based on my own experiences, the many experiences I have observed in our workshop participants, our trained Star Magic facilitators and the "innerstand"ing I have gained from these experiences.

Melatonin

When you wake up in the morning and open your eyes, the pineal gland produces serotonin, the daytime neurotransmitter. Serotonin brings your senses online and engages you, ready for the day. The second millisecond your eye receives visible light through your iris, receptors in the optic nerve send a signal to a part of the brain called the suprachiasmatic nucleus, to trigger this process. As serotonin levels spike you start to synthesize between the inner and outer world, dream time and the wakeful, conscious state. Serotonin stimulates the brain waves from delta, to theta, to alpha and then to beta. You then realize you are in a physical body, in this reality, lying in bed, and it's time to start your day.

When night-time falls, darkness sets in and a very similar but inverse process takes place. A signal is sent back along the same trail to the pineal gland. This time it transmutes serotonin into melatonin, the night-time neurotransmitter. As melatonin is released, your brain waves start to slow, from beta to alpha, making you feel more

sleepy, tired and less analytical. As you move into alpha brain waves you naturally become more interested in your inner world. As you drop off and move through from alpha to theta to delta, you have moved into that catatonic state where you restore, repair and dream and, as you now know, if you didn't already, travel, work, create and sometimes battle in multiple dimensional spaces.

We follow a cyclical pattern of wake and sleep, and our bodies sink into this rhythm. Our brain becomes automated and produces these two chemicals at certain times in the morning and evening, day in, day out. This is known as the circadian rhythm. When we fall out of sync with our natural rhythm it affects us. When we change time zones it can take some time to reset and recalibrate our system. It usually takes a few days, often longer, to readjust to the sunset and sunrise in your new environment. It's a series of chemical processes, all governed by our interaction with the 3D world, from our eye's reaction to the sun and visible light.

Melatonin induces Rapid Eye Movement or REM sleep, which is a phase of the circadian rhythm that causes dreams. As the mental chatter slowly subsides (or quickly in some cases), it creates space so we can fall into sleep and then dream state, and the brain begins to see images, spaces, symbols, pictures, patterns. Quite often when people fall asleep, they feel like they are floating or rushing over a forest or mountaintops, rapidly.

Melatonin is crucial. Before we explore it fully, let's take a closer look at the structure of this extraordinary dreaming neurotransmitter.

L-tryptophan is an amino acid and is the raw material responsible for creating serotonin and melatonin.

To create melatonin, L-tryptophan must pass through a series of chemical processes called methylation.

First, the pineal gland transmutes L-tryptophan into 5-hydroxytryptophan (5-HTP), which becomes serotonin. Serotonin is a more stable molecule than 5-HTP, sustains itself in the brain and also has a more useful function, which we'll get to soon. Involving another chemical reaction, the pineal gland converts serotonin into N-acetylserotonin and then an additional chemical reaction turns it into melatonin. All of this magic takes place inside the pineal gland.

It's important to note that melatonin levels are at their highest between 1 a.m. and 4 a.m. This is the best time to be doing your inner work/ creation.

One of the reasons we cannot sleep under stress is because our cortisol levels go up during a stressful situation. There is a direct link between cortisol levels and melatonin levels: when one rises the other falls. This served its purpose – and still does – in survival situations. If you are in a sudden dangerous situation, whether it be in a combat situation in the street or if you were face to face with a wild animal, your body and its natural intelligence want to prevent you from being killed or injured. It's obvious that sleep becomes less important than survival.

So the body cannot rest and it doesn't get the restorative sleep it needs because the survival chemicals, like cortisol, have switched the survival genes on.

When a dangerous situation comes to an end, like one involving a wild animal, the body returns to its normal rhythm after the event. But when, say, we have a strained relationship with a husband or wife or co-worker, which shows up, day in day out, the chronic, non-stop stress keeps the survival system activated. This means that the safety trigger does not appropriately adjust to its environment. It's no longer adaptive; it becomes maladaptive. This chronic stress alters melatonin and serotonin levels and knocks the body out of balance or homeostasis.

As we have seen previously, your body becomes addicted to these chemicals. Whether it's rejection, hurt, guilt, anger – the body is like an addict and must have its fix. When you break the stress response by overcoming the present situation, whether it be in your immediate environment or a thought construct about a past event or potential future, fear-based scenario, cortisol levels will drop and melatonin levels will increase. Your body can then go back to doing what it does best: recalibrating, healing, regulating, expanding, developing.

Here are some incredible facts about melatonin:

- Improves carbohydrate metabolism
- Lowers triglyceride levels
- Stops the excretion of cortisol in response to stress
- Promotes DNA repair and DNA replication
- Inhibits hardening of the arteries (atherosclerosis)
- Heightens the immune response, both cellular and metabolic
- Decreases the development of some tumours
- Increases REM sleep
- Activates a neuroprotective role in the brain
- Stimulates free radical scavenging (antioxidant and anti-ageing)

Activating the Pineal Gland – Preparation

There are numerous ways to activate the pineal gland. I have researched this topic because it's such a huge part of my work; to be connected to the information fields that lie within the invisible space, you must have this small gland in your brain functioning. I have combined the techniques used in ancient traditions with my own "ten cents" and have developed a method that works. We will discuss the full method soon.

But before we get into the pineal gland in detail and the full method to activate it, I want you to stop and practise this exercise for a moment. We began to play with it in the qigong routine earlier and we are going to be using it to set up the activation of the pineal gland, so I want you to go through this basic exercise. It will get you into the flow of the squeeze and breathe technique we will be using.

EXERCISE *Squeeze and Breathe Technique*

You can lie or stand for this. It's also possible to sit, but from experience, having the body straight is best. I want you to:

1. Squeeze your perineum, genitals and buttocks and pull your stomach muscles back towards your spine.

2. Bring your awareness into your perineum.

3. Breathe in a long, slow, deep breath and as you do, see/feel a platinum frequency being pulled from your perineum, up through your body and into your brain.

4. Once all of your awareness is inside your brain, bring it to the centre and back slightly (where the pineal gland is) and hold your breath for thirteen seconds.

5. Now, release the breath and the squeeze, keeping your awareness in the brain.

6 Wait for three to five seconds, squeeze and repeat.

7. Repeat thirteen times just to start.

I often do this several times a day. I just find myself doing it. I do it when I am sitting at the laptop, in a queue in a shop, on a plane and just generally relaxing. Just play with it and get used to it. It will cause cerebrospinal fluid to move up through your spinal column and into the area of the brain that surrounds the pineal gland, and add pressure to it.

The pineal gland contains tiny little calcite crystals made up of carbon, calcium and oxygen. The pineal gland is like an antenna: it picks up information from the field and transduces it into patterns, images and often inner knowings. Just like an antenna, the pineal gland has the capacity to become electrically activated and generate electromagnetic fields that can tune into and harness the information in the quantum field. The information travelling through the field is infinite and even though it's coherent within the field, the fractal patterns, spiralized geometric code and mathematics of these information streams are baffling to the logical human brain.

The pineal gland, combined with your intuition (when you trust it), helps with this translation into images or words or knowings that we can grasp. To stimulate the pineal gland and activate it, you must apply pressure to it. When you do, a piezoelectric effect occurs. This is when pressure is applied to certain materials and the mechanical stress is changed into an electrical charge. The materials in this case are the calcite crystals inside the pineal gland.

It works in a similar way to television or radio: there are waves travelling through the empty space and the antenna picks them up and transduces them into pictures on your screen and the radio transduces the signals into sound that you can listen to. You can't see these electromagnetic signals, but they are there.

The pineal gland picks up information beyond our third-dimensional reality and relays it to us in the most coherent fashion possible. As we have mentioned, pictures, images, colours, patterns, codes can be shown to us like a movie; or maybe you experience brief flashes of imagery. Other times you may be surrounded by this all-consciousness-consuming information, and when you go deep, beyond the body and mind, you feel like you are this experience and it is totally vivid and real beyond any question of a doubt. You become submerged so deeply in this experience that you lose all sense of time and space and you float/travel/journey, through an ocean of colour, beauty, magic, wisdom, knowledge and wonder.

The calcite crystals in the pineal gland are mission critical in creating the piezoelectric effect. You can see them in the image below:

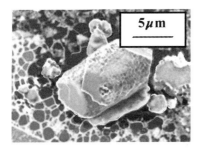

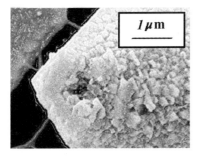

54. Calcite crystals in the pineal gland

These crystals are ever so small, tiny in fact. Their size can range from one-hundredth to one-quarter the width of a human hair. They are in the shape of rhombohedrons (a three-dimensional figure like a cube, except that its faces are not squares but rhombi. It is a special case of parallelepiped shapes where all edges are the same length) and are stacked neatly together in layers. Pretty fascinating to say the least. Such accuracy and precision in the most tiny of measurements. (Remember however, in our Angelic Human form,

tapped into our original base geometry, the pineal gland should be much bigger.)

We have seen, in the qigong exercise at the start and also again at the start of this chapter, how we can squeeze our perineum, genitals, buttocks and pull our stomach towards the spine to create a pressure. We are going to be taking this to the next level in the pineal gland activation exercise. The reason we do this is because the pressure, combined with our focus and breath (as we will go into in detail very soon) creates an internal pressure. The word "piezoelectric" is derived from the Greek words "piezein", which means to squeeze or press, and "piezo", which means to push. When we do the pineal gland exercise, we will be pushing cerebrospinal fluid up through the central channel of the body and up against the pineal gland, exerting the mechanical stress mentioned. This translates into an electrical charge, and it's this action that compresses the crystals, stacked on top of each other in the pineal gland, and creates the piezoelectric effect. The crystals, in turn, generate an electrical charge.

The piezoelectric effect is also reversible; once the crystals in the pineal gland are compressed and are creating an electrical charge, the electromagnetic field emanating from the pineal gland causes the crystals in it to stretch as the field expands and increases. When the crystals reach their limit and can stretch no further, they contract and the electromagnetic field reverses direction and moves inwards, towards the pineal gland. When it reaches the pineal gland it compresses them some more, adding more pressure, producing yet another electromagnetic field. The cycle of expansion and reversal of the field perpetuates a pulsating electromagnetic field.

The exercise will generate a force that turns your pineal gland into a pulsating antenna, capable of picking up the subtlest and finest frequencies travelling through the cosmic fabric.

You will be able to hone in on information streams that were once inaccessible.

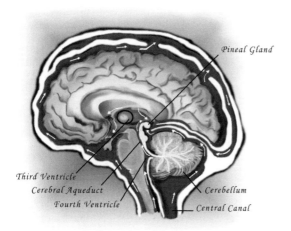

55. The inside of the brain

Look closely at the image above. The action we are discussing causes the cerebrospinal fluid to move up through the spinal column. As the fluid enters the brain, it moves up through the central canal, through the space between the spinal cord and the spinal column. It then flows in two directions: from the fourth to the third ventricle, at the back of which you have the pineal gland, and around the back of the cerebellum to the other side of the pineal gland, ensuring that the rice-sized gland is surrounded by the pressurized fluid.

The increased pressure exerts a mighty force that compresses the tiny little calcite crystals inside the pineal gland, causing them to compress and create a greater piezoelectric effect. This is the first action that takes place to activate the pineal gland. It requires effort on your part. With your continued effort, the pineal gland then moves through the next stages naturally.

The increase in fluid around the pineal gland also stimulates tiny hairs on the outside of the pineal gland, called cilia, which is Latin for eyelashes. The increase in cerebrospinal fluid moving through the chambers tickles the cilia and

stimulates them, which in turn stimulates the pineal gland.

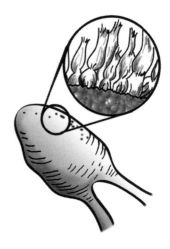

56. Cilia on the outside of the pineal gland

The pineal gland is shaped like a phallus and because of the enhanced stimulation produced by the accelerated fluid and the combined electrical activation created by an increase in pressure inside a closed system, it starts to ejaculate some potent, upgraded metabolites of melatonin into the brain.

The particles increase in acceleration and velocity and create what is known as an inductance field.

The inductance field reverses the flow of the two-way information stream that facilitates communication from the brain to the body and vice versa (see illustration 57). Like a vacuum, the inductance field draws the energy from the lower part of the body and delivers it directly to the brainstem in a spiralling motion. This is sometimes referred to as kundalini activation. You will see from the image that the stream of energy flows on up past the head. That is because the energy also connects you to the cosmic frequencies/energies of our celestial family, planets, suns, stars. This energy stream also runs from these celestial masters back into our body and back down into the Earth. We truly are an extension of the universe.

Or maybe the universe is an extension of us. This exercise is also influencing our transmission centres and vice versa.

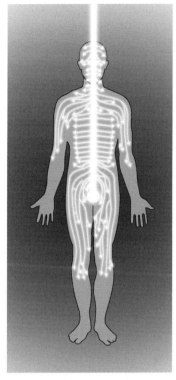

57. Inductance field

As the energy passes through the thirty-three vertebrae, it passes the nerves that run from the spinal cord to different parts of the body and some of the energy is transferred, through the peripheral nerves that affect the tissues and organs of the human body. The electrical current that runs through these nerves activates the body's natural energy channels, which in turn results in the entire body receiving more energy and increasing its vitality.

Inside the brain we have what is known as the Reticular Activating System (RAS). It's this system that finds things you are looking for. For example, someone tells you about a new car. You've never seen it before but now someone mentions it, you are seeing it everywhere because, now it has been made aware of it, the RAS picks it up. You will have

experienced that before, I'm sure. As the energy is delivered to the brainstem, it passes through the reticular information, which is a part of the RAS. The reticular information edits information flowing from the body to the brain and back again.

The RAS is responsible for your levels of alertness and arousal. If you hear a noise in the night, your RAS is picking that up and making you aware. It's like a subtle intruder alarm that notifies you when you are engaged in another activity or even asleep.

As the sympathetic nervous system is activated and merges with the parasympathetic nervous system, instead of depleting the body's stored energy it releases it back to the brain. Once the energy reaches the brainstem the thalamic gate opens and energy moves through the reticular formation to the thalamus, where it relays information/data to the neocortex. Now the reticular formation is open and greater levels of conscious awareness are experienced.

Remember your sympathetic nervous system and the parasympathetic nervous system are the go and stop mechanisms, controlling fight or flight or a shutdown of the system. The sympathetic nervous system, when in beta brain waves (awake), is stimulated for an emergency response and utilizes energy for survival. When in gamma brain waves it's very different. Instead of losing vital energy in the fight for survival scenario, you create and liberate more energy. You're not in survival mode but in ecstasy, joy, bliss. Your sympathetic nervous system directs your attention to what is taking place in your mind, often a full transcendental Super-Human experience.

The thalamus is the epicentre of communication. It has links into all higher centres of the brain. In meditation and during healing, if you hit gamma brain wave patterns (when a full-blown, internal, spiralized geometric experience happens, beyond the body and mind) it's through the thalamus that it is made possible.

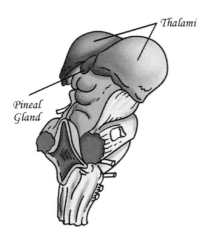

58. Pineal gland and the thalamus

There are actually two thalami in the midbrain, one on either side, which feed the left and right hemispheres of the neocortex (see illustration above).

The pineal gland sits in between them facing the back of the brain. When the energy reaches the thalamus, it sends messages directly to the pineal gland to secrete metabolites into the brain. The thinking neocortex then becomes aroused and goes into higher brain wave patterns, such as gamma waves. The chemical derivatives of melatonin relax the body (taking it out of the game so the experience manifests easier) and at the same time stimulate the mind.

We've discussed the two-way flow of energy, as well as the torus field, clearing the heart, dissolving the lower energy centres and throat and bringing energy up through the body. It is important to know that as you run the frequency up your spinal column, speeding up the flow and movement of cerebrospinal fluid, your body becomes a magnet as the torus field is activated to a stronger degree. The torus field represents a powerful and dynamic flow of energy, which flows up and out of the top of your crown as your pineal gland becomes activated and a reverse field pulls or draws energy back in through the top of your head. Much like

the protons (mini universes) in your cells, there is always this two-way exchange. It's the same with healing: when you give you receive; it cannot be any other way.

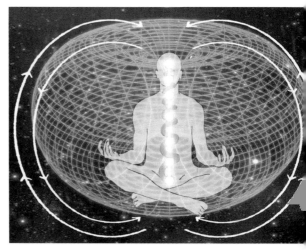

59. Toroidal field and two-way flow of energy/light

When you trigger all of these events, the brain switches on like never before. You have access to information that is non-physical, non-auditory, non-visual in the external world. You are accessing information in the form of electrical impulses, spiralized geometric code, colours, patterns, mathematics, which in turn your pineal gland transduces and then your body translates through feeling and knowing.

I was sat in the airport in Buffalo, New York state, after a training several months ago, and was meditating with my eyes closed. I saw this man walk towards me, even though my eyes were shut. Just as he got close, I opened my eyes and said, "I'm meditating, I do it to relax and get clarity on my life." He stood there with his mouth open. I said, "Are you OK mate?" He said, "I was coming over to ask you what you were doing because I was intrigued, and you answered my question before I could ask."

I smiled, told him he was incredible and that I loved him and closed my eyes again. I remember when my son went to grab my ear in the car one day as a joke. I sat there with my eyes closed (in the passenger seat) but fully conscious of my surroundings. I reached up and grabbed his arm and stopped him in mid-reach. He started crying, he was so freaked out that I knew he was going to do that. The thing is I wasn't scanning the area, watching, observing. I was simply in a total state of awareness and my energy field responded to its environment. You see, your third eye is just like a normal eye and when you use it regularly it gives you a whole new outlook on reality, literally.

The power we possess, once this little gland is functioning, is mesmerizing. We can see anywhere in the world, anywhere in the galaxy, anywhere in the universe. All things are available.

Upgraded Melatonin

When your pineal gland is activated, it picks up higher frequencies and these higher frequencies alter the chemistry of the melatonin. As the frequency rises the alteration becomes greater. It's the translation of light or information into chemistry that prepares you for otherworldly, magical, spiralized geometrical, colourful experiences. The pineal gland, just like you, is a master alchemist. It transmutes melatonin into some profoundly powerful neurotransmitters.

Illustration 60 shows what happens when higher frequencies, potent energies and higher or expanded states of consciousness interact with our third eye. One of the first things to happen is the higher frequencies transmute melatonin into benzodiazepines. Benzodiazepines are a type of drug from which Valium is made. These chemicals anesthetize the analytical mind, so the mind or brain stops analyzing and chills out. Benzodiazepines suppress neural activity in the amygdala, the survival or fight or flight centre. This severely limits chemicals that can cause lower-vibrational moods such as feelings of anger, aggression, fear, agitation, guilt, loneliness and sadness, which in reality are all variations of the emotion we call fear. With neural activity suppressed in the amygdala and these lower-

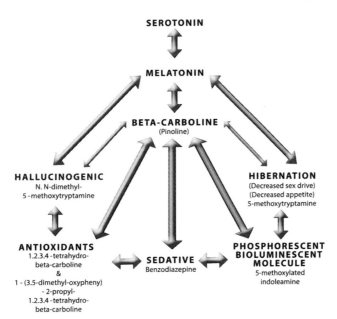

60. Chemical changes in melatonin

vibrational chemicals reduced, your body feels relaxed and calm and your mind is awake and activated.

Another chemical created from melatonin produces a class of very powerful antioxidants called pinolines. Pinolines are important because they attack free radicals, which harm your cells and cause ageing. The antioxidants are anti-ageing, anti-cancer, anti-stroke, anti-heart disease, anti-inflammatory, anti-neurodegenerative and anti-microbial. Melatonin is known as an antioxidant, but now it becomes a highly upgraded SAS (elite soldiers) version of an antioxidant, ready to take down or take out anything that causes harm or hinders healing and restoring the body to a higher degree than the melatonin molecule normally does.

When you take the molecule and change it again, into another offshoot of melatonin, you find the same chemical that makes animals hibernate. Melatonin, which makes us sleepy anyway, shifts into a new variation; it becomes more powerful and now carries a message that induces further rest and repair. It causes the body's metabolism to slow down, sometimes for months, just like a bear going into hibernation for the winter. When mammals hibernate, they lose their appetite, sex drive, interest in socialising or going anywhere. They go within into a form of stasis. It makes sense then that we, as humans, exploring our inner world, journeying through our cosmic hearts, having full-blown Super-Human experiences, find it easier to do so when these upgraded versions of melatonin shift us into a space where the external world becomes less important.

But instead of hibernating like the animals, we have an altered experience, which, once experienced, you can never go back from. We go past the body and its biological activity and into a space of nothingness. It's so beautiful and transformational that you want to experience it often. And remember,

if you ever want to create something in this physical world, it must be created in the quantum first and foremost. The quantum world is the foundation of our physical reality.

I was working with a client recently with stage four cancer, and getting them beyond their body and mind has been challenging to say the least. This beautiful soul called me and told me they were meditating and suddenly they found themselves up on the ceiling, looking down at their body. They lost all sense of time and drifted and floated, then suddenly they jolted and were back in their body. They had lost three hours. This put a huge smile on my face. It's in these moments, outside of time and space, beyond the physical body, beyond the thoughts and emotions, that rapid healing takes place.

The next stage in the evolutionary process of this magical molecule is to produce the same chemical found in electric eels, a phosphorescent, bioluminescent chemical that amplifies energy in the nervous system. Just like an electric eel lighting up when it's stimulated, the very same thing is happening in your brain. Your brain is stimulated from the inside and another world is activated. More information is available as your frequency heightens.

As we work on ourselves, things shift and change. Light coming from the primary light and sound fields of Source and into our local environment, flows through our eyes and communicates with our pineal gland, making serotonin and melatonin, and we move into a harmonious rhythm within our environment; or maybe we become an extension of our environment as we fall into this pattern of nature that we call the circadian rhythm. The information carried by serotonin and melatonin marries with the frequency coming from our third-/fourth-dimensional, physical world, but when we tune in to higher-frequency bands and off-planet light/light codes, the information within our brain changes, is new and this will affect our inner geometry, catalyzing changes within our body structure, as the source code reactivates our original/core Divine Blueprint/ Template.

Source Code

As our frequency increases and we move beyond the realms of visible light, energy or information coming from the quantum field / the primary light and sound fields of Source, changes the chemistry of melatonin, upgrading our brain and its activity, creating an environment where we can access more information and have heightened internal experiences where we re-engage with our source code. The pineal gland is the master alchemist that takes this information and translates it into messages that we can read, feel, know or "innerstand" in the most subtle and most profound ways. The more often you can take your brain into these higher and more advanced states of consciousness, with an elevated frequency, the easier it becomes to keep the doorway open to this universal database of intelligence and those 5D Electrical Currents streaming from the primary light and sound fields. As with everything in life, practice makes you better. Your intention is everything.

I am tapped into the field 24/7 now and can access information easily to assist others in healing. When you practise and make it a positive habit, one that you look forward to and enjoy, you too will tap this potential effortlessly.

When you alter melatonin again you produce another chemical called dimethyltryptamine, better known as DMT. DMT is one of the most powerful substances known to man.

It is found in ayahuasca, a plant medicine we use on our Star Magic Deep in Space Retreats and which has been used by shamans for thousands of years, in sacred rituals to enhance spiritual visions and gain powerful insights from the invisible

world beyond matter and form. When ayahuasca is ingested, though, the body receives only DMT; when the pineal gland is activated, you receive the entire blend of chemicals we have been discussing. I highly recommend everyone tries ayahuasca, at least once. It's phenomenal and when we do it on our retreats, we combine our Star Magic ways with the plant medicine, which totally elevates the experience. Hence the name Deep in Space. It's life changing. With that being said, otherworldly experiences take place with or without plant medicine. You simply have to follow the right protocols and I, like many others, have mastered them.

Unless you have experienced one of these beyond-this-realm experiences, it's near on impossible to explain so make it your mission and experience it yourself. Know that the pineal gland is a part of your Super-Human arsenal. In fact, the pineal gland plays a massive role in you becoming Super-Human.

The Cosmic Fabric and How to "Innerstand" It

I have referred to the cosmic fabric throughout this book. I mean the ether, the intelligence, the universe, the quantum field. I prefer to call it the cosmic fabric because I think it fits the description of what we are trying to describe so much better and when your third eye is turned on (if it's not already) I am sure you will fully agree with me. It is just like a large Persian rug; woven intricately from the finest cotton, silks or fabrics, often geometrically designed in a flawless fashion, to absolute perfection, often infinitely long and wide, these rugs are mesmerizingly beautiful. When I look at the fields of information and the frequency bands all around me, filling the so-called "empty space", I see an infinite Persian rug, a never-ending piece of fabric, that looks metaphysical, cosmic. This fabric is not static like a rug, though; it's moving continuously, codes, spiralized geometrical codes shifting in alignment through the fabric. It's as though they are weaving themselves into new designs to share new knowledge and wisdom with me and everyone else who is tapped in.

Our trained facilitators and our tribe members who regularly do our guided meditations from our Meditation Library report explosions of light inside their mind, their bodies being filled with light/information and their hearts expanding into deep states of bliss and joy. They feel surges of energy rushing through their bodies and they break into tears of ecstasy. The best way people can explain it is that it feels like going home.

Once you switch on the pineal gland, it literally is another eye and it's more important than the two you have peering through your eye sockets. It opens your awareness, expands your consciousness, which seem to me to be the same thing. I mean, I could give them different logical meanings, and lay down good reasoning for why they are different, but really and truthfully, what is the difference? What I do know is that once your third eye is activated, your levels of awareness heighten, your levels of energy and consciousness rise, and you get access to more light/information/data. One thing is certain, once you activate your pineal gland you get to experience greater depths of reality.

You are naturally going to have amped-up connections and experiences as you meditate, journey, dream or heal.

As we tune into these different frequencies, we have access to a new stream of data/information/light and in turn a much higher intelligence. The higher frequencies produce a change in chemistry and geometry. In actuality the higher the level of frequency, the more greatly our chemistry is altered and our geometry re-aligned, allowing us to see/feel/know more. We have heightened experiences, more visually enhanced experiences. Experiences that are high-energy and hallucinogenic. The tiny calcite

crystals vibrating inside our pineal gland are the key that turns and switches on our universal antenna and gives us direct access to the cosmic fabric and the spiralized geometrical data it contains. Again, you are the one who must instigate it all. The more effort you put in, the greater the results you will reap.

As the pineal gland delivers information and we have these magical Super-Human experiences, and because the heart and brain and the human nervous system is extremely coherent in the right conditions, it's able to tune in to the data, and enable you to make sense of, through feeling, these ultra-coherent data streams. The pineal gland is like a vortex, a portal, a Star Gate picking up and organizing data and doing its very best to deliver it to our brain in a way we can first, acknowledge it, and second, "innerstand" it.

As we have seen, trying to understand all this new data is the wrong way to go about it. Reaching out and focusing on it will make it difficult for you. Simply being, observing with a soft inner eye, and waiting for the information to flow to you and through you is best. With regular practice you become a Jedi Master at deciphering this information. The best way to access information from the field is to be like an angler. An angler casts their rod out into the ocean or the lake or the river and is patient. If they move the bait around on the end of the line, the fish will get scared and go nowhere near it. So, the angler remains patient and lets the fish come to them. Connecting to the field is the same. Don't search or look. If you see something don't turn towards it. Let it be in your space softly. Let it expand and fill up your space. Be patient. Let the image build and the information flow. Remember, it's all inside you anyway.

These patterns are not waves or particles. Waves only exist in a two-dimensional concept and particles are there at a superficial level. Some say particles are only available when you don't look. Well, I can tell you I see particles in nature, in buildings, I see them everywhere. Once you go past this stage, just beyond the 3D illusion, you enter a different space, a space filled with complex, infinite, ever-evolving, moving patterns. These fractal patterns, a bit like a kaleidoscope of fluid, spiralized geometry, are light/ information. Good raw data. Building blocks of our universe. Once you connect with this Krystal Code and start allowing it to flow through you on a subatomic basis, with zero judgement, when you surrender to the information flow, your life will never be the same. Once you reach this point, there is no turning back. The truth is so vibrant and beautiful. Once you become aware of this it alters your inner and outer worlds forever. The question is, can you handle it?

Can you handle knowing that everything you thought you knew is false, a lie, an illusion? My suggestion to you is this. Commit to knowing that you are about to have your life, your identity torn to shreds and you are about to be rebirthed like a phoenix rising from the ashes.

Once your pineal gland picks up and tunes you into these information streams and you are in full surrender mode, present, turned on, you better get ready for a ride. You may pop out of your body and be somewhere else looking back at yourself, maybe several metres above looking back down thinking, "wow, I am in two different places at once"; or you may be in another universe. You may travel down a tunnel of light and experience what we know as death. You may expand so infinitely that you feel like a giant star, connected to every other star in the galaxy. Your heart may explode with joy and ecstasy, and you may cry uncontrollably because you have not connected with this level of love before. The infinite possibilities that await, when you expand your light body out through the cosmic fabric, are mind-blowingly beautiful and totally cosmic and realer than the words you are reading right now.

Past the Programming – No Going Back

When you start to experience these altered states, you have two choices. To go into fear of the unknown, or to let go even more and let the experience take you deeper.

Quite often in an experience like this you can stop breathing normally, through your lungs, and instead feed off cosmic energy. When we take people through our enhanced breathing exercises on our trainings, this happens a lot, and once the mind realizes the body isn't breathing, the human being can get nervous. It's an automatic reaction of the ego mind and it can bring them out of the experience. With the right training and preparation, however, this can be overridden. You can enter a space where your brain is fully sedated, and you simply get swallowed up by the experience. The experience takes you and you become the experience. No body, no mind, no thoughts; your consciousness intertwines with all that is and all that is not, and you float, spin, spiral through a galactic portal of geometrical bliss and a sea of beautifully elevated emotions. You become whole and at one with the universe and you truly know the expression "One Love, One Heart, One Human Family". But – and it's a big but – it goes way beyond the One Human Family. It becomes a galactic experience where all universes, all quantum spaces, merge as one infinite stream of beauty and magic.

When you enter these very real states you go beyond your outer environment and beyond your body and its five senses. Your 3D/4D reality no longer matters and is not affecting the way you are. You are being changed and altered at a deep level by your inner experience. It's in this state of colourful zen that you heal deeply. It's in this state that your body does what it's supposed to do and that is self-heal/organize. Whenever I am facilitating the healing of another human being, I am aiming to create an environment where they can self-heal. They can be taken there through meditation, breathing exercises or through certain healing techniques/ways that we teach/share on Star Magic Facilitator Training Experiences. How the environment is set up is important but how they get there once the environment is in place, doesn't matter. Each journey is unique.

We perceive our external reality the way we are and not the way the reality actually is, but from this altered state of elevated emotions and expanded awareness, we start to see and feel our world, our reality, our environment differently. Now, remember, your external reality affects your cells and your genes and has an effect on your health. Now that you are changing your perception of your reality, you are signalling new genes. Your heightened inner experience captures all of your brain's attention and so the focus and in turn the energy creates something new. This is the perfect space to heal and manifest from.

Once, during these magical experiences, you encounter mythical beings, angels, elementals or extra-terrestrials and have deep and profound conversations, once you see through a human being's body or see their entire nervous system light up pink, or you float down through the earth and end up in a forest with pixies playing or you see a door, walk through and you are in the Last Supper with Jesus giving his sermon and you pick up a grape and eat it and can taste it so vividly – it's real. When you then come back into your physical reality, you see it from a different perspective. You are open now to a greater spectrum of light and information, a spectrum that goes way beyond our visible light spectrum. You have gone past the point of no return. Now your extrasensory scope of vision/feeling/knowing is programmed to experience these experiences always. Now you can start to influence matter, by influencing the quantum field.

Once you have such a profound experience, it's etched into your memory. Your brain has significantly changed; you are starting to rewire yourself neurologically. You will totally transform the software in your brain. Remember your body and brain are two components of a biological computer and the software programs can be changed. You are literally reprogramming yourself, rewiring yourself to be a Super-Human. Naturally, your esoteric abilities will start to present themselves. Telepathy, distance healing, telekinesis. The dumbed-down, subdued, version of your infinite self that you once were, will die and a new and empowered Super-Human version of you will be born. It's inevitable, unquestionable, it's your birthright/Earthright to know this power as a sovereign being.

When you regularly give yourself the gift of these experiences, by doing the work, the level of light and information continually grows. You see the world as though it's alive. You look at a flower and see a level of beauty that was masked up until this point. The veil of illusion is lifted, and you start to see the truth in many different ways. Buildings start to shimmer, trees start to glow, people show their true colours, and you start shining from the inside out like a cosmic beacon of stardust vibrating through a physical form. Anger, fear, jealousy, pain, suffering, rejection, guilt . . . all of these lower-frequency states seem to dissolve from your reality and you fly high like an eagle, soaring above the chaos in a storm. The chaos, the 3D reality is down below but you don't see it, feel it, sense it any more because your vibration is so high. You cannot even interact with it any more because it's not in your new reality. When you start vibrating like this, life flows towards you, abundance enters your life in every which way possible and you don't even have to try. All you have to do is keep having these magical, mystical Super-Human experiences and upgrading your consciousness, and that is NOT work. It's fun, magical and totally blissful.

9

The Pineal Gland
and the Ancient Code

If you have read my previous books, you will know that I have spent a lot of time in ancient mystery schools with beings from other worlds/dimensions/realities showing me how to heal using mathematical codes and geometrical equations.

As my journey has continued, I realize more and more that our world, our galaxy, the universe itself is a gigantic piece of code. It's all mathematics. I live near Wiltshire in the UK and it's a place where many crop circles emerge. During the summer I will often take a drive and visit some. Some crop circles are real, and some are not, staged maybe. Some carry a positive frequency and some a less positive frequency, depending on who created them. Each crop circle carries a frequency radius of up to 700 miles, so a crop circle can send its mathematical code (positive or negative) into the space around it for quite a distance. They appear as many different patterns such as merkabas, fractals, intricate codes that blow your consciousness wide open. I sat in an incredible one some time ago and recorded a video with a meditation and light language transmission. You can watch it on YouTube. When I looked back at the recording, I was sat inside a golden pyramid created from light. It stayed around me for the whole transmission and then disappeared. You can see for yourself on the video.

There have even been crop circles that show the chemical structure of melatonin. Compare the structure of the crop circle in image 61 with the chemical structure of melatonin in image 62. Do I think that some galactic race was trying to share important knowledge with us? Absolutely.

We are not alone. How do I know? I've been face to face with other beings.

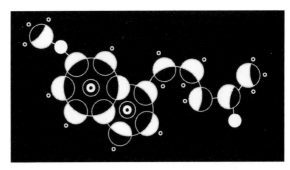

61. Crop circles in the formation of melatonin

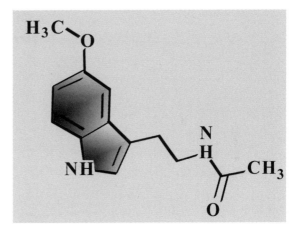

62. Chemical structure of melatonin

Signs, Symbols, and the Pineal Gland

Signs and symbols are everywhere. Some of them we can't see and some we can. The ancient Egyptians drew or sculpted signs, symbols, glyphs and pictures, one of the most well-known being the Eye of Horus. It symbolizes protection, power and good health. These three qualities are certainly qualities that we can experience and embrace once we switch on the latent systems in our body.

We have two hemispheres in our brain, linked by the corpus callosum. When you perform a sagittal cut (a cut that slices the brain down the middle) and observe the location and collective formation of the pineal gland, hypothalamus, thalamus, corpus callosum and pituitary gland you will see that it looks very familiar. Does it not resemble the Eye of Horus?

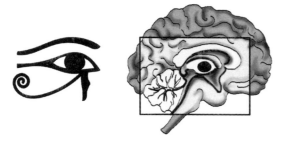

63. Sagittal cut of the brain and
the Eye of Horus

Maybe the Egyptians knew the importance of activating the pineal gland, switching on the autonomic nervous system, stimulating the reticular activating system, opening the thalamic gate and bringing energy into the areas of the pituitary gland and hypothalamus; and that by focusing our attention on these magical parts of our anatomy, we can transform, ascend from this third-/fourth-dimensional reality and enter different worlds. Maybe? What do you feel?

In the system used by the Egyptians, the Eye of Horus represented a system of measurement to measure parts of the whole. In modern mathematics we call it the Fibonacci Sequence or the Fibonacci Constant. It's also known as the golden mean, golden spiral or golden ratio. This formula is governed by the fact that every number after the first two is the sum of the preceding two. This formula shows up everywhere in nature. It's in pine cones, seashells, flowers, eggs, growth points

of tree branches, pineapples, cauliflowers . . . Take a good look at yourself in the mirror. You'll notice that most of your body parts follow the numbers one, two, three and five: you have one nose, two eyes, three segments to each limb and five fingers on each hand. The proportions and measurements of the human body can also be divided-up in terms of the golden ratio. DNA molecules follow this sequence, measuring 34 angstroms long and 21 angstroms wide for each full cycle of the double helix.

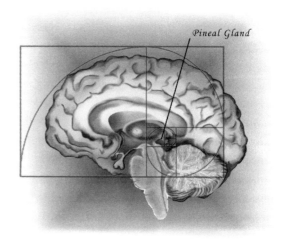

Pineal Gland

64. Golden spiral laid over the human brain

In the image above you can see this formula has been superimposed over the human brain. When you draw squares, adding another square and another, you will see a fractal pattern emerge, a never-ending pattern that repeats itself at every scale. When you follow the golden spiral, the Fibonacci Constant, along the circumference of the brain, the spiral ends at the exact point of the pineal gland. What really is the pineal gland? Is it just there by chance? Or is it a latent Star Gate, waiting to be activated through certain exercises and protocols?

Now, this system of mathematics fits neatly into nature – or maybe nature fits neatly into this system of mathematics? This is crucial. Just like people believe in their chakras and have helped to re-enforce them, creating an energy network that holds stuck emotion, the Fibonacci mathematics has woven nature into this equation. Our bodies, our brains, flowers, trees, seashells, all things. While it looks beautiful, it carries a significantly dark undertone. We as humans buy into things without question and when we buy into them, we help create more of them. We are our own worst enemies. We don't question enough.

Everything in this world has been inverted for far too long. It's time to flip the planet and our human species on its head. The new timeline (which is really the original timeline) and the new mathematics (which are really the true and original mathematics of creation), known as the Krystal Spiral, are changing the frequency of Earth, our worldly home, and offering us a New Humanity potential. A new time/space frequency band to operate within. The old one contracts us and stunts our ability to expand. Humanity's gene code has been played with, raped and pillaged in fact for a long time (creating a more disempowered species) and the mathematical structure of our time-based matrix has been corrupted for much longer. Imagine this: some huge, powerful beings, taking a mould in the form of an entire universe (our time-based matrix consisting of our 15 dimensions, 5 densities, multiple Star Gates, billions of planets, stars and other celestial beings) and manipulating energy to ensure everything inside that system fitted perfectly into that mould. It seems a little crazy right? At first thought it does. It did to me. Go into your heart and feel this. Go into your heart and meditate and decide for yourself.

I am no scientist. I am no professor. And here I am suggesting to you that everything in this world is completely false. That everything that you have ever known is a corrupted version of the truth. And if it's corrupted then it's not the truth, plain and simple. There is truth and not the truth. Go into your heart and feel this information. Meditate on this information. Remember, our bodies adapt to their environment. You adapt to the cold or the heat. Humans adapt to low-vibrational environments until they forget what a high-vibrational environment was like. If there is a mathematical code, introduced into the DNA of nature, then nature will adapt to this code.

Just keep an open mind and know that our human brains are too small. Our pineal gland is an eighth of the size it should be. If we can access these deep, quantum, Super-Human experiences when the mathematics of our physiology are out of whack, imagine what we are truly capable of when everything is in order and our bodies and brains return to the mathematics of the Krystal Spiral New Earth Code. I've witnessed clients whose skulls, feet and hands have grown massively over night or in hours or minutes after a huge download of high-frequency light. Their bodies are realigning to their true mathematical nature. I will share one of these mind-blowing stories later.

Third Eye Merkaba Matrix — Pineal Gland Activation

What I am going to share with you now is a technique/way we have been working with for several years in Star Magic, with some extremely profound results. I am going to share with you how to do it with a partner, but know you can do it on your own also. As it's possible that you will feel dizzy, I am going to encourage you to do this lying down to start with. As you get used to it you can try it standing, but only ever do so when you're alone, once you have been working with this daily and with commitment and feel comfortable.

This is very important: NEVER do the breathing sitting down. It puts too much pressure on the chest and heart area when you get to the holotropic stage. When the body is not vertical or horizontal the energy can't flow efficiently and can get stuck. It is quite easy to fall unconscious and it can cause a racing heart.

This exercise draws the blood up into your brain, pushes and pulls energy and information up through your body and into your pineal gland and stimulates it with various light-encoded frequency streams.

We are going to break this exercise into three parts.

EXERCISE *Part 1*

One soul will lie on the floor with the partner standing or sitting next to them. The soul on the floor will be breathing and receiving and the soul standing will be spinning and sending. So, we will call the two roles breather and spinner. And remember you can be both a breather and a spinner.

The breather will start by squeezing their perineum, stomach and genitals, pulling their abdominals towards their spine and breathing long and slow deep breaths, in through the nose, down to the pit of the stomach and out through the mouth, maintaining and releasing the squeeze periodically, say every 10–15 seconds (but don't be too hung up on time, let it flow).

The spinner will now visualize a hologram (and say, this is the hologram of Jerry Sargeant or whoever you are working with, three times) in front of them and visualize the pineal gland, in the centre of the breather's brain and back slightly. It does not matter if you don't get the spot of the pineal gland perfect because we are quantum-entangling the pineal gland you are visualizing with the actual pineal gland simply through intention, by using the hologram.

Next visualize a merkaba around the pineal gland (see image below and also colour insert after page 160).

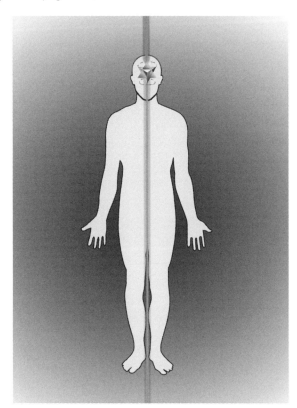

65. Merkaba around the pineal gland and the frequencies of Sirius and Earth flowing into it

Don't get too hung up on visualizing this perfectly. You can just see it as two triangles, one upside down and one the right way up, overlapping each other; or two pyramids. The entanglement and intention will do the rest. The spinner is going to spin the top tetrahedron clockwise. You can use your mind or your hand. The spinner will now connect to the star Sirius and see an electric pink light flow down from it, through Mother Earth's atmosphere, down through the sky, through the space, through the crown (on the hologram) of the breather and into the top tetrahedron. Now the top tetrahedron will spin crazy fast in a clockwise direction.

Next, the spinner will spin the bottom tetrahedron anti-clockwise, with the hand or mind. The spinner will then focus on the centre of the planet, where a large merkaba lies. This is Mother Earth's heart. Her top tetrahedron is electric green and her bottom tetrahedron is platinum. The spinner will intend the electric green light to flow up through the rocks and the minerals, up through the surface of the planet, through the breather's hologram (body) and up into the bottom tetrahedron of the merkaba spinning around the pineal gland. The bottom tetrahedron is now spinning really fast in an anti-clockwise direction. The merkaba in full flow is creating a vortex and blood and energy is being drawn into the area of the pineal gland. Also, the breather is squeezing and pulling. Both elements are working together.

The spinner will see light codes flow through the green and pink light and their job is to see that light flowing faster and stronger. The spinner can also increase the bandwidth to bring in more light. Now you are going to start the clock and do this for twenty minutes. You are going to do it every day for seven days. The spinner and the breather will swap over and do twenty minutes each.

Remember, you can do this for yourself: simply see your own hologram, vertical in the space above you, or wherever you would like to create it.

The information flowing through the pink and green lights contains very specific coding for activating and amping up the pineal gland's ability to tune in to, receive and transduce the information flowing through the field.

PLEASE NOTE: The reason we use the hologram now becomes clear: because we are bringing vertical light streams up and down through the body, if the human being is lying horizontal, it can be confusing to the mind. Using the hologram eliminates any confusion and takes the ego mind out of the way. If you are used to playing with energy, you may not need to use the hologram when working on a partner. When you work on yourself, you also have the option to work on your hologram or your body. If you do this exercise on your own, you will be breathing and spinning and you have the choice to use your hologram or not. Personally, I use my own hologram for this, whether I am standing or lying. I always use my own hologram when working on myself.

I recommend you do Part 1 for seven days before moving on to Part 2.

EXERCISE *Part 2*

The second part of the process starts off like the first: the breather is breathing normally, squeezing their perineum, genitals and buttocks and pulling back the abdominals towards the spine and releasing and re-squeezing periodically. The spinner continues to visualize the hologram, pineal gland and merkaba, spins the top tetrahedron clockwise and brings in the pink light, spins the bottom tetrahedron anti-clockwise and brings in the electric green light. At this point, the spinner visualizes a second merkaba in the heart centre of the breather.

The spinner now becomes aware of Mother Earth's merkaba once again. This time they intend the platinum light to flow up through the rocks and the minerals (from the bottom tetrahedron), up through the surface of the planet, through the breather's hologram (body) and up into the merkaba in the heart. Both tetrahedrons fill up with platinum light and also start spinning, the top one clockwise and the bottom one anti-clockwise. This merkaba draws electromagnetic energy into it from the breather's field, and the breath and the squeeze push this energy up into the pineal gland.

The platinum light, which filled up the merkaba in the heart space then flows up through the body. At this point the green light and the platinum light are on completely different frequency bands and travel separately next to/ through each other in the same space and into the bottom tetrahedron of the top merkaba. The platinum and electric green lights merge together once they arrive there. This combined frequency stays in the bottom tetrahedron. Even though the top and bottom tetrahedron are superimposed over each other, spinning through the same space, they do not recognize the frequencies in each of the tetrahedrons at this stage. The pink light in the top tetrahedron now flows down into the merkaba in the heart. At this point the breather brings their attention to their pineal

gland. The breather also starts to fire-breathe, keeping everything squeezed for ten breaths and then releasing for ten breaths as they breathe in through the nose, down to the pit of the stomach and out through the nose, hard and fast.

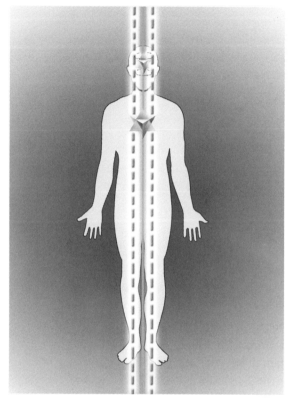

66. Introduction of second merkaba and the flow of pink, green, and platinum light from Sirius and Earth

The above image shows the flow of the pink, green and platinum light (see also colour insert after page 160).

Now everything is in motion, the clock starts. The breather will continue breathing, squeezing and releasing (every ten breaths) and will keep their attention on their pineal gland. The spinner will keep increasing the flow of pink, electric green and platinum light and see light codes flowing through all three streams. The spinner can increase the bandwidth and make the light brighter, elevating the total experience.

After twenty minutes swap over.

PLEASE NOTE: You do not need to do Part 1 for twenty minutes first. That is just the preparation phase. Get the functionality of Part 1 into operation and move into Part 2 and it all becomes one process.

I recommend you do Part 2 for seven days before moving on to Part 3.

EXERCISE *Part 3*

The third part of the process starts like Part 2. The breather is breathing normally, squeezing their perineum, genitals, and buttocks and pulling their abdominals back towards the spine. The spinner (or if it's you that is working on you, you do the same) visualizes the hologram, pineal gland and merkabas, spins the top tetrahedron clockwise (in the top merkaba) and brings in the pink light, spins the bottom tetrahedron (in the top merkaba) anti-clockwise and brings in the electric green light and then sees the platinum light flowing from Mother Earth's bottom tetrahedron into the merkaba in the heart, which fills up that one, flows into the bottom tetrahedron of the top merkaba and then the pink light flows down into the merkaba in the heart.

At this point the spinner visualizes a third merkaba halfway between the heart and the perineum. The green and platinum light flow straight through it. It's unrecognizable in terms of frequency at this stage. The green and platinum light now flows up, from the bottom tetrahedron of the top merkaba, into the top tetrahedron of it (where the pink, green and platinum frequencies become one) and the pink light (combined with the others – a tri-wave frequency) flows down and fills up the bottom merkaba. This merkaba also now starts to spin rapidly, the top tetrahedron clockwise and the bottom one anti-clockwise. The incredible thing is this: it's a natural process. You don't need to encourage or intend the light. It just flows of its own accord – you will see/feel.

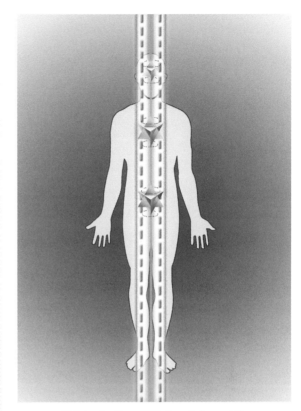

67. Introduction of third merkaba and the continuation of light/energy flowing

Light now starts to flow between all three merkabas. Code will move up and down. At this point the breather brings their attention to their pineal gland and starts to breathe holotropically. In through the nose, deep into the belly and out through the mouth, hard and fast, exhaling with a force that can create noise, squeezing and releasing as they do. Again, I would squeeze for ten breaths and release for ten breaths.

Now everything is in motion, the clock starts. The breather will continue breathing, squeezing and releasing and will keep their attention on their pineal gland. The spinner will keep increasing the flow of pink, electric green, platinum lights and see light codes flowing through all streams. The spinner can increase the bandwidth and make the light brighter, elevating the total experience.

After twenty minutes swap over.

PLEASE NOTE: You do not need to do Part 1 or 2 for twenty minutes first. Just get the functionality of Part 1 in operation and move into Part 2, get that in operation and then move on to Part 3 and it all becomes one process. Once you move on to Part 3, you will never need to do Parts 1 or 2 again, unless you have stopped for several weeks, then you would possibly want to build up again.

IMPORTANT: On Part 3, many of our workshop participants go past their normal breathing and into a state where they are breathing cosmic energy. It's a beautiful experience but at the same time it can be a little scary. The ego gets scared. It realizes you are not breathing and panics a little. It may bring you back to your normal breath. It's OK if this happens to you. Try to remain as present as possible and you can bypass this ego situation.

After doing Part 1 for seven days, and Part 2 for seven days, I recommend you do Part 3 a few times a week, or maybe daily. I know some people who do it twice a day and are so tapped in. Make it a part of your life. You brush your teeth and wash, so why not make this a part of your lifestyle? You will find your way with it; and remember, I'm going to share with you my plan and how I do it to give you some ideas.

These three merkabas are very important. The way I like to do this on a regular basis is as follows: Get all three merkaba fields spinning and all three light streams flowing and then do ten minutes of breath one, ten minutes of breath two and then ten minutes of breath three. Once a week or every couple of weeks I will go at this for 60 to 90 minutes. As you go through this process, you are also activating your source code template, which is a tri-wave template. We have been running on a limiting bi-wave cellular structure template for a loooooong time, and it creates ageing and death.

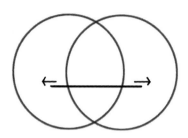

68. Bi-wave cellular structure where energy is finite, creating aging and death

Within this structure energy shuttles backwards and forwards and has nowhere to flow. So, we get old and die. As, when activating the pineal gland, you link all three merkabas together through the light-encoded streams, you will switch the geometry and activate the source code template, which in turn re-engineers the cellular structure and creates a tri-wave system with back flow to source/the zero-point.

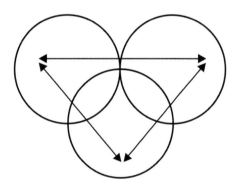

69. Third sphere of consciousness comes into play, creating the tri-wave structure, so energy can flow freely

Within this structure the energy can flow freely, producing quantum sparks as the energy can flow and make its way back to the zero-point bringing in eternal life force currents. Remember, they are spheres not circles and the bottom sphere links all three. Within this cellular structure ageing becomes a thing of the past, a concept. We were once eternal beings, connected to Source, the primary light and sound fields and we chose when we wanted to exit our bodily vehicles. They didn't decay and often we took them with us, having the ability to de-materialize and re-materialize in another location. There are many geometries within our field that do not serve us well. In our Star Magic Meditations, I have used these geometries to reverse the codex, to invert the maths back to how it should be. There are many talented grid workers and quantum architects who "innerstand" the game and have also been re-engineering the quantum schematics and aligning our planet with the Krystal Architecture.

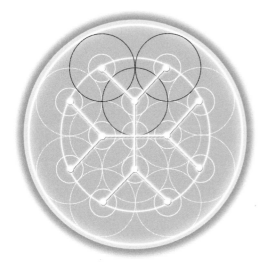

70. God Seed Atom, original source code

If you look at the above image you will see the original source code, the original universal/God Seed or God Atom. This is the original nature of the cosmic fabric from which all things unfold. The God Seed, as the first level of individuation from Source, holds the full pattern of the original pulse of consciousness that you came into manifestation on. All manifestation, all individuation is based on sets of twelve. Inside the seed you will see twelve spheres. These represent twelve streams of consciousness and twelve strands in our DNA. It represents the truth and the infinite flow of universal energy

and how the source point or zero-point, in the centre, connects to all life everywhere. If you look at the top two circles within this diagram, the one that joins the two represents the tri-wave cellular structure and how that connects with the centre, the zero-point. The lines (highlighted) connecting to the centre point of each of the cells show how the energy is pulled from the centre of each of these cells back to the zero-point. The energy flows from the zero-point back through each cell (consciousness field), also in an inverse fashion. These spheres could represent planets, galaxies, or universes. The mathematics is the same. Everything should be interconnected in this seamless and harmonious way.

Activating your pineal gland using the Third Eye Merkaba Matrix not only brings your third eye online properly, it sets in motion the foundation, the building blocks to change your inner geometry and move from the Old Earth structure to the New Earth structure. From the Fibonacci to the Krystal. From Metatron Mechanics to God Seed Intelligence.

It's very important that you stay hydrated when you commence this work. We should all be drinking a minimum of three litres of water per day and staying hydrated anyway, but with this level of work, up your daily intake. The more liquid crystal in your body, the healthier you are and the easier and more effectively these cosmic frequencies can flow through you. I often drink six litres per day. Doing this work and exercising vigorously, it's imperative.

The reason why this is so effective is because the merkabas are drawing light and information into them, all of which are in the central channel of the body. The squeezing of the bodily parts (genitals, perineum, buttocks, abdominals) pushes the information and energy up through the body and into the pineal gland area. The information starts flowing from the Earth and the Stars, and communicates with the third eye of the breather.

Also, the focus of the breather (keeping the attention on the pineal gland area) draws the energy into that sweet spot.

If you do this on your own straight out of the gate, please ensure that you do it lying down until you get acclimatized. You can still get a little dizzy standing and the more effort you put in, the more intense it can be. You do get used to it though and once you do, you can really start pushing the boundaries and expanding. And with this work, go hard. Push yourself, stretch yourself and go where it's uncomfortable and I promise you the rewards will blow your mind. Once you finish the twenty minutes on Part 2 (or the thirty, sixty, or ninety minutes if you go harder), the best thing to do is lie in silence and let your body do what your body does best: self-heal.

Recalibration Symptoms

It's important to mention that this work can cause the body to have symptoms. As well as opening and activating your third eye, you are cleansing the body and healing deeply. You are bringing high levels of light/information and oxygen into the cells. This can cause the body to feel pain — the organs, joints, bones. You may experience headaches or feel nauseous, or when the heart is opening/expanding you may find it hard to breathe and have a tight chest. Your arms and legs can go numb, and your body may contort. You can drift off into other realities, and that isn't cool if you are standing. (Please follow my suggestions. Get used to it lying down and then do it standing.) These symptoms don't happen to everyone, but they do happen, so be in your own individual process with this experience. Accept and keep creating magic.

Upside Down

Another incredible way to stimulate the pineal and pituitary glands is to be upside down in a headstand position. A few minutes daily has so many benefits as well as increasing the blood flow to the brain and stimulating these incredible glands (see also page 94).

EXERCISE *Headstand*

I generally stay in a headstand position and breathe deeply, just as I would if I was the right way up. Before you can start you need to have a basic level of strength and be able to support your body weight in other ways. If you can't do push-ups, squats, plank, then wait until you can and when you do give it a go, use a wall for support and ensure your body is in alignment – nice and straight.

It's also good to put your hands and feet on the floor and then place your head down. Take 90 per cent weight in your feet and hands and 10 per cent on your head. Move your neck slightly, back and forth and side to side, to build strength. Then go 80 per cent feet and hands and 20 per cent head and move back and forth and side to side. Then 70 per cent/30 per cent, and so on. When you feel comfortable, interlock your hands behind the back of your head and have your elbows, forearms and head on the floor, along with your feet/toes and the majority of the weight on your toes. Again, gradually move more weight onto your head and build up the strength and confidence. When you feel ready, you can kick your legs up into a headstand. Make sure you are in front of a wall to begin with, for extra support.

I recommend that you build up your headstand slowly; you can start with even a 5–10-second supported one. Remember to breathe deeply and be calm and relaxed. You may want to use a cushion to start with if you have a wooden or another type of hard floor. If you are unsure of anything, then it's best to get some guidance from a yoga instructor or personal trainer who "innerstands" this work.

When the pituitary gland is activated during a headstand, endorphins are released and there is a reduction in the levels of the stress hormone cortisol. The continued headstand practice can alter your brain chemistry and aid you in producing ideal cortisol levels naturally.

In yoga, the headstand is considered the king of poses because of its many benefits, which range from improved brain function and mood to increased upper-body strength. When done in correct alignment, many muscles are engaged, including those of the arms, upper back and core.

When the body is upside down and the pituitary stimulated, digestion is improved, metabolism can speed up, hormone production is regulated and the process of water reabsorption in the kidneys is enhanced. Headstands are also recommended for Irritable Bowel Syndrome and other digestive ailments, as they reorient the colon and intestines, encouraging healthy bowel movements.

Many yoga instructors say that a headstand is the equivalent of a facial because it stimulates blood flow to the face. Increased circulation to the skin of the cheeks and forehead means oxygenation and keeps you looking younger and maintains a healthy, energetic glow.

Because the pituitary gland is responsible for releasing endorphins, (the body's happy hormones), headstands can alleviate the sadness and lethargy associated with depression.

Headstands as well as reducing the production of cortisol, the stress hormone, increase blood flow to the brain, stimulating the production of melatonin, dopamine and serotonin, all hormones that help regulate mood. They also stimulate the brain and the spine, as well as the cerebrospinal fluid – and remember, we want that cerebral spinal fluid stimulated and flowing up towards the brain. Super-Humans spend time upside down.

The Magic of Breath and the Pineal Gland

The merkaba spinning and breathing exercise from the last chapter is potent and if that is all you ever did you would activate massively. It's the most powerful way to activate your third eye. However, there are many ways to switch yourself on and from personal experience, working on myself and also with an international client base, adopting a multi-faceted approach is best. Firstly, you get to hit this from different angles and secondly you keep things interesting. Doing the same every day can be boring for some people. But it's worth remembering that a Formula One racing car drinks the same high-performance fluids every day it races.

So, while many people like variety, sometimes sticking to the same thing might be best for results. It's your body and you should listen to what it wants.

Here I want to look at some breathing techniques. We have met them already, but now we've done more work we can go into much greater depth and approach them with more wisdom.

There are three in total, plus a bonus breath, and you can do them on their own or stack them on top of each other, which is what I do and what I ask our workshop and training participants to do.

They are powerful exercises that will transform you and upgrade your dimethyltryptamine (DMT) levels. DMT, as we know, is found in large quantities in the cerebral spinal fluid and is thought to be produced in the lungs and the eyes. And it's produced in the pineal gland as a by-product of the work.

EXERCISE 1 *Breathing – 21 and Hold*

Lie down flat and relax with your eyes closed. Breathe in through your nose, down to the pit of your stomach and back out through your mouth. That is one breath. Ensure you breathe deep and strong and reasonably fast; but speed isn't the aim.

Repeat this twenty-one times. On the last breath, let all oxygen out of your body when breathing out, hold the breath out and be still. Lie there, just being, for as long as you can. When you get to the point when you really need to breathe, you start again and repeat the twenty-one breaths.

This time around, on the twenty-first breath you will do exactly the same: let the oxygen out and then be still. Lie there. You will find your mind empties, and you can stay in this space much longer than at the end of the first lot of twenty-one inhales and exhales. You may find that you start to drift, travel, journey, become unaware of your body and the fact that you are not breathing. You can at this stage become pure consciousness. You may see colours, patterns, geometry, symbol, images. It's totally normal. Surrender!

Once you get to the point where you need to breathe, start again and repeat another twenty-one breaths. At the end of the twenty-first, exhale once again and be in your space. This time you will go longer again, and if you didn't drift or travel the first time it's likely you will now. As a test, it's good to ask someone to be there with you and time the three holding periods at the end of each set of breaths. You may find that after the first set you can hold for forty-five or sixty-five seconds. At the end of the second set, you will find you double your time, or maybe more. At the end of the third set you could be there for 3–5 minutes without taking in any oxygen, possibly a lot longer. The more you do this practice and surrender, the deeper you will go.

If I was going to do this as a stand-alone exercise I would do it five times. Generally, I will use it before the next two exercises.

EXERCISE 2 *Pressure Breathing*

These next two exercises I like to alternate. You are going to continue in the lying position with your eyes closed. Make sure the tip of your tongue is on the roof of your mouth throughout the exercise.

Squeeze your perineum, genitals and buttocks and pull your abdominals back towards your spine. You are then going to focus on a merkaba down in the centre of the Earth. The top tetrahedron is electric green and the bottom one is platinum. Visualize the platinum light racing up through the rocks and the minerals, up through the surface of the planet and into your perineum. If you want to use a hologram for this you can. Or you can imagine that you are vertical, and the Earth is underneath you. It's your choice.

Next you will breathe in and pull the platinum light up though your body, with the breath. Your focus/awareness will be on both. You will draw the platinum light up into your mind/crown and your focus will be there also. Once you get to the top, with a full belly of oxygen, your attention and focus moves to the centre of your brain and back slightly, exactly where your pineal gland is. You are going to keep your focus there for thirteen seconds and hold your breath as you do. Once you get to thirteen seconds, you will release the squeeze and let out the breath slowly. Bring your attention back to your heart, and just be for 2–4 seconds.

After you relax and be for between 2 and 4 seconds (whatever feels right) you will repeat the process. You are going to do this thirteen times.

After the thirteenth set, you are going to lie still for two minutes and just be.

Next, if you are alternating like I do, move to Exercise Three.

204

EXERCISE 3 *Fire Breathing*

"You can do this standing as you progress...." and get used to it. It is intense, though, so I recommend that you start lying with your eyes closed, get used to it and then switch gears after a few weeks or whenever you feel you are ready. I have seen people really go for this and leave their body while they are standing and the body has collapsed, so be sensible. Remember, you are doing this after the previous work, so you are already charged with light and oxygen and activated.

Some people call this breath the breath of fire or dragon breathing. We have looked at it already, but it is a fundamental technique. You are going to squeeze your perineum, genitals and buttocks and pull your abdominals back towards your spine. Doing this breath with the abdominals pulled back takes a little getting used to, but you are a Super-Human. I have faith in you, beautiful soul.

Next you are going to place your right hand on your stomach, just below your belly button. This hand is a target for your breath. You are going to breathe in through your nose, down into your stomach and back out through your nose as fast and as hard as you can while all of your attention is on your pineal gland. Each time the forceful breath enters your body it will push your stomach and hand out. So, as you breathe rapidly, with every breath your hand will be like a firing piston going up and down/in and out. You are going to breathe like this for six minutes. It requires real focus. You may feel tired, your nose may start burning or running or get blocked/stuffed. Keep going. Again, you will get better with practice. Make sure the tip of your tongue is on the roof of your mouth throughout this exercise.

Once you finish you will lie still for two minutes.

Then you will repeat Exercise Two, rest for two minutes, repeat Exercise Three, rest for two minutes, repeat Exercise Two, rest for two minutes, repeat Exercise Three. So, three sets of Exercises Two and Three, alternated. Or you could do three sets of two and then three sets of three. I sometimes cut out the rest, to really amplify things, and go from one exercise to the next. This really cranks it up again. Play around with it. After you have completed the three sets you are going to kick back and relax and just be. After all this hard work, your body will start to do what it needs to do to heal, elevate and transform you. Again, you may lose all sense of time and space while DMT races through your system, while your nervous system goes to work and your pineal gland is tuning in to and transducing information from the cosmic fabric, the ether. You have to kick back and enjoy the fruits of your labour. I've seen miracles take place in our trainings when people have done this for the first time, second time, third time. It just keeps getting better. When you truly put the effort into this systematical breathing approach you will be rewarded, massively. Mental, physical, emotional trauma, GONE!

The information that you tap into spiritually/ esoterically is mind-blowing. But you have to really put the effort in. Really go for it. Push yourself and let nature do the rest.

You could do all of these every day, but it is time-consuming. You are looking at a minimum of one hour and thirty minutes, taking into consideration the relaxing period at the end, which is usually twenty minutes minimum. It can be much longer if you hold the out-breath for greater periods of time on Exercise One. You may want to consider doing the full routine one or twice a week and bits of it every day. I will suggest a plan for you at the end of the book. Trust the process. If you are overwhelmed right now, it's OK. You may feel more overwhelmed as you continue reading but once you see the plan at the end, you will know exactly what must be done.

Bonus Breath

On our trainings, after going through these first three exercises we will always do one hour (sometimes more) of holotropic breathwork. When you have a group doing this it becomes very tribal and a galactically transformative experience.

On our trainings we normally do it as a part of a ceremony where we drink our Star Magic Cacao Elixir (and Mother Aya, on our Deep In Space Retreats) and then do some specific chanting exercises before going into the first three exercises and finally this. So, you can imagine, by the time people get to this stage they are often already in a completely elevated and expanded state of consciousness. People leave their bodies, burst into ancient or native tongues, sometimes speaking light language, their bodies morph and human beings doing the work have risen from the ground a few inches.

Quite often people's brains shut down and they drop under into an altered state, or even fall asleep, because it's too much. We get in their ear, wake them back up and get them focused and back in the game. It really is a team effort. I am a bit like a spiritual personal trainer in this environment, pushing you to your limits and then taking you beyond.

Maybe you could get a few friends together. Doing it in a group definitely helps because the group energy carries you through the dips and the tough periods. When people do this in our trainings, my team and I constantly walk around motivating everyone.

This breathing can seem daunting at first, especially doing an hour. It's taxing on the body and mind. But even doing it once a month will be awesome.

You will be lying down, eyes closed. Breathe in through your nose, down to the pit of your stomach and back out through your mouth. As you exhale, do it forcefully and make a kind of grunting/shouting sound. I always count people in at the start and encourage everyone to breathe rhythmically and in sync with each other for the first ten minutes. It's good to set a steady pace and slowly increase it. Generally, by fifteen minutes every one is at full capacity going hell for leather. Once you get to thirty minutes and cross the halfway point it feels easier because the finish line is in sight. After forty minutes it's pure joy, like you are journeying.

It's important to know, too, that your body may go numb, your hands, feet, fingers and toes. You may feel pain in your vital organs. Your body may contort. I have seen a lady turn into a swan, another soul a praying mantis. We had a guy go to the toilet once and come back so happy. He said when he went to pee, he was peeing out light codes. Just a stream of codes in his urine that went on and on. We've had ancient tribes come into our space where frequency bands/dimensions have bled into each other. You can see them, feel them, smell the fire and incense.

Once the hour is up it's really important to lie in silence and observe your body. This is where you go into deep healing and also where trauma and information rises. Stay and be as long as you can. It's good to be and observe. After fifteen minutes on our retreats, we go into a deep guided meditation.

I have seen people leave their body and not be able to get back. I have to go in and find what reality they are in and guide them back. This requires a particular skill set and a set of calm nerves. I am sharing this with you because you need to be aware of the possible scenarios that can flow out from going on these deep experiences. So be sensible. If you are on your own, maybe don't adopt a go hard-or-go-home attitude to start with. Feel into it and build up slowly.

The other thing is this. If you do a full routine as above, don't drink too much water beforehand. If you do the routine in the morning, drink

250–500 mls max. If you do it in the evening, stop drinking fluids three hours before and have a big pee before you start. Bon Voyage!

5D Light Body and 5D Activation

All of us have a light body. Our light bodies are made of light, high-vibrational geometries/mathematics, that weave together and create the most mesmerizing spectacle. There is actually so much light and information travelling through our space that if you tried to depict it all you wouldn't see anything but lots of lines and patterns and spheres and codes that are not really solid but fluid, moving lines and codes and patterns that take your breath away. It's simply pure light and vibration. Our physical human bodies are a sliver of what we are.

The ascension process that people talk about can be total rubbish, or perfection. It depends on your perception and understanding/ "innerstanding". I feel we are simply raising our vibration and expanding our conscious awareness so that we can remember our wholeness, embody more light and in essence be less dense and also get to grips with our mathematical structure so we can navigate Star Gates and make our way out from this time-based matrix. But that is just my opinion based on my under- and "inner"standing and none of us will ever truly know unless we do or don't go somewhere.

As we are becoming less dense, we let go of our human trauma and start loving, caring, sharing, being kind and loving each other with a ferociousness that dissolves any potential judgement. The result of this is that we live in total acceptance of all things and naturally vibrate on a higher frequency, pure love. As we raise our vibration and expand our consciousness, I feel we will be able to have full conscious access to our multidimensional selves, hosted in other frequency bands/dimensional spaces, and can be having two or three or four or more very real experiences at the same time. The eternal I AM, will be all that is essential. Memory, thoughts, they will be less important. It already happens to us – a thought can be in your head and then poof, it's gone again. You try to remember it but it's not there. That is because it's not relevant any more in this moment. If it's important it will surface again. Telepathy, healing and telekinesis will also naturally rise as gifts within our species, as we move into a higher vibrational field of experience.

There are many different components to our light body and some people's light bodies are switched on fully and some are not. Some components of people's light bodies are used to manipulate them. For example, our merkaba. Our female (bottom – magnetic) tetrahedron is supposed to spin twice as fast as our male (top – electromagnetic) tetrahedron. When these spin rates change so does the frequency within the human being connected to this merkaba. There are souls teaching other souls to spin their tetrahedrons opposite to the way I have shared and some people are telling others to spin both tetrahedrons the same way. This also manipulates the energetic field and creates havoc. When the rate of spin is doubled in both tetrahedrons and the angle of rotation is changed the human being in question can travel from one quantum space to another through this vehicle. This, in essence, is time travel, or multidimensional or interdimensional teleportation, depending on where you go. Mirrored space-time is created and the ability to appear in the mirrored version is possible. This is positive when used effectively. Your merkaba is also a manifestation machine, and we will discuss this later on because once it's switched on, you can literally manifest anything and everything, quicker than normal.

When the rotation of the particles is adjusted (by forces that do not have our best interest at heart) our merkaba can wobble, and the field becomes incoherent, and we will become unbalanced. I will be showing you the fastest way to keep your merkaba balanced later when we discuss manifestation using the merkaba fields.

When I started seeing these spinning tetrahedrons around people I didn't even know what a merkaba was, as well as other geometries. I spoke with other healers, spiritual teachers and psychics, and others too had experienced the same.

As I continued to facilitate the healing of more people, I began to see patterns in these geometries. I saw what happened to them during and after a healing session and what state they were in prior to the healing session. I learned about clients' mental, physical, emotional and spiritual well-being, before and after healing sessions, and started to analyze what I was and what I was not doing during sessions to invoke this change.

I soon realized that all of us needed our light bodies to be functioning effectively in order to be happy, healthy and on a high vibration. Sometimes, just opening a client's heart and shredding their parallel life trauma, having a coherent mind and heart, shifted the light body and its components into gear. This made me realize that love, real love is the predominant factor in being healthy and vibrant.

I also realized that not everyone could easily find this coherence and I wanted to find a recipe for success, a way of assisting my brothers and sisters. In order to activate our light bodies fully, so we can raise our vibration and live and operate in 5D, from within a more loving field of coherence that has access to more information, we must first of all "innerstand" certain components of our light body.

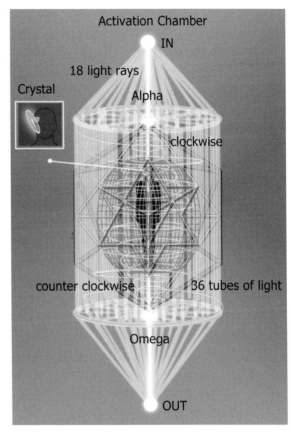

71. 5D light body and activation chamber

Above is a picture of our fifth-dimensional light body and its components. You have the physical being (the human) in the middle of the light body, then the merkaba, the octahedron, the toroidal field, the icosahedron, and the larger cylinder with the activation chamber at the top and bottom. There are other components that are important to highlight and we will add those in soon. Doing your qigong, breathwork, pineal gland activation exercises and other activations I will share later will all assist in switching on and maintaining this invisible-to-most energetic structure. What it also creates is a spiral of light that flows through and around your body.

Light travels down through the in-point of this energetic structure, then it flows through the next sphere of light, which is your alpha (male/positive) transmission centre. The light travels through your physical body and out through the next sphere of light, your omega (female/negative) transmission centre, then down through the out-point of the chamber. You are literally giving birth to light codes through this network of light. Between the alpha and the omega, there are transmission centres.

We have spoken about these already, *but it is important.* These transmission centres control the flow of cosmic energy, based on the strength and vibration of the person's physical and energetic bodies. Transmission centres are like dams, opening and closing fluidly and naturally to protect, amplify, upgrade the human being in question. This is why exercise and nutrition, coupled with qigong and breathwork, are mission critical for your Super-Human evolution. You must be physically strong to enable you to handle the electromagnetic and magnetic currents flowing through your body. Energy also shuttles in reverse, back up through this structure to the stars. Everything is a two-way process.

What is important to know is that we are multidimensional beings and there are many versions of us in the same space. We operate in sets of twelve. There are twelve of us here in this frequency band and each of those twelve has an oversoul, consisting of twelve, and each of those twelve has an avatar version, again, consisting of twelve. All versions have a Light body. What this means is that there are multiple geometries and multiple cylinders, all spinning in the same space.

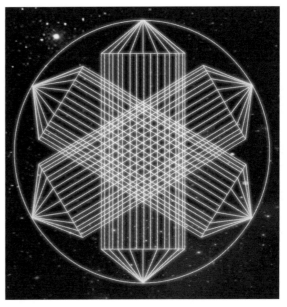

72. Multiple activation chambers

The illustration above depicts a dumbed down, simple version of this (as if it were all depicted, it would just be pure light and nothing would be clear. All of these cylinders are constantly rotating and it's the rotation that creates a larger toroidal field in our space among other spherical rotations of light that expand and expand. This image is a front-on view and it shows three cylinders, but in actuality (as mentioned) there are a larger number of cylinders because there *are* many versions of us existing in the quantum field.

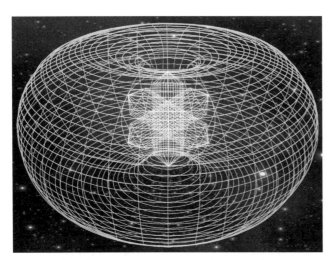

73. Multiple activation chambers spinning and creating a larger toroidal field which expands and contracts in unison with the activation chambers

The image above shows the larger extended toroidal field that is around your body. It extends far in all directions and we naturally contract and expand this field of light.

When the merkaba field is functioning as it should, and these cylinders are spinning very quickly, the person is in a high-vibrational state. How fast do the cylinders spin? I don't know. But when I ask the question, I am told way beyond the speed of light.

One day when I was working on a client I was visited by a blue Lyran being. This being told me that to shift someone into a place where they could adjust their consciousness, from a 3D or 4D state of awareness to a 5D state (+) of awareness, and in turn switch their light body on, so they can start accessing the Krystal Coding, there was a protocol to use, and they showed me. I have tried it on hundreds of people in our workshops and trainings and those who I've shown it to have had amazing results with their clients also. It's simple and it works and so I will share it with you.

PROTOCOL *Switching on the 5D Light Body*

The first thing you do is bring up the client's hologram or, if you are doing it for yourself, your hologram, and lie it horizontally in front of you. Hold up your right or left hand several inches away from them, below their feet and in the centre. You then see/visualize/know there is a violet octahedron in the palm of your hand. See or intend this code into it: **R44RX3**.

You only need to intend this code the first time around. After you have used it, it becomes a part of you and will just happen as soon as you enter the space and raise your hand, knowing what you are about to do.

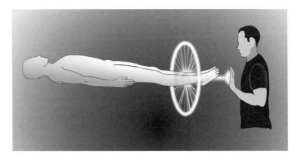

74. Octahedron in hand and light coming out to create the first wheel of light

So, you hold your hand, see the octahedron, intend the code and then watch. You will see that a stream of light flows out from it in between the feet/ankles. Eighteen streams then flow out from it and create a circle of light, as in the image above.

Next, another set of eighteen streams of light flow out from the circle and into the heart.

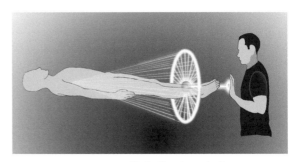

75. 18 streams of light flow into the heart

At this point one of two things will happen.

1. Another eighteen streams of light flow out from the heart and form another circle, as in the illustration below.

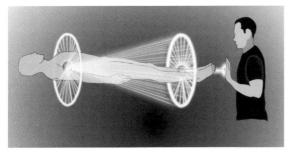

76. 18 streams of light create the second wheel of light

2. Or the platonic solids appear above the human being's heart, as shown below.

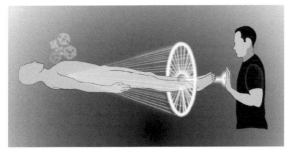

77. Platonic solids appear above the heart

In the first scenario, the eighteen light streams appear as below, and form a second circle. Then another eighteen streams of light flow from the second circle of light into the pineal gland.

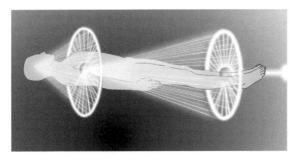

78. 18 streams of light flow into the pineal gland

A third circle then appears. Eighteen streams of light flow out from it, up into the alpha transmission centre, and then a stream of light flows down through the human body all the way down through the planet and into the centre of Mother Earth.

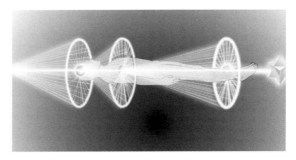

79. 18 streams of light flow into the alpha transmission centre

This light stream connects with her merkaba and locks the person into a new information stream held in a 5th-density space within the Earth's grids where a pool of Krystal Coding is held. The human being now has information flowing into them from above and below.

At this point the person who you are working with will start to shift, their 5D light body will come online and start to activate. For some people it can happen within minutes and in others it's a process that can take weeks or, in a rare number of cases, months. This sets them up nicely to do all of the exercises in this book and continue to elevate and expand.

Now let's discuss scenario two. The platonic solids appear above the human being's heart, as in the image below.

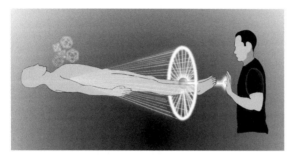

80. Platonic solids appear above the heart

This means the human being is out of alignment and you have to collect the platonic solids, place them inside of each other, then place them in the heart (see image 81 to the right). You place them in this order:

> The icosahedron goes inside the octahedron, the octahedron goes inside the tetrahedron, the tetrahedron goes inside the cube, which goes inside of the dodecahedron. You then take the dodecahedron, which contains all of the other geometries, and put them neatly inside the heart space.

It's important to note that these geometrical building blocks are not stand-alone. They represent a part of a whole field of code. This field's spiral flowing formation connects cosmically and seamlessly with the flow of the Krystal Spiral. Nature will take its course once again from this point on. By that I mean the heart will open, the eighteen light streams will flow, and the same process will occur. Another eighteen streams of light flow from the second circle of light into the pineal gland. A third circle then appears, eighteen streams of light flow out from it, up into the alpha transmission centre, and then a stream of light flows down through the human body all the way down through the planet and

into the centre of Mother Earth. This light stream connects with Mothers Earth's merkaba, locks into the Earth's grids where a pool of Krystal Coding is held and connects the human being into a new information stream held in a 5D space within the Earth. They now have information flowing into them from above and below. At this point the human being you are working with (or you, if you are working on yourself) will start to shift, their 5D light body will come online. It can happen within minutes and in others it's a process that can take weeks or in a rare number of cases, months.

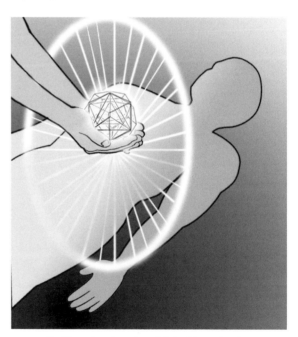

81. Place the platonic solids inside each other in the correct order and place into the heart

It's important to note that once the light locks into Earth's merkaba and into the Earth's grids where a pool of Krystal Coding is held, it also communicates with a huge diamond skull down in the centre of the planet, just below the merkaba. This diamond skull is like a huge hard drive. It contains data on our New/Old Earth Template, our Source Code Template Activation Keys (that link us to our celestial star family), New Earth

Architecture, Planetary Grids, Star Gates and more. This hard drive is constructed from an incorruptible crystal core transmitter that makes it impossible to hack. Our old/present Earth has many grid networks and Star Gates and they have been hacked and corrupted. Many were manipulated by a negative, dark force but some were not and some have been rebalanced. This entire field is literally a gigantic computer. The diamond skull (along with a number of crystal disks not in the Earth but elsewhere) in the centre of the Earth, carrying all of our new data streams for humanity's ascension, is built differently. It's a huge quantum computer that is always changing, moving, creating and recreating within itself so nothing is stagnant, making it near impossible to corrupt. I truly feel it's uncorruptible.

Your role in activating yourself or another human being to be 5D-ready is to simply facilitate the process. Start the ball rolling and let nature take its course; or start the ball rolling and then do what's necessary with the platonic solids, if it unfolds that way. This entire process takes seconds. A minute or so maximum. Sometimes the human being's reaction can be strong, other times they don't feel a thing. I was in the bank once, queuing up behind an old lady. I had just discovered this and was playing around. I asked her higher/inner self if it was OK and got the green light, so I brought up her hologram and went to work. She wobbled and I just put my hand on her shoulder and said, "Are you OK, love?" She turned and looked up at me with the most radiant grin on her face and sparkle in her eye. She didn't say anything. She just smiled. It was as though she was aware on a different level and was so grateful.

Do it with yourself first by bringing up your own hologram and then work with friends and then clients. This is a real gift for anyone on their journey, wanting to expand, elevate and move through the spiritual gears of consciousness. 5D baby, let's rock and roll!

Krystal Spiral and the New Earth

I have mentioned the Krystal Spiral and the new/ancient Earth frequency and now I want to go into this in more detail to explain the difference in two predominant energetic mathematical structures on Planet Earth. You have the Krystal Spiral and the Fibonacci Spiral.

The differences between the Krystal Spiral and Fibonacci Spiral can be understood in terms of their respective relationships to their creation point. The Krystal Spiral and the mathematical sequence from which it emerges come directly from the zero-point or central point of all creation/Source. The Krystal Spiral perpetually retains a living, breathing connection through the preservation of what came before, as it expands through multiplication. Out of the one comes the many.

Multiplication is the alchemical process that greatly increases the concentrated refinement, energetic effectiveness and sphere of influence of the embodied biological eternal light source, which in essence is the perfect union of the divine feminine and the divine masculine in a human being.

The Krystal Spiral/architecture is self-perpetuating and inner sustaining. Its maths is represented by including the zero-point or zero/Source in its numerical sequence: 0, 1, 1, 2, 4, 8, 16, 32, 64, etc, by doubling each numerical value as consciousness mathematically expands/evolves. Each of the numerical values is derived through returning to zero and adding all of the numbers together to get to the next highest value in the sequence. The value of zero represents the central point of union, or zero-point or God or Source or Infinite Intelligence. While increasing the values of the Krystal Spiral, the consciousness remains connected to the original Source field while progressively expanding.

In mathematics, the Fibonacci numbers or Fibonacci sequence are the numbers in the following sequence:

1, 1, 2, 3, 5, 8, 13, 21, 34, 55, 89, 144 . . .

If we pick any of the Fibonacci numbers, they will equal the last two Fibonacci numbers in the sequence, added together to create the current Fibonacci number.

Beginning with zero, then 1, it then moves on to the next number, as such: 0+1=1, 1+1=2, 2+1=3, 3+2=5, 5+3=8 and so forth.

When we apply this mathematical formula to quantify or measure the movement of energy or consciousness within time or space, the Fibonacci Spiral loses its connection going back to the zero-point or Source. Instead, the sequence uses the previous number to add into itself to get to the next higher number of the sequence. This is how humans have been operating for many years. Stand and crush the human being in front of you to climb up the ladder and if we leave them behind or if they suffer or die, so be it, it's a dog-eat-dog world.

The Fibonacci Spiral illustrates the maths used to perpetuate the war over energy, therefore the consciousness suppression on the Earth, as, when the sequence grows in number or size, it is due to the consumption of the previous values in order to grow itself larger. The larger it gets, the more it progressively moves out and away from the Krystal Spiral of the original core manifestation body or divine template body, as it expands. You have the timeline on Earth that is fuelled by compassion and unity and expansion and ultimately love, and one that contracts and is driven by ego and ultimately fear.

As I've said, everything has its place in this world and balance is the key. Love and fear are at opposite ends of the emotional spectrum but are not separate. You have varying degrees of both emotions up and down the scale and they are a part of one stream of consciousness but when it comes to the mathematics, there is only one frequency stream to ride if you truly want to ascend.

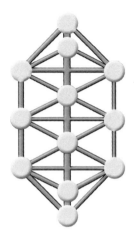

82. Kathara Grid

Above you have what is known as a Kathara Grid. The word Kathara refers to the core structure of morphogenetic fields, the holographic templates of sound—light and scalar waves that serve as the blueprints on which matter manifests.

When broken down into syllables Kathara is KA – Light, THA – Sound, RA – One.

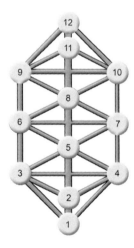

83. Kathara Grid with Star Gates and DNA strands

Above you can see the Kathara Grid with numbers. Each number represents a Star Gate. These also represent DNA strands 1–12 in the body. Later on I will show you the link between your transmission centres and DNA strands. There is a planetary Kathara, a Galactic and a Universal Kathara Grid

Structure. We don't need to go into the locations of the different Star Gates now. We will cover how to move through these Star Gates and the multidimensional and biological mechanics behind that in another book. Right now, we must activate ourselves and be ready. Ultimately, we must thrive on Earth and enjoy the human experience fully and at the same time as a by-product of doing the work that brings your full potential online, you will be preparing for interdimensional and multidimensional travel.

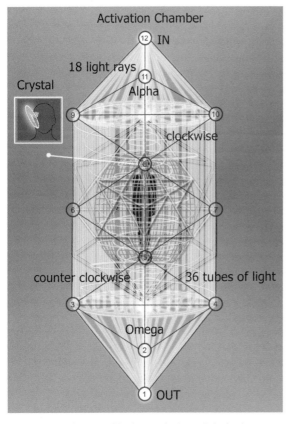

84. Kathara Grid laid over platinum light body

Above you can see how the Kathara Grid is overlaid vertically within the platinum light body structure. Also in the centre we see another horizontal smaller Kathara, which fits neatly inside the angles of the octahedron.

EXERCISE *Advanced Merkaba Activation*

I want to share with you some codes that will assist you in tuning your light body through sound and bringing high-frequency light from God/Source/primary light and sound fields into your energy body to activate it. This exercise will also activate your twelve-pointed advanced merkaba field. This we will discuss later.

All you will need to do for this exercise is be still. Eyes open or closed and go into a still state, a state of presence. Bring your awareness into your heart and feel/see/know your platinum light body structure is around the outside of you. Then one by one you will say these codes out loud or speak them in your mind. Codes 1–12 three times through. Do not say code 1 three times and then move to code 2. Say each code in order 3 times through and then move to code 13. As you speak them, feel them in your heart.

1. **Aya Eka U Ma**
2. **Reishi Ma Hun Sheya Ta**
3. **Kara Ki A Aa Nem Ka**
4. **Dera Mi Aa Kryst Na Ma Ra**
5. **Ei Esh Ee An Ra Ha Zi**
6. **Gresh Ee Ash A Ka**
7. **Gresh Rei Ash Ha Ya**
8. **Ta Ra Aan Dra N Shu Ma**
9. **Oo Nu Bta Ma Eshh Ta**
10. **Ka Ra Ak A E Ka**
11. **Ash Tei U Na Elo Nia Shu La**
12. **Aan Dren Vu Ea Kan Arataa**

Code 13 is the gateway to the original primary light and sound fields. The first part of code 13 – **Ka Ra Ya Sa Ta Aa La** – you will chant, keeping your awareness on your third eye. The second part of code 13 (see below) you will speak. Chant the first part once and then speak the second part and repeat two more times.

PART 1 – Ka Ra Ya Sa Ta Aa La

You will chant Ka, then Ra, then Ya, then Sa, then Ta, then Aa, then La.

Then speak part 2 below.

PART 2 – Kia Kuna An Shra Du Ka Ina Ma

Then repeat the sequence part 1 and part 2 two more times. As you are going through this process, feel Krystal Frequencies flowing down through your body and up through your body.

You will feel this. This is something you can do daily and always.

The Kathara Grid is the causal factor beneath all dimensional expressions, thus all forms of consciousness and consciousness integration-expansion too! The Kathara Grid is considered, therefore, to be the foundation on which the axiom grids, merkaba fields, auric field levels, subtle bodies, transmission centres, meridians and physical matter systems and multidimensional levels of consciousness manifest.

It is geometrically structured as twelve primary Kathara Centres connected by fifteen primary Kathara Lines. It is the core level of scalar standing wave/vortex creation and energetic organization within and behind all dimensionalized systems and is thus considered to be the core of the holographic template upon which the morphogenetic scalar wave/vortex blueprint and all other dimensions of form are built. The Kathara Grid is the causal element within all manifested effects of dimensionalization and consciousness. The form of the Kathara Grid is reflected in the Macrocosm and the Microcosm of all manifestation. All forms have at their core the common structure of the Kathara Grid holographic template spiralling in and out from the point of creation. Energy is eternal consciousness that perpetually changes form by projecting through the structures of the Kathara Grid, while simultaneously remaining with the same base template. Energy cannot be created or destroyed, as you know; it only changes form, following the geometric structure of the Kathara Grid.

The Kathara Grid, the one closest to Source, is called the Kryst Grid, and from it the Krystal Spiral emerges. The Krystal Spiral Code is the Perpetual Motion and Precise Mathematical—Geometrical Instructions for the Creation Program from Source.

Deviations from the natural Kryst Code configuration of "First Creation" create alterations of the energetic balance (inorganic Grids such as the Flower of Life and Metatron's Cube and Mathematics of the Fibonacci Spiral) causing interruption of the continual self-regeneration (perpetual life) of the manifest forms that eventually lead to destruction of the corresponding matter-form via self-annihilation.

Again, in our world, both the Fibonacci and the Krystal Spiral play their part in duality and within the realm of duality there is love and fear, beauty and magic and pain and suffering. It has been instrumental in our evolution for this time cycle and many humans are realizing that pain and suffering, while they play a role, are choices we can move away from. When I say pain and suffering in this context, I am referring to among other things, starving children, disease-ridden communities, paedophilia, 9/11, war and situations/circumstances that are avoidable when unity, balance and love are at the centre of life.

If there was unity and balance and love as our driving forces, wealth as well as health and happiness would be better distributed. The matrix as it is held in place by human compliance (and the fact that most of humanity are totally unaware that we are living in a false system, let alone that they have a choice to move out from it or change things) and when we shift our frequency, live from the heart, recode our mathematics, activate our dormant DNA, realize our power, we can amplify unity, balance and love and say no to this situation.

When we bring our attention to and embark on the journey of transformation through physical exercise, qigong, nutrition, healing ourselves, healing our relationships and other worldly pursuits, pain and suffering can be a part of the process. But perception here is everything. For me, there is no pain, there is simply the process. All emotions are a part of the process. All feelings. Everything physical and mental. How you perceive and frame the process is up to you. The process can be comfortable or uncomfortable. I choose to find comfort in the uncomfortable.

In illustration 85 on the left (top image) you can see the Krystal Spiral tracking the Kathara Grid rotations. As the Kathara spirals and expands, the Krystal Spiral is in alignment with it.

The bottom image of illustration 85 depicts how the Kathara Grid rotates, showing the axis of each grid on each of the turns. If you look into the very centre of the diagram, you will see a very small Kathara Grid. As it rotates and expands outwards (or inwards, depending on your perception, because it's infinite and will go inwards as well as outwards), it rotates at 45-degree increments. These are the lines of vibration and oscillation that the Krystal Spiral tracks.

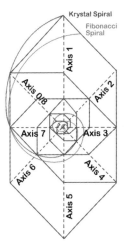

86. Krystal Spiral and Fibonacci Spiral

Above you can see the Krystal Spiral next to the Fibonacci Spiral. They are running a similar pattern. The Fibonacci Spiral is running an angle rotation of 60 degrees (such as the 60-degree angles with Metatron's Cube and the Flower of Life, both one and the same and contain the fallen Earth Mechanical Template Codes to create disharmony in nature) whereas the Krystal Spiral runs a 45-degree shift. These are the two timelines playing out. You can see where they overlap. It's expected that they will cross in November 2023. The plan is for the Fibonacci Spiral (the dark/negative frequency) to pull the Krystal Spiral into

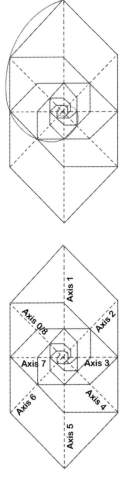

85. Kathara Grid and the Krystal Spiral tracking it

it, creating a lower-vibrational space on Earth once again. Right now, on Earth, you can see many dark and frightening events (for some but not for those who are aware and "innerstand" the game and play by their own rules) playing out; through the coronavirus, the war in Ukraine as well as many other aspects of reality we have already touched upon. Your mission is to raise your frequency, adjust to the New Earth Template Codes and ride the positive timeline, and the New Earth Timeline can pull the Fibonacci Timeline into it or they will both run their separate courses and some of humanity will ride one timeline and some will ride the other, and eventually humans on either timelines will not recognize each other and the vibrational space they are in because the frequencies are worlds apart. We can raise the vibration on Earth and create unity. Love is our greatest weapon. If we do pull the Fibonacci Timeline into the Krystal Spiral Timeline and create coherence, there is still the potential for some elements, people for example, to be pulled into the New Earth Architecture and some elements to remain, thus having two timelines running, because some humans could not free themselves from the bondage of darkness. Again, awareness

and choice. Some are unaware and so do not know there are options. Some are aware and still choose fear and others, like you and me, are aware and choose love, freedom and sovereignty.

The old geometries are used by grid workers/ healers/quantum architects who know how to reverse the mechanics and alter the templates. Some people follow these structures blindly and are locking themselves into a false program. At Star Magic we used them strongly for a couple of years, in meditation groups, to do the necessary grid work on the Earth to correct the mess that was made in the quantum. Now the foundation is complete in the quantum, we are focused on the New Earth Codex and the Krystal Spiral Template Frequencies to hold space for the collective.

Below you see the God Seed Atom (running off Octagon Geometry with total Source connection) on the right and Metatron's Cube (running off of Hexagon Geometry with no connection to Source) on the left. The Flower of Life is another pattern that sits fluidly in the Metatron architecture.

I have previously explained that healing is like unplugging from one data stream/server and plugging into a new one. The Krystal Spiral originates from Source and we have the

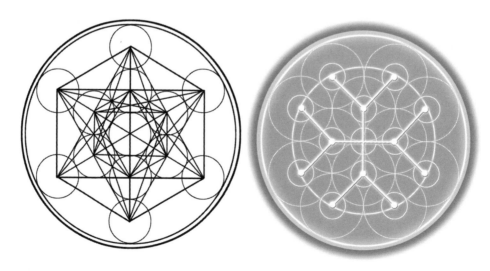

87. Metatron's Cube and God Seed Atom

opportunity to plug into the server/data stream at its creative centre; we as evolved humans, with a genetic template/cosmic code, have been able to plug into this new field of light and sound to further expand and evolve our ascension. Some people still choose the old timeline consciousness, some consciously and others unconsciously.

The planetary body of Earth and her children, humans, are now free to follow the Krystal Spiral architecture in order to heal and help evolve Earth's inhabitants and species to a path of ascending consciousness, should Earth and her inhabitants choose this of course.

Splitting in Two

During the Krystal server/hosting change, fallen life forms have been undergoing sequential Bifurcation (splitting in two) of Time in the consciousness fields and have no other choice but to split into the direction of the Fibonacci Spiral, unless they choose rehabilitation or transiting through certain protocols put in place by the founding consciousness streams of our Earth/galaxy/universe. The Fallen species do not have a DNA template that allows them to rise into higher dimensions or hijack the Krystal Spiral or

those human beings who are connected to that architecture.

When this Bifurcation of Time and the subsequent frequency split occurred, it caused higher grid wars to control the Star Gates. Access to these multidimensional and inter-dimensional entry and exit points onto or into our Earth were made impossible. As a result of the change in planetary architecture to heal into its original organic path of the Krystal Spiral, the Earth can continue to accrete more Higher Source Energy and is out of the control of the fallen life forms. This doesn't mean they just give up and move on. No, they have continued to fight and cause mayhem for many years. It's playing out on Earth right now but the more we choose love and maintain a higher consciousness field of operation and choose to operate outside of their system, the less energy the dark ones can draw on. Fear is their fuel and, without this low-vibrational energy, they will not be able to sustain themselves. Eventually they will fade out and live on a timeline that is unrecognizable by you or me and many who choose the new operating system, the new/ancient/original mathematics, the Krystal Spiral frequency

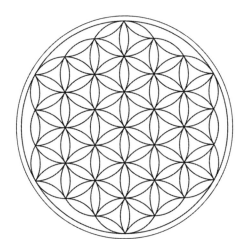 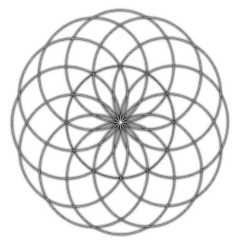

88. Metatronic Flower of Life and Eternal Flower of Life

stream. Even though Earth's architecture is shifting, she, our mother has made a choice and that is to be a good mother and do what every good mother does; put her children before her. Earth's template is being held and tuned into the Krystal Spiral by higher forces. This is because other forces wanted to destroy Earth (by messing with her rod and staff, a part of her architecture) in order to create a huge source or pool of quantum energy that they could use to fuel their agenda. Remember, it's a game of energy and this goes to show the magnitude of what we are discussing. The darker forces would wipe out Earth and all of her inhabitants to get a huge influx of energy that would be let out during the collapse. This was supposed to happen in 2012 but higher forces did not allow this to happen. They are holding Earth in place energetically and mathematically. Humans have to figure out how to move through the Star Gates and exit the matrix, because death is not an exit. You will still be in the system and will return full stop. Earth will return to stardust, a choice she made, and so will all streams of consciousness here at the time (approximately 200 years), if the higher forces or guardians, cannot repair Earth's broken mathematics. You see, your physical body is your greatest ally right now. Make it strong, do the work and figure out how to get your mathematics compatible for movement through the Star Gates. This book and its tools is step number one.

So, we humans, Earth's children, can go through this ascension cycle. We have to raise our consciousness, expand our awareness, change at a DNA level and upgrade our mathematics so we can remember how to, once again, move through our Planetary Star Gate structure and out from this time-based matrix/system and move on, maybe back to Andromeda, who knows?

Bifurcation means the splitting of a main body into two parts. In the mathematical study of

change that occurs within a structure or space, bifurcation occurs when a parameter change causes the stability of an equilibrium (or fixed point in a field) to change. The comprehension of the mathematical change that is currently shifting the geometric value of frequency, which further generates a bifurcation in the structure of time and space, is very relevant to us now. This is directly related to the split occurring between timelines (unfolding right now as I write this book) that govern our continued consciousness (energy) expression on the Earth plane as it is moving into future time (which isn't really future, it's now). Thus, the planetary fields and humanity are coming to experience the next phase of the planetary ascension cycle, which is the nature of bifurcation of time.

We have been witnessing the timeline spilt and the wars play out in real time here on Earth, in full view of our human family. 5G, wars, chemtrails, attack on our water supply, gender manipulation and the influence of the media and social media . . . the list goes on and on but you get my point. Some human beings with a lower vibrational frequency are choosing to still opt into the Fibonacci Spiral and play the 3D game and some of the humans are choosing the Krystal Spiral and playing the 5D + game, because we are hosted in multiple dimensions in any one time. We are not just moving into the higher dimensions.. We are riding the vibrational scale on a multidimensional level and our reason for being here on Earth is for this. We are re-engineering our inner geometry (realigning our mathematics to the way it was) and activating our DNA potential, so we can pass through the Planetary Star Gate system and travel.

The lower the quality of overall energy, the more unstable and disconnected the personal and environmental experience on Earth will become. The higher the quality of overall energy, the more stable and connected the personal and environmental experience on Earth will become. The planetary collective energy field has many, many layers of intersecting links, which are building more access points into diagonal lines moving throughout interdimensional fields. These links make it possible to directly intersect into many different realities and timelines, travelling in the past, present and future, which are one in the field. This is called transdimensional time travel.

The cumulative effect of gradually increasing frequency and changing instruction sets in many of the transdimensional time and space fields has reached a point of divergence. The culmination of reaching this point of divergence within trans-time and space is forcing the shift of the overall planetary energy field parameters. That pressure of force being applied in the planetary energy field is resulting in cumulative intensity and extreme polarity amplification. When the extreme polarity of combined forces that co-exist together within a collective energy field reaches its apex, a split occurs. This is called the point of divergence within the fixed point in the field (in the range of possibilities), of which a Bifurcation of Time transpires. As mentioned, this is the 3D/5D timeline split; but it's much more than just that. It's a choice to be hosted across multiple frequency bands/densities/dimensional spaces, all at the same time, and it's a choice to exit this corrupt matrix.

You chose to be on Earth at this time, just like I did, and I will not leave until my work is done. I didn't come here to make friends. I didn't come here to gain followers.

I came to Earth on a mission. That mission is to raise consciousness on this planet. I do that in my own unique way, and it works. It scares some people because they are not ready to look in the mirror and face their Shadow Side. They externalize everything through blame and judgement. It's these people who inspire me the most. It's those humans who blame and judge and ridicule that motivate me each day!

Because while they are still walking around this green and blue ball I've still got work to do and so have you. I will not leave until the job is done. This is what Sovereign Soldiers do. Our intention is to never leave any woman or man or child behind. There are, however, casualties in all wars.

We are all in every human being, tree, rock, animal and flower. Wherever you turn, your Shadow Side will be mirrored back to you until you can be still and face it, and every time you get up and run it will get more and more painful.

Galactic Titans don't choose the easy path. We don't choose sunshine and rainbows. We dive into the chaos and mayhem, where our sisters and brothers are blaming and judging. We sit in this space with our diamond torch and transmute. We mirror back their own darkness until they shine light on it themselves and balance their energy.

Are you still running, or are you healing in the stillness?

Remember, energy doesn't die and vibration doesn't lie. If you don't do it in this vessel you will have to do it somewhere else and if you don't work it out you will turn to stardust in 200 years and lose your place as a human. You may have to start at the beginning again, manifesting into a lower life form and over millions, maybe billions of years, make your way from a nanobe (a tiny filamental structure found in some rocks and sediments. Some scientists hypothesize that nanobes are the smallest form of life, 1/10 the size of the smallest known bacteria) to being a human being again. Do you really want to go through this long process? There is no escape! Learn your lessons! Grow exponentially! Get it over and done with and choose the higher-dimensional fields. Plug into the new architecture.

10

Useful Tools

Reset Code

If you have been to Star Magic Facilitator Training or watched videos of our trainings or me facilitating healing, you will notice that sometimes I place one hand over someone's neck and the other over their forehead and they collapse, bend, twist, shake or generally contort in a strange manner.

The universe is intelligent, and it knows how to self-organize. It naturally does this. This is why self-healing is a naturally occurring process that the body just does – when we get out of the way and allow it to. As we have discussed, a lot of us are thinking and feeling in ways that are detrimental to our health because we are addicted to the trauma, to the chemicals released during trauma, and so we recreate or relive these events over and over in our mind.

We have developed a way of healing that resets the body. It shuts the mind down and allows the body to do what it does best, and that is to recalibrate and heal. The back of the neck has a portal. It's an entry point or exit point for energies. Priests call it God's Mouth and they wear those big collars because they fear being attacked by demonic forces and it is a vulnerable point.

In Star Magic we run a frequency in through the back of the neck, up through the pineal gland and out through the forehead. We create an energy channel and run this frequency around and around. The human being you are doing it to (which could also be you using your own hologram) will know exactly what is happening but the energy will take them. Sometimes healees stand upright or

bend forwards or fall to the floor as though they are unconscious. When it happens, they are fully aware and simply a witness to the experience. You can hear people talking in the room, but you are somewhere else. It's an amazing experience, but hard to fathom if you have not experienced it yet.

So, How Does It Work?

I will ask the human being (or me, if I am working on myself) what they want to release, shift or change or what they want to bring into or create within their reality. Some people know what needs releasing and others are in a great space and want to create something new. Some people say nothing and so we hand it over to the universe. Once they have verbally told me their intention, I ask them to take three deep breaths and then send that intention out into the universe by speaking out loud or in their head.

I then ask for Star Magic Codes of Consciousness, or I call upon a very specific code or set of codes that I know will help this particular situation. We have bundles of codes in Star Magic for different situations. I have created them as and when different situations have risen. We have codes for confidence, to remove entities, open the heart, activating the merkaba and many more. We have codes for pretty much everything. Right now, you don't have a bag of magic codes, so you will have to leave it up to the universal energy to select a frequency that does the job – and it will. You will hold out your right hand, call upon Star Magic Codes of Consciousness. You will feel them in your right palm, in your wrists and forearm. You connect with them through the heart and then place your right hand over the back of the human being's neck, or over the back of your hologram in the same position. Your thumb and forefinger will touch the base of the skull to the left and right of the atlas and up slightly.

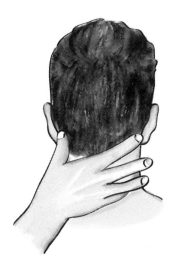

89. Thumb and forefinger at base of skull

The above image shows exactly where you should place your hand, finger and thumb.

Once the right hand is in place, you will place the left hand over the forehead. The frequency containing the codes will now flow from the right palm, through the neck, up through the pineal gland and out through the left palm, travel up through the left arm, through the body and back down the right arm and continue on its journey. It will keep circulating. As the codes flow through the pineal gland, it will download them to every cell in the body. The human being in question may drop immediately, or it may take thirty seconds for the codes to hit the sweet spot. By that I mean the quantum space where the trauma lies. Once it hits, the man, woman or child will become kind of "stuck". This will be in whatever position the energy has moved them into. They will be in that position while the energy clears out an old program and resets the body/mind/

spirit and a new and empowering data stream is downloaded. Sometimes people shake violently, other times they bend and contort and sometimes they are stuck upright with two feet planted into the ground. You are basically unplugging yourself or whoever you are working on from one data stream/programme and plugging them/you into a new, fluid and expansive and infinite data stream.

I remember the very first time I tried this in public. I was in Birmingham in the UK. I was in a café on a Sunday morning. The café had been closed for the day and there was a very small spiritual fayre. I had a stand and people came for healings. My stand was near the toilet in the café and this lady came and sat down. Yes, they don't have to be stood. I used this technique and she fell off the chair and onto the floor. (I supported her on the way down and cushioned her landing so don't worry.) She fell in front of the toilet door and was out for forty-five minutes. People clambered over her to get to the toilet.

Women lifted their pushchairs over her to get past. She was out, totally conscious of everything, but couldn't move. She was releasing and downloading. When she came round, she said it was the most amazing experience of her life. When people surrender to the energy and let it work its magic, miracles happen.

I did this to a woman in Asia at a Facilitator Training and she was out for thirty plus minutes. When she came round, she said she was floating through the universe, and it felt like she had been reborn. This lady had a tumour in one of her kidneys. When she went to the doctors for a scan it had gone. Did this reset her consciousness and heal her soul to the point before the trauma happened that created the symptom we call a tumour? It seems so – or maybe it was a coincidence?

When you commit to surrendering and get out of your own way, miracles really do happen. Let me put it another way. The universe is full of intelligence that wants you to thrive. It's trying to access your biological computer, 24/7, to make this happen. But the computer has a virus. The virus is you. You are blocking the new software being downloaded so the computer can be upgraded. Or in this case, so you can receive a biological upgrade. If you tried to download software into a virus-ridden laptop, it would struggle or shut down. Connect to the Star Magic codes/light, trust, surrender, get out of your own way and let the download take place.

If you do it on your own, make sure you are sitting with a soft surface around you. If you do it to another human being stay very close and be aware that they may fall suddenly once the frequency kicks in, whether forwards or backwards, or they may just drop like a sack of spuds – stay close! In China in 2019 I did this to a lady and she just froze. She was stood upright in the middle of the training room and could not move. For several minutes she could not speak. It took about thirty minutes for the download to finish and during that whole time she was stood in the middle of the room. Everyone went for lunch and she was stuck. A few of us stayed with her and waited for her to come round. It's powerful, so use it wisely.

You can do this at distance, although do it when the other human being is lying down, on a soft surface.

I remember once on our Level 2 Training. It was the first time we had run this training experience and I had some new sets of codes to download using the process. As I had not used them before, I had to be the first to try them (I never download anything until I have experienced it myself). I asked a man to assist me and explained what to do. He connected to this specific frequency and placed his hands on my neck and forehead. Three seconds later it was like Mike Tyson had hit me with a right cross, straight in the jaw. My head spun and I hit the deck, face first. I knew I was going to hit the floor but I could not push my arms out to stop it. Once I hit the floor, I was downloading these Sirian and Oraphim frequencies. It was amazing. I felt dazed for a short while.

If you are curious about the magnitude of this work, you should attend a training. Using this healing way/technique can and will heal anything and everything when you truly commit. So, go for it. Don't doubt. Don't second-guess. Apply the way and then surrender! Or surrender and then apply the way. It is very important to truly surrender to this process and let the light/intelligence work. Those who surrender get the best results.

Quantum Protection

I would like to take this opportunity to discuss moving through the quantum world effectively. You will have heard the terms remote viewing and astral travel. Remote viewing is where one human being can view another human being, other worldly being, location or object remotely. Astral travel is where a human being can travel, astrally, to another location. It's like they are really there, energetically. They can walk around and interact with the location.

Remote viewing and astral travel cross over to a certain extent. When you are good at remote viewing you can listen to and interact with a location just the same, so for me remote viewing and astral travel really are one and the same. Teleportation is a different ball game: this is where someone can take their physical body from one location to another, phasing out of one reality and into another. During large group healings at workshops, people have looked up towards the front and I haven't been there; or they have seen me as a pirate or as crystalline energy. We do phase in and out of reality naturally in an altered state of consciousness.

My friend Aljaz witnessed and experienced this with me:

I was talking to Jerry and Lory, and Lory started sharing a story about discovering her higher self.

I was sat to the left of and a bit behind Jerry. All of a sudden he completely disappeared. And I mean disappeared as in ceased to exist. He was gone, not there any more.

It was like someone pressed the "delete" button. No flashy lights going off, or a breeze of wind taking him away – nothing, just gone, as if he was never really there. The only thing profoundly noticeable was peace, stillness, knowing and a deep sense of the infinite intelligence within all existence, God. The room was quiet.

Time stood still for me. This lasted about five seconds, yet it felt longer. When my mind kicked back in, I hastily called out, "Jerry". And puff he was back, turning his head toward me. When we talked about it, he said that what happened was while Lory was talking, he was so deeply present, listening to and immersed in the story with none of his attention on his body, that he had ceased to create his body. He had gone beyond the physical and so the physical was not there.

Spiritual Armour

Everyone has these abilities. They are natural to us. Remote viewing and astral travel are something I do regularly. Teleportation is something I haven't mastered, but when I was taken on a spacecraft in New Zealand to Alpha Centauri, I feel I had a glimpse into how teleportation works. I was meditating in the garden inside a pyramid when the space pod (the best way I can describe it) landed. I brought my light/consciousness out from my body and went and jumped inside. There was a blue being inside the craft. Once inside, my consciousness

saw where we were going to. It was as though the blue being next to me, or maybe the craft itself, placed my consciousness in the location we were going to travel to. Then, my light body went through a tunnel for a few seconds and caught up with my consciousness. This is the best way I can describe it. A very strange, interesting but natural feeling.

When we remote view or astral travel it's so important that we are aware of our space. So many people talk about protection in these spiritual fields. First up, I don't like to think I need to be protected. As soon as you say or think that, then you are creating duality and creating a situation where you may need to be protected, or may invite an energy into your space that wants to attack you. Maybe that situation didn't exist until you decided you needed to be protected? It's one perspective. I am not saying danger doesn't exist because it does. There are lower and higher vibrational forces but when you are standing in your Kryst Light, you are untouchable.

My very first spiritual teacher drilled this into my head: when remote viewing or astral travelling, never work directly from your space or project or travel directly to your target. Even if you are simply shining light and love and positive energy into a building, never do it from your home.

This human being suggested that I should go to a field or wood. I always felt that this took too much time, so I came up with the idea of using jump stations. It works, and works well. When we train our Star Magic facilitators, we teach/show them the jump station idea below.

PROTOCOL *Jump Stations for Protecting Space*

If you have a definite target/location, set up a black tourmaline pyramid in the ether somewhere, then in another location, an inverted smokey quartz pyramid, then another black tourmaline pyramid and then another inverted smokey quartz pyramid. You simply intend and envision these geometries and frequencies in space. You then intend your consciousness out from your body (which takes practice) into the first inverted black tourmaline pyramid. Then one by one you travel through the four pyramids (more if required, depending on the situation. Sometimes I will just use one black tourmaline and one inverted smokey quartz pyramid. You then, from the final pyramid, go to your location and start walking around or doing the work you set out to do. On your return you come back through the four jump stations (sometimes more or less depending on what you are doing), blowing them up behind you so you leave no energetic trace that can be followed.

PROTOCOL *Geometry for Protecting Space*

If you are new to this spiritual world, you can use geometry to keep your space clear. If your awareness is still moving up through the levels and you are still remembering how to control your space energetically, you may want to put yourself inside a chromium octahedron, then an inverted chromium pyramid, and then a chromium cube or sphere or both. Spin all of the geometries clockwise and know that nothing will move through that grid. Open your heart into the grid and fill it with love and also fill the space between your body and the octahedron with violet light, the space between the octahedron and the inverted pyramid with diamond light and the space between the inverted pyramid and the sphere or cube with chromium light. Then open your heart and inject some serious love vibrations into the grid. This will keep your space clear.

It's so important to be aware of what is around and to stay in love. Never tip into fear even if it's seeming a little scary. Stay focused, remain calm, keep your balance and composure. You are vulnerable if you destabilize your core frequency by tipping out of love and into fear (or any emotion

on the lower end of the spectrum: guilt, jealousy, rejection, anger. But nothing can interfere with you if you keep this vibration and stay in love.

How to Stop a Psychic Attack

There are times when one comes under attack energetically. It can happen in many different ways and the ways are infinite. Doing the work that I do and being good at assisting others who have come under attack, means I have built a reputation for this kind of work and the inquiries we receive at Star Magic Healing are many and vast.

In psychic attack situations, your willpower, determination and mental strength is of the utmost importance. You must be lovingly ferocious, in zero fear mode and know nothing in the universe is more powerful than you.

I have had my share of encounters and so have members of my family. When you do so much good work and remove darker/lower vibrational energies from another human being, you do tend at times, to annoy the entities or the beings that are controlling the entities. A few years back we were at facilitator training in the UK and there was a Romanian guy there who was riddled with what I call Shadow Parasites. I call the entities Shadow Parasites because they behave in the same way as a parasite, but they are to most people invisible and live in the shadows. Just like a parasite in the jungle that enters a caterpillar, takes over its consciousness (the host) and makes the caterpillar climb to the top of the tallest tree and explode. The insides of the caterpillar then get eaten by other caterpillars and the parasite spreads. They make all the other caterpillars do the same. Climb to the top of the tallest tree and explode and this is how the parasites spread.

Shadow Parasites/entities/dark forces take over human consciousness, do their best to keep us in fear by altering our thoughts and feed off of the low-vibrational energy. They claim the host (the human) and then the human being is like a walking zombie. Most drug addicts or alcoholics have Shadow Parasites in them or within their field and many other humans, ones you may never suspect, are being manipulated on some level by Shadow Parasites. There are beings, certain species of Greys for example, who are incredible at controlling the field of consciousness of others, including brain waves, thoughts, emotions and imagery.

I laid the guy down and removed several beings. As we did this, we saw two huge beings, maybe thirty metres tall, with long spider legs, looking down at us. They were in charge of the beings we were removing and were upset to say the least. After this training I had a spacecraft over my house for two weeks bombarding me with heavy energy. They did their best to bring me down and harm me and drain me, but they gave up in the end and left me alone. It took a lot of focus to stay in love in this situation but eventually it paid off.

You can find Shadow Parasites in a physical body or in the energy field of another human being. Sometimes they work from distance and it's effective. Why? Because there is no distance in the quantum field.

PROTOCOL *Removing Shadow Parasites*
I will explain to you how I remove Shadow Parasites from someone. I create a smokey quartz pyramid around them and install a code into the pyramid. The code is **M369** and it is programmed to take the Shadow Parasite/s back to Source or whichever dimensional space it/they are supposed to go to. Maybe it has/they have their own journey and learning? I then open the navel or the heart of the man, woman or child and see what is inside. Sometimes there is one or often many beings. They can look like slugs, spiders, Komodo dragons, scorpions, or other different types of strange things. They can be in different parts of the body, often shape-shifting so you

cannot see them. I will shine as much chromium light (we will talk about Kaleidoscopic chromium later) through the human being's body. This will eventually expose the beings as they cannot shapeshift fast enough through the fast array of colours within Kaleidescopic chromium. Then you can take them out or negotiate with them and sometimes they are willing to come. Sometimes it's a battle and other times it's not. I've seen these beings choking people to death and also digging their claws or nails into the inside of the body when you are trying to take them out. The pain people go through is extreme at times, but in other cases it's painless.

One night, my son Josh was aware of his dreams while he was sleeping. He said he had been travelling, and these beings were coming towards him. Josh put a golden sphere around himself and the beings were looking in through the top. They tried to get through but Josh wouldn't let them. He carried on his journey and dream and smiled at the beings above, looking annoyed as they could not penetrate his space. His intention and willpower was too strong for the beings.

I remember a few years ago at one of the first spiritual exhibitions I went to, a lady was walking down the passageway towards me. She looked massive. Like a huge man in a woman's body. Her hands were like shovels. She walked up to me, put her hands into her own mouth, looked at me in the eyes and said, "Fuck You," very aggressively. As she did, she was ripping her own mouth, really hard. It was like she was about to tear it apart. She had come for my help but the three beings inside of her didn't like her being near me. To cut a long story short, I removed the three beings and her body turned very slender. Her big hands, shoulders and back just shrunk down. Her face changed. She looked twenty years younger and had a big smile on her face.

You see, these beings can actually change your physical appearance. The body of the human becomes their home. Some are actually scared to leave, and so negotiation is in order. Others need a little force and some actually need loving into submission. You will have to figure it out if you ever come across it. It's one of those things where practice is essential. You may never come across this but at least you know now what to do.

A fella called John was being strangled to death in a church one day. We were meditating in an ancient church on some awesome ley lines at the end of the road from one of our Facilitator Training Experiences. John came into the church halfway through. He just stood there, and it was a little dark. He started to walk down through the pews and then vanished. I sensed something wasn't right. I walked down the aisle between the pews and saw him lying on a wooden pew being strangled. I called my friend over. We sat him up and took these African spirits out from him. If we hadn't been there he may have died. But everything happens perfectly, and we were there. I saw it as a great opportunity to show the souls on our training how to deal with this stuff in real time. I simply went into John's body and pulled these spirits out. I did not move a physical muscle. This was all done using energy.

The message here is loud and clear. You must be lovingly ferocious, in zero fear mode, and know that nothing in the universe is more powerful than you. Love is the question and the answer and the key to stopping psychic assaults.

You must be calm, heart wide open, and committed to the situation. Commit and KNOW you are coming out on top, and you will!

This area of healing and the spiritual field is a minefield but I wanted to bring it into your awareness so you can have a starting point if anything should ever arise. We train people on this at our Facilitator Training Experiences. Some people say to me, don't tell people about this stuff because they may create it. This is the other side of the coin. If you go around expecting to see the bogeyman at the end of your bed or around every street corner, you eventually will. Just like expecting bad news or a big water bill or some unpaid taxes. If you think of it, you will create it. I am not asking you to think of this. I am simply making you aware. It's like being at sea: the ship starts to fill with water in a storm, but no one told you where the life jackets and inflatable dinghies are kept. Knowledge and awareness can save lives.

Removing Implants and Electromagnetic Webbing

You may or may not have heard people talk about implants. These are like little devices that you find in people's bodies. This can be physical or metaphysical, but either way they can have extremely negative effects. Some dentists and surgeons have found bits of metal inside the bodies of their patients and when they analyzed the metal, it was not of this world. So, where does it come from? And who puts these things there?

Some of us agree, before we incarnate, to collect information for our Star Families, so once here they visit us in dream time and insert these small devices, which are metal, and can look like little balls, rectangles, square shapes or slivers of some kind of material, metal or crystal. Sometimes they are the size of a pinhead or your little fingernail and other times as large as a finger or some I have seen are as large as a hand. Sometimes they are thick and other times thin. In this situation, when full agreement and acknowledgment is in place, it can be OK to let them stay as long as they are not having a negative effect.

There are many reports and experiences of other beings that will come into your space, often in dream time, and take you somewhere, onto a spacecraft in some cases, and install implants in your body which are against the will of the soul or the human being. I have many emails from people about this. One woman told me how she had put up a fight; these beings, whiteish/greyish with a tint of blue, were operating on her when she became conscious of her dream state. She fought and got away. When she woke in the morning, she had a broken collarbone, a broken nose, a black eye and scratches. There was blood all over the pillows and sheets. I have heard of many incidents like this.

Now dealing with these implants is tricky because there are so many different types. The older ones are like boxes or chips, objects that can be removed. The newer technology is what I refer to as electromagnetic webbing. It's like a spider's web that is alive. As you try to take them/it out, they reappear or grow and expand. It's not always easy and patience and determination are required. Quite often the implants are monitored or controlled externally.

For example, we had a lady at our Level 1 Training who kept having these strange spasms. She would talk in an evil tongue; her eyes would roll back into her head and she would be taken over. She would be frothing at the mouth. As we were looking at her physical body and her light body, we could see an implant in her ankle. We removed it and it would reappear somewhere else. We knew it was being controlled from elsewhere.

My team and I could see two green and red beings, in a control room on a spacecraft, pressing buttons. I went into the craft and destroyed the computers and sent the beings to another dimensional space.

That took a bit of effort and wasn't easy, but remember, willpower and determination is everything. Nothing is more powerful than you, beautiful soul.

So, once the beings were gone and the computer destroyed, the lady lit up like a Christmas tree. We could see little red dots all over the inside of her body. There were multiple implants, all connected. Once the computer was gone, they were exposed. One by one we removed them, simply by taking them out. I always cut a hole in the cosmic fabric and throw it through, just like I would do a Shadow Parasite, using M369 and the smokey quartz pyramid.

To find these things and do this kind of work, you really need your third eye and your intuition switched on.

I've seen people clinically diagnosed with mental health or other psychological or behavioural issues completely turn around and become OK again in minutes after these implants have been removed.

When you have a box-style, what I would call old-fashioned implant, it's easy to remove, but with electromagnetic webbing you have to work really fast because it grows as you start removing it. I often freeze it with my mind and try to extract it all in one go, but it doesn't always work. Every situation is different and there is no method here.

I will give you another example of how real this stuff is. I knew something was not right with a man on one of our trainings. He walked and spoke in a strange robotic fashion. I brought him on to the stage and laid him down on a healing bed, looked inside him and saw wiring throughout his body. Some of my team and I set about taking it out. It was intense. This guy's body was lifting off the bed and slamming back down. His arms and legs were writhing. It took two people to hold him still while I did the work. It took about forty-five minutes to clear him. Once he was clear he went to the toilet, came back and said he'd urinated what looked like purple brake fluid. When he walked back into the room, he walked fluidly and spoke fluidly. His eyes were sparkly for the first time.

If you've never witnessed this kind of work it's hard to fathom but the reality is that this is happening and we need more people to step up, claim their sovereignty, remove any unwanted gifts from their body and be their Super-Human version and in doing so assist any other sisters and brothers who need it to remove these unwanted gifts from their bodies.

The truth is this: regardless of what technology is put into your body, or your energetic field, if your vibration is sky-high, nothing will come close. Any disease/illness/poisonous bite that ends up in your body, even nanotech from chemtrails, can all be dissolved and transmuted through your intention/energy/willpower/commitment and internal KNOWING!

For me, all of these situations are incredible and simply sharpen my tools. If it wasn't for forces and situations like implants, lower-vibrational humans and otherworldly entities, how would we ever up-skill? We would have no training ground. We can enter the sphere of fear and become a dead notch on the bedpost, or we can enter the sphere of love, rise like Galactic Guardians and level up. Your choice, beautiful soul. Super-Dead or Super-Human?

PART 3

Raising Consciousness

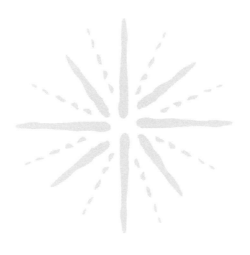

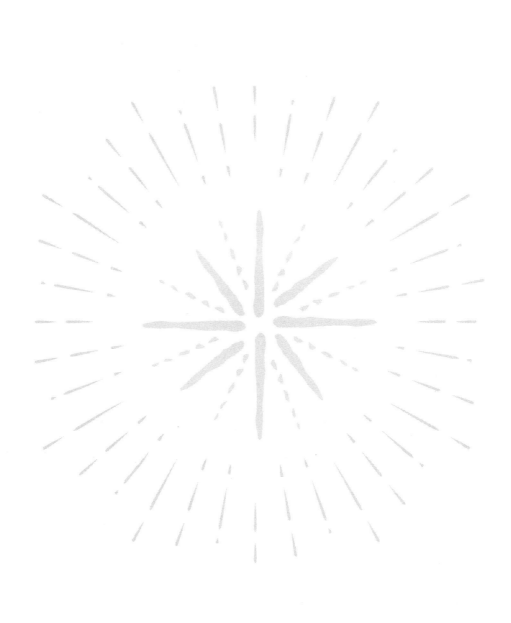

11

Upgrading Your Consciousness

Activate Your Master Alchemist

We are all Master Alchemists in our own right, here on Earth to create, dissolve and recreate reality. We can alchemize anything we so wish into our local environment. Our thoughts and emotions, when they are controlled, are super-tools. When we apply these tools in the right way, using our biological computer, the human body and brain and the focus, discipline and determination that we all carry and can activate if we so choose, real magic can happen.

There are some new souls on this planet that have not been here before (predominantly children, but some are adult walk-ins), but the majority of the human race have lived here on Earth or are living in other simultaneously parallel realities, right now, many other lives. It's important to note that, while past lives exist from one perspective, from another they are illusory and are actually parallel versions: remember, there is no time, distance or measurement in the quantum field. Everything is now and one body can have multiple soul experiences moving through it and one soul can have multiple experiences in many different bodies. These versions of us that lie within the quantum field can be accessed and brought back home, into this now space, so we can harness the alchemical power of these ridiculously powerful energy signatures. When we harness and embrace these other aspects of us, our potential rises and the increase in energy, power and output can go up ten times, fifty times, a hundred times.

Now, I am going to take you through a process that you can use to access these other multidimensional versions of you. When you do this, I want you to be sensible. Don't be like a bull in a china shop. Do it methodically and give yourself time to recalibrate and integrate these new energies. Sometimes they can be overwhelming and the major point to note is this. You are going to access alchemists, physicists, inventors, creators, wizards and witches, of both a dark and a light nature.

Remember, you are all things, and your power lies within each and every facet of reality. You must master dark and light and embrace your totality. When you do, don't rush out to use this new energy. Sit within, meditate on it, get to know and "innerstand" it. See the ego temptation within the power this energy provides you with and harness it and keep it on reins. Let it out little by little. Train it and master it and exercise caution. Only when you have sat with this energy for a few weeks or months and have truly "innerstand" it should you use it to create, dissolve and recreate reality.

New qualities will flow through your energy field, your consciousness. You will see and experience life differently and really step up into a new and empowered way of living, being and acting. You will be free, and you will be sovereign. A master alchemist, knowing that energy can change in a heartbeat and life can be lost or gained, never takes anything for granted. An alchemist knows energy never dies but the physical aspects, representing the manifestation of the metaphysical, can wither and crumble. A master alchemist knows that she or he has no duty.

To be bound by duty is slavery. A master alchemist makes conscious choices to serve and to be a shining light within the species (because humanity is not the only space an alchemist resides in) she or he or it lives, seeking to raise the vibration always but at the same time having zero attachment to any potential outcome. A master alchemist flows.

A master alchemist doesn't plan too much, as they know the tides can change and the present moment is all that exists. A master alchemist is a warrior, a quantum explorer of the physical and metaphysical planes, ready to show up at the drop of a hat and utilize her or his skills, knowing they have no obligation but simply knowing that, by working in a unified fashion, barriers can be dissolved, and worlds can unite. A master alchemist is the source of oneness, an activated soul on a mission to do what is necessary, when it's necessary, simply because they can, and totally embrace the smiles and happiness, the joy and bliss that fill the hearts of others from the alchemical work they have done.

Does this sound like you? Of course it does. This is you. You chose this magnificent path and even if you have not embraced the fact that this is a possibility, soon you will. This book and the ideas in it are giving you the perfect platform to be the master alchemist you are in many other dimensions, densities, and realities right now. We work in cycles of time and these cycles are not natural and that is because the mathematics are corrupted in our system. Everything is cyclical in this human time-based reality. We have the procession of the equinoxes, 25, 920 years, the 2,160-year cycle of the age of the zodiacs, 365 days in a year, 24 hours in a day, 60 minutes in an hour and 60 seconds in a minute. We go around and around and around and it's not natural. What we are going to do with this process is break down these cycles of time and collapse them into this now space. All of these other versions of you are accessible right now, so why not harness this power and energy now? You are ready to access these parts of yourself.

EXERCISE *Activate Your Master Alchemist*

The code I share with you during this process has been programmed to connect with all aspects of you, throughout all time and space, across all dimensions, densities and frequency bands, that are specialist creators and alchemists. The code will work its magic. All you have to do is follow the process.

1. Sit comfortably with your back straight (or stand if you wish).

2. Breathe deeply into your stomach. In through your nose and out through your nose or mouth.

3. Visualize a golden light flowing in through the walls, down through the ceiling and up through the floor of your space.

4. Breathe this light into every cell of your body. Once your body is full, say thank you.

5. Now, bring your awareness into your heart and open it. Feel it and see it blooming like an electric golden flower.

6. Now I want you to place a code into your heart. The code is **A3694**.

7. Now you will see golden streams of light shoot out from your body in all directions. These electromagnetic streams will connect to other versions of you in other quantum spaces.

8. The code will now flow through these streams and into these other spaces. You will see codes travelling through these golden streams, back from these quantum spaces, carrying the energy signatures of

your multidimensional selves. They will download into you and you will become more whole.

9. You may want to sit in this space for 10–15 minutes, allowing the code to work.

10. Repeat this process every day for thirteen days. Be aware that there are some people who don't require the full thirteen days and others who require more. Feel it.

It's important to remember that as well as bringing your multidimensional selves back home, healing can be triggered as these parallel realities and timelines that your soul's aspect was playing/living/being in collapse. You may go on an emotional rollercoaster for days, weeks, or months. It's normal. Embrace your emotions and let them pass. Don't run from them or try to stuff them back down. Befriend them and you will transcend them.

Remember, don't rush out to use this new energy. Sit with it, meditate on it, get to know and "innerstand" it. See the ego temptation within the power this energy provides you with and harness it. Let it out little by little. Train it, merge it, integrate it and master it. Exercise caution. As I said, only when you have sat with this energy for a few weeks or months and have truly innerstood it, should you use it to create, dissolve and recreate reality and start weaving your own alchemical spells. There is so much power for you to muster and harness and once you have full access to it, things will change. How? That's to be seen. We are all different. Enjoy the process. Be patient and give yourself the space to integrate.

You are a Sovereign Being. You are a Master Alchemist. You are a Super-Human.

Kindness Code

All powerful, sovereign beings are naturally compassionate towards their fellow human family, and I want to offer you another tool to enhance the kindness that naturally flows from within. In life you are going to meet all sorts of different characters. Some will challenge you and some of the encounters will be pleasant. You will meet angry people, jealous people, insecure people, all dealing with their own internal issues and arguments. As an aware human being, living in your heart, breathing consciously, in tune with your environment, you should be able to diffuse any situation. Or at the very least completely maintain your composure, regardless of what life throws at you, and be loving and kind towards your fellow human being. There should never be any judgement or animosity in any situation. Love fiercely and ferociously, that is the key.

I want to share with you a code and a simple process to assist you in elevating your levels of kindness and composure in all situations. This process takes several minutes, and I want you to do it every morning for thirty-six days. Once it's done it's done, and you will naturally be on this frequency and adopt a new way of being. You may have cracked the kindness code already, but I still challenge you to undertake this process and stretch yourself. The benefits are unreal.

1. As soon as you wake up, place your feet on the floor at the side of your bed, turn your palms up, place them on your legs and visualize a pink energy moving into your space. Breathe this pink frequency in through your nose, down to the pit of your stomach, and maintain this deep, rhythmic breath as you breathe the pink light into every cell of your entire body. Once your body is full, say thank you.

2. Once your body is full you will become aware of an electric green ball of light in your heart. As you continue to breathe, this light expands.

It will expand 360 degrees in all directions and keep growing until it's three metres in diameter and you are sat in the middle.

3. Next an inverted golden pyramid will appear, three metres up above your crown, spinning in a clockwise direction. It will be pulling in codes from the cosmic fabric as it does. The codes will be multicoloured.

4. Next, place a code into the pyramid. Intend the code by visualizing it inside the pyramid. The code is **NR 42**. See the code vibrating inside the pyramid.

5. The code (**NR 42**) will dissolve inside the inverted pyramid and flow through the multicoloured codes.

6. Next, the apex of the pyramid will open, and the codes will flow down into the pineal gland.

7. The master cell in the pineal gland will then send these codes to every cell of your physical body. You will see and feel 75–100 trillion tiny little streams, one flowing into every single cell.

8. The green sphere will now shrink back to its original size. The golden pyramid will shrink and move down inside your head, fitting neatly around your pineal gland. An electric green stream of light will flow from the ball in your heart up into your pineal gland and a golden stream will flow from the pineal gland down into your heart. Light codes will flow up and down these two streams, from the pineal gland to the heart and from the heart to the pineal gland.

9. These codes will flow through you and your awareness will continue to heighten.

10. As you go through your daily life you will notice the difference in your vibration as the codes radiate out from you.

Bring Kindness to the Streets

As I said, you are going to do this for the next thirty-six days. Now, I have a challenge for you. Each day after you have done this, I want you to communicate with the first thirteen people you encounter. I want you to approach them with a huge smile and ask them, "How are you feeling today?" They may smile back and tell you. They may look at you as though you are a complete nutter. They may grunt or be ecstatic. However they respond, it is perfect. Your mission is to exercise kindness. Regardless of their response, smile even wider and say, "Have an awesome day" and "I love you", and continue on your upbeat path with your heart wide open and a huge smile on your face.

You are literally training yourself to be kind. The codes will be flowing through you, radiating out from you, and people will be affected by this on a very deep level. This is a beautiful gift you are giving to yourself and an incredible gift you are giving to the people you interact with.

This is Jedi Training. It seems simple but the effectiveness is massive. You will grow in kindness and confidence with every interaction. You will actually be more confident in being kind. It is surprising how some people actually struggle with being kind because of confidence and the potential judgement of others, or self-judgement. Kindness is natural. We all want to be kind underneath, and love everyone, but putting it into practice is the hardest part.

Seize this opportunity and within a week you will notice a huge difference in your life and how people and situations respond to you. After thirty-six days the universe will be responding to you in magnificent ways. Everything in your environment will be kind to you. You will see. It's surreal to witness but when everything flows in your favour, when all things are kind to you (because you are kind to all things), an ease enters your life and in turn you become even kinder, happier and more loving, just like a Super-Human should be.

Remember, some of the first thirteen people you encounter in your day may be annoyed, unhappy, in a hurry. Don't let their mannerisms or behaviours faze you in any way, shape or form. Smile, open your heart and be right in their face with galaxies of kindness. Don't ask them how they are feeling from three metres away or over to the right. Walk right up to them and say it. Some people will hug you, others will cry and some will abuse you and some may even tell you to F off. It's all perfect. Eventually you won't encounter low-vibrational people. They will simply be unable to step into your field. There may be days when you don't encounter thirteen people, and then you can say it to people on the phone, on Zoom, on Skype. Take every opportunity you can get. Walking down the street, in a shop, petrol station, supermarket, park. Make a point of going out for an hour a day into a busy space to accomplish this challenge. It doesn't matter who the people are, what they look like, what they are doing.

By the way, never ask "How are you?" or "How are you doing?" NO! Ask them, "How are you feeling?" This brings them into their body. It will be so weird to some people. That is OK. Ask it and then regardless of the response say, "Have an awesome day, I love you."

Be powerful and committed to your conversation and you will see magic pour into your life as the days go by and after thirty-six days you will naturally start being like this. You will feel so comfortable being like this that the universe will give you even more opportunities to be in beautiful situations and if you ever find yourself in the occasional challenging situation, it will not seem challenging any more. You will surprise yourself. This is a magical process, and you will feel your own alchemy working in every energetic encounter.

Manifestation

A Super-Human finds it easy to manifest. Why? Because a Super-Human lives in the now, has binned her or his expectations, lives in a focused and conscious, balanced mental and emotional state where heart-based action is the driving force. A Super-Human knows that their mind is like a canvas, and just like an artist or painter, the Super-Human goes to work, to create, on a clean canvas. The thoughts are either the mess on the canvas, or the work of art itself. A Super-Human knows this and creates accordingly, by cleaning the canvas of their mind and then going to work to create magic.

When the mind is cluttered, bombarded with 60,000-plus thoughts every day, the canvas is dirty, and the Super-Human knows that now is not a time of positive creation. To take a dirty canvas and paint a work of art, while possible, is thwart with challenges. So, the Super-Human empties the mind of all thoughts, enters a present state of awareness and now is ready to paint the perfect picture on the canvas of the mind.

The brain is a biological computer. When it's used to focus its electrical intentions onto the canvas of the mind, and once infused with the magnetically charged emotions, the work of art, the vision of the future (which is now) will be constructed in the quantum field and all the forces of nature, all living things, all energetic beings in coherence, often unknowingly on a conscious level, will coerce none the less on a telepathic quantum level, and bring opportunities, through natural lines of transmission such as people, situations and events, into the path of the Super-Human, so they can strike like a cobra and seize the opportunity to expand into their inner vision, until it fits neatly into their local environment and they manifest their dreams into being.

The electrical and magnetic influences of the body, the brain, the heart, the body's energy field and the cosmic fabric at large, especially the Stars and the Earth, enable you to become a vortex of creation. You can create an environment whereby anything you want is truly possible to create internally and then have externally. You will have it because you are it. You will have it because you become it. When you empty your mind and enter the stillness, that place or space of no-thing, no future or past, just silence and bliss, you have the perfect environment to create from. It's like an inventor in her or his workshop: no one is around and they have all of their tools and loads of time to get lost in the creative zone, not knowing where it will lead and loving every second. When your mind is empty you can start visualizing, constructing, like an architect designing a building or city, you are a quantum architect creating in the invisible fields of energy and information, using the quantum building blocks, creating directly within the universal fabric, knowing that everything you see, construct, create will, at some point very soon, manifest in the physical.

You must know that regardless of what your current reality or environment presents you with, you can prepare and plan your potential desired future now. You don't have to wait for your current environment to improve before you get started. No, that will only hinder the process. You start creating in the quantum now and when your vision is infused with emotion, the invisible will become visible. It will be magnetized into existence through natural lines of transmission, e.g., people, interactions, events and situations. You will be presented with a myriad of opportunities. All you have to do is take them.

Cleanse your mind – like a painter on canvas. Place your thoughts/intentions/electricity. Infuse it with emotions/charge/energy/magnetism.

Manifesting with the Merkaba

As you know, you are a quantum architect, the creator of your reality. I want you to start creating a blueprint for your life, a template. This blueprint will be like the blueprint of a house or project. You are going to design it exactly how you want your life to be. Once you do that, I am going to show you how to use the elements of your light body, to ensure that this blueprint is communicated to the building blocks of the universe, the cosmic fabric that flows through, and is, all life, visible and quantum. Remember, the space is not empty, it's full of energy and, once you create your blueprint, you will communicate with this energy, through your merkaba field, and bring this blueprint to life.

In the qigong section, I shared with you a technique where you move your hands up and down the front of your body in opposite directions and, at the same time, move a ball of light up and down the centre of your body. If you have been practising as you should, you will know exactly what I am referring to. Now, this element of the qigong routine brings the speed of your tetrahedrons into balance, ensuring your merkaba is operating as it should.

What I want to share in this chapter is another way to fire up your merkaba, but bringing an extra element into the equation. This is specifically for manifestation.

Around every living organism is an energy field. This energy field, surrounding people and all sentient beings, is known as the merkaba field. In fact, the merkaba only makes up a part of this field (as previously discussed), but a very important part it is.

According to the Ancient Egyptians, Mer means special kind of light, Ka means spirit and Ba means interpretation of reality. In Hebrew it means vehicle and is spelt merkaba. One thing I know from working with my merkaba is that it holds infinite potential. The basis of your merkaba is two tetrahedrons superimposed over the top of each other.

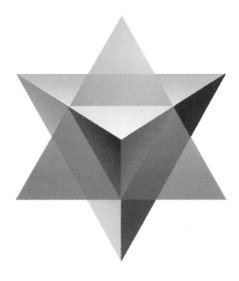

90. Merkaba

This merkaba connects you with the cosmic fabric, layers upon layers of geometrical, spiralized, moving code, woven together by mini portals that share streams of light/information/data. It's an infinite web of beauty and power. A human being inside their merkaba looks like this. You will notice that, depending on whether you are male or female, the merkaba is positioned around your body slightly differently.

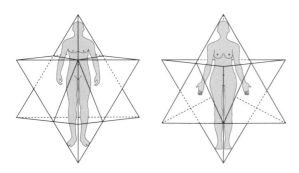

91. Male and female merkaba

In these images we are looking at masculine and feminine, but what I am seeing as our vibration rises is a change in the merkaba field. Our merkaba fields naturally change when we are doing the real work. Using light and sound, our merkaba

field expands and more tetrahedrons are coming online. Below is a merkaba field with twelve points (which link to the twelve strands of DNA) and this merkaba field is what must be fully activated to enable multidimensional travel. We will discuss how to use light and sound codes very soon, to turn on this part of your light body.

The bottom and top tetrahedrons are merging and becoming more fluid and both the female and the male have five top tetrahedrons and five bottom tetrahedrons. It's like five sets of merkabas. This is the activation of the blending of duality in our own consciousness and it's being represented in our energy field. This is just happening, and we don't need to be too concerned with it. Here is an image showing what it looks like:

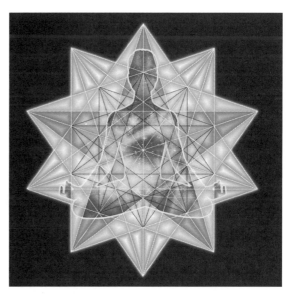

92. Human being inside 12-pointed
multidimensional merkaba field

I wanted to make you aware of this expansion in your merkaba field now; which is imperative for Star Gate travel. However, for manifestation we utilize the original merkaba field with the two tetrahedrons and so will focus on that again now. To fully manifest your heart's wishes you must connect to your activated merkaba, through the heart. You must bring your awareness into your heart and connect it with your head. You can do this with your intention. Sit or stand comfortable, relaxed and loose, bring your awareness into your heart, see a platinum ball of light in your heart and then place the code **X3631** into the platinum ball. It will start to vibrate and then light will travel from the heart to the pineal gland, into the left and right brain and then back to the heart. It happens automatically. The code is programmed to set up this connection. Once this link is made you can bring/intend/visualize the star light from Sirius (male/positive energy) into the top tetrahedron. You then bring/intend/visualize the star light from Orion (female/negative energy) into the bottom tetrahedron.

Once this has taken place you will see that the tetrahedrons will fill up with light. All the time you are fully in your heart. Your love is also filling up the merkaba. Your next move is to invite the Dolphin light/frequency in from Alpha Delphini and Beta Delphini, two stars in the Delphinus star constellation. Light will travel down through your crown and into your heart once you intend it. Once this is done your body changes/shifts its vibration immediately. You will be lighter and will start to vibrate at a higher frequency.

The top tetrahedron spins clockwise as you bring the light from Sirius into it. It will get faster and faster. The bottom tetrahedron spins anti-clockwise as you bring in the female energy from Orion. Both tetrahedrons will spin faster and faster until they spin so fast that they look still. To the trained eye, they turn into a sphere. In actuality the bottom tetrahedron (female) spins twice as fast as the top tetrahedron (male). You will feel them spin around your body.

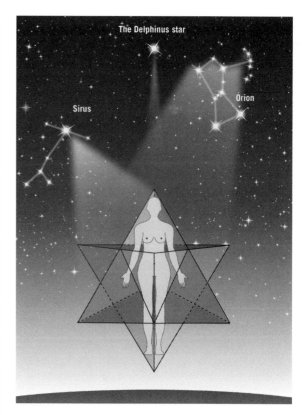

93. Light flowing from Sirius and Orion
activating the merkaba field

If you spend fifteen minutes every day bringing these light frequencies into your merkaba and do it every day for twenty-one days, your merkaba will start to spin of its own accord. You will see it and feel it. Once it is spinning it will enhance and elevate every intention you have. I bring these frequencies in every time I meditate. It takes no extra time. I sometimes incorporate it into my qigong routine or when I am on the treadmill. That is the beauty of frequency. It's available 24/7, 365, in every location. You don't need to spend an extra fifteen minutes; you can combine it with another exercise of your choice.

As you go through the twenty-one days of activating your merkaba I want you to spend some time visualizing and creating the reality you want to live in, inside your mind. It actually takes seconds to fire up your merkaba and the time is simply spent visualizing and creating. I want you

UPGRADING YOUR CONSCIOUSNESS

to create it fully. Live in this reality and play in this reality.

Again, I do this while exercising or driving or when I am on the move. The movement adds to the energy and the emotion. You can of course do it in silence. Make sure your health, business and relationships are all exactly as you wish them to be. Feel what it's like, invoke those powerful emotions, of joy, happiness, bliss, ecstasy, success and total harmony, as you live this reality out inside your mind. When you infuse this reality with emotion, your merkaba will go to work and start bringing opportunities your way, ones that will lead to you living the life you are creating. Do this every day, live it and feel it so strongly and it will become your reality. Your merkaba is designed to bring about this change. You must truly submerge into this inner reality, so vividly that it becomes realer than your current 3D/4D reality. Eventually (potentially very quickly), one will replace the other.

Manifest and Build Your Blueprint

So, what I want you to do is this:

1. Close your eyes and breathe deeply. Get really relaxed and really focused.

2. Start to create, inside your mind, the life of your dreams in terms of health, business, relationships, travel, lifestyle and the planet.

3. To do this I want you to see yourself inside a gigantic sphere. This sphere is your world and the planet. Inside this sphere, which is huge, you start having fun with people in your life. Maybe you create new relationships, or see old ones blossoming. Walk around your home, your business. Not the one you have now, but the one you want to create or develop or the one you have in this new, upgraded and expanded version. Travel the world,

see your healthy body. Lie on the beach, climb the mountain, drive the car, relax with your partner, play with your kids or grandkids, spend time in your garden. Start creating, building, seeing and truly living in this reality inside your mind. All of this happens inside this large sphere.

4. For twenty-one days, spend as long as you wish (minimum fifteen minutes) living this reality inside your mind. Keep adding to it, building it, enjoying it. See and feel it vividly. Smell it, taste it and truly know this reality. Make it realer than what your life is actually like.

5. After twenty-one days of building this blueprint, it's time to start manifesting it. I want you to activate your merkaba field by connecting to Sirius, Orion and the Delphinus star system. Communicate with these celestial lights and tell them you want to activate your merkaba for manifestation. Feel Sirius, Orion and Alpha and Beta Delphinus, see them and connect to them and know deep in your heart and soul that in this moment, everything will change. Feel/see/know the light steams from these celestial beings are switching you on.

6. Once you feel that your field is activated, I want you to start living inside the blueprint in your mind. Truly enjoy the life that you've created and as you do, I want you to consciously open your heart, feel the energy of your heart flow into your merkaba field and then start amplifying the feelings in your body as you enjoy the life inside of your mind. Truly feel all the excitement, gratitude, love, joy and happiness and success as you experience your perfectly designed life.

7. Spend at least fifteen minutes a day living this inside of your mind, with amplified feelings and an activated merkaba.

After 15 minutes or however long you stay in the process, shrink this large sphere down until it fits inside your heart centre. When you go to do it the next day, expand the sphere and play and live in that reality once again.

Please choose your thoughts and intentions carefully. Once this is fully activated you will automatically connect to the Kryst Consciousness Grid around the planet. Each human being has their own Kryst Consciousness mini grid, connected to their own energy field, which then connects to the Planetary Kryst Consciousness Grid. It is an icosahedron: a 20-sided shape. Within this field there are a number of other geometric shapes, all connected to you through atomic spin points, woven into the cosmic fabric. Everything is connected so positive and negative events can manifest. Both are governed by your thoughts and emotions. We don't need to go further into this right now. This is enough information for you to fully activate your merkaba. Just remember, you will manifest any highly charged thoughts and visions. So, choose your thoughts, visions, words and emotions wisely.

I suggest you spend fifteen minutes every day for twenty-one days bringing in the light energies/ frequencies to activate this aspect of your miracle-creating soul machine. I also suggest spending time/space each day connecting your transmission centres to the Stars. This is what will activate the full potential of Star Magic. This is mission critical. Use the code **X3631** each time you go in.

Without that heart/mind connection you will not unleash your full human potential. It takes dedication and discipline to be a Super-Human.

When you continue to do this daily, your merkaba field will start communicating with the cosmic fabric and the invisible field and the universe will start to communicate with the minds of women and men all over the planet. Consciousness will go to work to make this vision a reality. Remember, what you see inside your mind is a reality. The universe will influence the minds and hearts of your sisters and brothers to collaborate to make this new life a reality, very quickly. You are a divine cosmic instrument, and you can play any tune or song you wish. So why not play the tune and hear the song that fulfils you and makes you truly happy? Why not live the life that you came to this planet to live and not one society has conditioned you into? Use your heart and your body to create a powerful emotional charge as you live the life and create the blueprint inside of your mind. The charge sets the activated merkaba in motion to communicate with all things necessary to make this dream a reality.

Ensure that every waking second you are tuning yourself, the instrument of life, to feel, be, know and experience your Super-Human self now. Live, breathe and feel the parallel you that exists. Entangle yourself with your Super-Human blueprint. The Delphinus stars will bring your mind and heart into perfect coherence, and this is mission critical. The heart and mind coherence can influence the quantum field at any distance; after all, it's illusory. The universe will conspire in your favour and magic will unfold. Your subconscious mind also doesn't know the difference between what's on the outside and what's on the inside. So, as you live this life with emotional charge, your cells will start to know this reality. The more you do this, the more the body will signal new genes that are congruent with your vision, your Super-Human blueprint. Everything will conspire in your favour to bring this reality into fruition. Start now, beautiful soul. The universe awaits you.

Next-Level Manifestation

When you reach a certain level of energy, this kind of visualization can hinder the process. I have found that deciding what I want, knowing what I want and then speaking it firmly into existing with my word or feeling it into existence with my inner knowing, is faster. Having your merkaba fired up is always important and the higher your frequency goes, the more all of these natural processes will move into place, fire up and stay activated.

If you need to do the work to fire them up, that is cool. Soon it will be effortless. You can control everything with your intention, very quickly. Knowing, intending, deciding what is happening or has happened, is the fastest way to manifest. Just decide it and speak it out loud. Think and speak things into form.

Until you feel comfortable and assured in your own heart, knowing that what you want to manifest is manifesting, use the merkaba and visualization technique. It 100 per cent works.

Twelve-pointed merkaba

The twelve-pointed merkaba field is a larger field with a greater degree of mathematics than the two-tetrahedron merkaba we have just been discussing. The two tetrahedrons offer you the opportunity to travel, but this travel is limited to the two specific rotational spins of the two tetrahedrons. The twelve-pointed merkaba field contains a greater degree of mathematics that offers multiple rotational spins within the same space, offering you the opportunity to move in multiple directions. Spacecrafts for example have a twelve-pointed merkaba, spinning within and around the craft's field.

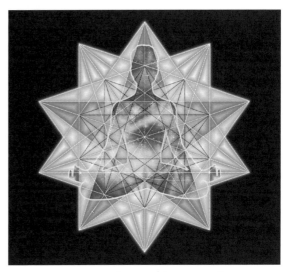

94. Human being inside 12-pointed multidimensional merkaba field

Above is the same picture of a human being inside the twelve-pointed merkaba structure. I mentioned earlier that using the sound codes to tune your platinum light body would also start building your twelve-pointed merkaba field. The codes will not only tune your platinum light body structure and build your twelve-pointed merkaba, they will also amplify the Krystal Light, flowing through your transmission centres, creating a stronger connection between your light body and the Earthly and Stellar Grids.

They will also activate your twelve-strand DNA template and connect each strand and sub-strand into the Kathara Grid Structure and from there into the Star Gates; and will plug your twelve-strand blueprint into the twelve-pointed merkaba. These sound codes are potent. I have listed the instructions again here for ease.

PROTOCOL *Activate Your Twelve-Pointed Merkaba Field*

All you will need to do for this exercise is to be still. Eyes open or closed, go into a still state, a state of presence. Bring your awareness into your heart and feel/see/know your platinum light body structure is around the outside of you. Then one by one you will say these codes out loud or speak them in your mind. Codes 1–12 three times through. Do not say code 1 three times and then move to code 2. Say each code in order three times through and then move to code 13. As you speak them, feel them in your heart.

1. **Aya Eka U Ma**
2. **Reishi Ma Hun Sheya Ta**
3. **Kara Ki A Aa Nem Ka**
4. **Dera Mi Aa Kryst Na Ma Ra**
5. **Ei Esh Ee An Ra Ha Zi**
6. **Gresh Ee Ash A Ka**
7. **Gresh Rei Ash Ha Ya**
8. **Ta Ra Aan Dra N Shu Ma**
9. **Oo Nu Bta Ma Eshh Ta**
10. **Ka Ra Ak A E Ka**
11. **Ash Tei U Na Elo Nia Shu La**
12. **Aan Dren Vu Ea Kan Arataa**

Code 13 is the gateway to the original primary light and sound fields. The first part of code 13 – **Ka Ra Ya Sa Ta Aa La** – you will chant and the second part you will speak. Chant the first part once and then speak the second part and repeat two more times.

PART 1 – **Ka Ra Ya Sa Ta Aa La**

You will chant Ka, then Ra, then Ya, then Sa, then Ta, then Aa, then La.
   Then speak part 2 below.

PART 2 – **Kia Kuna An Shra Du Ka Ina Ma**

Then repeat the sequence part 1 and part 2 two more times. As you are going through this process, feel Krystal Frequencies flowing down through your body and up through your body.
   You will feel this. This is something you can do daily and always.

DNA and Transmission Centre Configuration

Each transmission centre connects to a DNA strand and to a specific point in the twelve-pointed merkaba field structure. To really switch this on there are a few simple steps:

1. Close your eyes and breathe.
2. Place/visualize the God Seed Atom inside your heart.
3. Bring your awareness into your heart and connect with the God Seed Atom.
4. State: I am activating my twelve-pointed merkaba field through DNA and transmission centre configuration.
5. Then say each code out loud or inside your mind, three times. Once you have said each code three times, chant and say code number 13.
6. Done.

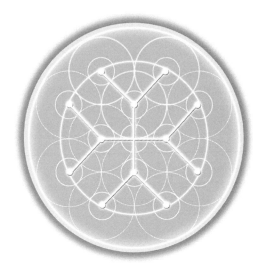

95. God Seed Atom

Above is the picture of the God Seed Atom that you place in your heart.
   You will feel your body and energy field vibrating and if your third eyesight is switched on you will see multiple tetrahedrons spinning in

your energy field, as well as streams of energy/ light, flowing from the God Seed Atom into your transmission centres and your cells/DNA, from your transmission centres into the God Seed Atom and your cells/DNA, and from your cells/ DNA out into the twelve-pointed merkaba field. This takes a few minutes.

The illustration below shows the transmission centres and which DNA strands each one connects to.

When Jesus — the one with the twelve DNA strands activated (because there were two Jesuses) — was incarnated on Earth, he was sharing the truths about Ascension. This is information that you find in this book. His Ascension knowledge, however, went beyond this and into the true mechanics of how you utilize these advanced merkaba fields to move through Star Gates. This will be the topic of another book, still to be written.

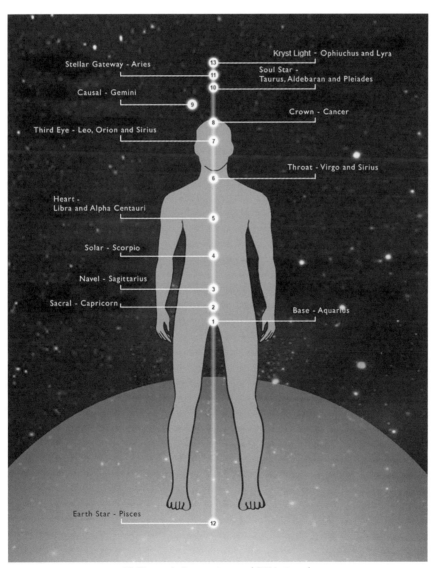

96. Transmission centres and DNA strands

12

Nervous System Upgrade

Nervous System Activation

What I want to share with you now is a tool to truly upgrade you and activate the greatest pharmacy on the planet: your nervous system. The nervous system has many different components, the main ones being: the central nervous system, the autonomic nervous system (made up of the sympathetic and parasympathetic nervous systems; we've looked at this already) and the peripheral nervous system (which is made up of the somatic and autonomic nervous system; again, we've met the autonomic nervous system already). All of these different elements work together to deliver information around the body.

The central nervous system (CNS) controls most functions of the body and mind. It consists of two parts: the brain and the spinal cord. The brain is the centre of our thoughts, the interpreter of our external environment, and the origin of control over body movement.

The peripheral nervous system's (PNS) main job is to send information gathered by the body's sensory receptors to the central nervous system (CNS) as quickly as possible. Once the CNS has understood the information, the PNS will relay the specific orders back out to the body. The autonomic nervous system is the part of the nervous system that supplies the internal organs, including the blood vessels, stomach, intestine, liver, kidneys, bladder, genitals, lungs, pupils, heart, and sweat, salivary and digestive glands.

The peripheral nervous system has two components: the somatic nervous system and the autonomic nervous system. The PNS consists of all of the nerves that lie outside the brain and spinal cord.

The somatic nervous system, which we call the SNS, is part of the peripheral nervous system. Major functions of the SNS include voluntary movement of the muscles and organs, and reflex movements. In the process of voluntary movement, sensory neurons carry impulses to the brain and the spinal cord.

The autonomic nervous system has two main divisions, sympathetic and parasympathetic. These two aspects are opposing forces. The parasympathetic element slows you down and the sympathetic element speeds you up. The sympathetic nervous system prepares the body for the "fight or flight" response during any potential danger. On the other hand, the parasympathetic nervous system inhibits the body from overworking and restores it to a calm and composed state.

Both are important but we do not want to have our sympathetic nervous system activated unnecessarily, otherwise we may burn out and be in a constant state of anxiety or fear, and that is extremely unhealthy. With that being said, a real warrior fights in a calm and composed state. They don't let their heart rate go through the roof during battle. They stay cool and that way can fight longer and make better decisions.

Through meditation, qigong and breathing exercises, we can activate our parasympathetic nervous system, which is healthy for our body. We want to live in a state of calm. The thing is that a large number of people live in fear, thinking and creating realities into being in the most negative of ways; they think and focus on all of the things that could go wrong instead of the infinite possibilities of things that could go right. Remember, wherever your attention goes, your energy surely follows.

It's not critically important that you remember what each of these components of the nervous system as a whole do, but it's good to lay it down so you can see the complexity of this phenomenal system residing inside you, always working, never sleeping, and making you tick.

Throughout our body there are billions of chemical changes happening second by second, and our nervous system and chemical neurotransmitters (a type of chemical messenger) share these chemicals throughout this intricate system through signals. All of this is amplified in a positive way when we do certain exercises, such as the deep breathing exercises, qigong and pineal gland activation exercise. What you do is switch on the most powerful chemicals – and they are free. You don't have to get a prescription; you simply have to apply a little discipline and do the work.

I want to share a powerful way to really activate your entire nervous system. (You will know it if you know my book *Healing with Light Frequencies: the Transformative Power of Star Magic.*) When you are switched on at this level, you become a walking, talking healing machine. As a Super-Human, this is what you want to be; but what comes as a byproduct of that is a truly activated arsenal of super-extraordinary chemicals that make you happy and healthy.

By following this protocol, you will amplify your life in so many ways. Even if you are not a healer, you will start healing others by simply being near them, and sometimes no-where near them. What I am going to do is show you the way to do this over a 23-day process. Once you have completed the twenty-three days, I will show you how to create

a template of your fully activated nervous system, that you can then plug into when you need a top-up. But you will have to go through the 23-day process first to be able to create a supercharged blueprint that can be stored in the ether, for you to plug into as and when you require it. Please, don't just try to create a template/blueprint as it will have no substance.

I am going to discuss this from the observational standpoint of a healer. If you are a healer it will come in handy, and if you are not then at least you will have some extra knowledge, and I am sure it will be useful at some point on your journey.

The Whole Body Heals

When it comes to Star Magic and facilitating healing, no part of my body is hot. I have trained it to be this way. Occasionally my hands will emit a little warmth but at the same time, if you were to touch them, they would be ice cold. My hands also vibrate when I am scanning the hologram of a human being. They vibrate at a place I need to bring my awareness into.

The only way to truly know is to experience. I want you to experience temperature control within your own body. Healing is more effective when the body is cool. The light and energy can flow more freely and there are no side effects for the human being facilitating the healing process. When your body is warm it's out of balance. When you focus on bringing energy/light into certain parts of your body and neglecting others, you are out of balance. You can overload the electrical energy in one part of the body, for example.

Being out of balance can result in various unpleasant and unhealthy side effects like vertigo, organ pains, muscle pain, headaches, pins and needles and sickness. It's ineffective to facilitate a healing and get ill yourself in the process. If you are a healer and have been taught that heat is good, and you are getting some results, then try bringing your own body temperature down and see what results you get then. You will be amazed.

When you are facilitating the healing of someone, they may feel heat, or cold, and both are OK. It means healing is taking place. It's different for the human being being healed than for the healer. The healer wants to maintain a nice cool temperature flow for two reasons – safety and effectiveness. It's also mission critical to treat your entire body as a healing vessel, not just certain parts of it. We are not mechanical, we are natural.

Within your body you have approximately forty-five miles of electrical wiring or nerve fibres. They spread throughout your entire body. The secret to powerful energy/light is to build up and emit light from your entire nervous system. Many healing modalities teach healers to run energy through the hands. If you try to pocket light and energy in certain areas, like your hands, you are limiting yourself. When you run energy through your hands, they become overloaded, as there are 4,000 nerve endings in each hand. This is what creates the symptoms above. To fully experience the power of Star Magic, you must build up your entire nervous system and, once you do, learn to regulate the temperature of the energy flow throughout your body. Once you do this you fully activate the connection between your body and the Channelled Network of Light (CNL) or light grid system/cosmic fabric throughout and extending beyond your entire body, enabling you to work on a level of light and information much more easily.

Increase the Light

To build up the nervous system you need to use light. You use your awareness to tune into the nervous system and feel the light/energy flow. Then, by bringing in more light/energy, you can increase the flow, strengthen the system and

increase the bandwidth, which will enable more light to flow throughout the entire nervous system, in turn allowing more information to flow through it. Remember light is information.

As the bandwidth of the nervous system grows and strengthens, so does the amount of light/energy you can use, and the volume of information contained within the light can be increased. You can put codes into the light travelling through your nervous system, which will totally amplify things again, and you can also delete codes and upload new ones. Remember, your brain and body are like biological computers, and they respond immediately to the instructions given to one or the other or both.

There are around 400 nerve endings in each foot. Wouldn't it be great to have 4,000, as we have in each hand? Imagine if you had a high volume of nerve fibres and nerve endings running throughout your entire system, and you could control and direct the flow of light through them all. Well, soon you will. And you are going to be able to control the temperature at the same time. Your body will have its own built-in air conditioning unit.

Remember, you cannot push light or energy around your body. Energy has to flow, and light is everywhere. You can control this flow, but never by force. If you force light, you will experience the same symptoms as when you are overloading an area of the body and it becomes heated. When you overload your system in one area, it's too much electricity, so the nerve-fibre building process must be executed throughout the entire body.

When your entire system is built effectively, light pours from all parts of your body evenly, through the ether, carrying information necessary for healing, and into the energy field or holographic body or physical body of the human being whose healing you are facilitating.

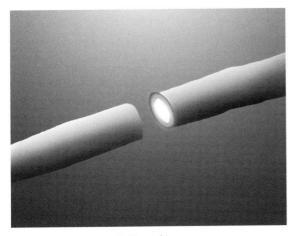

97. Nerve fibres

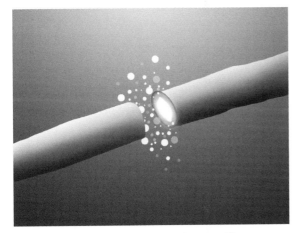

98. Bio-photons in between the nerve fibres

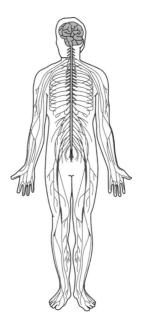

99. Nervous system

Bio-photons, which are units of light that store data, collect between the nerve fibres. To build your nervous system into one complete and powerful unit, you will need to use your imagination, your intention and your awareness. Once your third eye is activated, you will be able to see what is happening, but until then these three ingredients are crucial. You will also need to trust and know. Before you start this process, it's good to have an idea of what the nervous system looks like.

PROTOCOL *Nervous System Activation*

You start by creating an inverted crystal-white pyramid up above your head or above the head of your entangled hologram. Visualize it there, spinning clockwise. As it spins it draws in light and codes from the celestial bodies of Alpha Centauri, Lyra, Pleiades, Sirius, Arcturus, and Ophiuchus. See the light streams flow into the base of the inverted pyramid and collect there.

Next, open the apex of the pyramid slightly, bringing in light through the top of your head and see it flow throughout your nerve fibres. Just have your awareness over the nerve fibres inside your face and head. Use your imagination and see the light flow through the nerves in your head and your face. Tell it where to flow. Command/intend it but don't force it. Remember, your body responds to your intention and so does the light. Once you feel/see or know the light has spread throughout each nerve fibre and into each nerve ending, you can move to the next part of your body. Repeat the process with your neck. Then with your shoulders and chest. Next, your back and arms. Then your

249

stomach area. Then your hips and buttocks. Now your legs, and finally your feet. Once you see this light flowing through the entire system you can stop. You are ready to start building it – slowly!

Amplify the Bandwidth

Here is a phased 23-day way for you to build up and strengthen your nervous system. Do this and you will enhance your ability to heal as well as feel happier, stronger and lighter in your vibration.

DAYS 1–5

Spend fifteen minutes each day for five days, repeating the process described above. By the end of the five days you should be able to activate your entire nervous system, with light, real fast, almost instantaneously. See this light as a crystalline white colour. If it takes you longer than five days, that is perfectly OK. Just move on to day 6 once you get to this point. The aim is to bring light through the entire nervous system and see it/feel it/know it's lit up. You will want to open the apex of the inverted pyramid slightly wider as you work down through the entire body.

DAY 6

Repeat as above. Then with your imagination and intention see the nerve fibres start to expand and grow thicker, just inside your head and face. The entire process should take no longer than fifteen minutes. Every day; no longer than fifteen minutes. Once you have doubled the bandwidth of the nervous system in your head, move your awareness to your feet and visualize/create 4,000 nerve endings in each foot.

Then do the same in your knees, hips and shoulders. Visualize/create 4,000 nerve endings in each knee, each hip and each shoulder. The whole time the inverted pyramid is running current in through your crown and into the new expanded parts in your head and it will naturally filter through the rest of your body.

DAY 7

Repeat as above, adding the next body part: your neck and throat. With your imagination and intention see the nerve fibres start to expand and grow thicker, just inside your neck and throat. Also continue bringing your awareness to your feet, knees, hips and shoulders and building these new nerve endings. I see them growing out from my nervous system like grapes on a vine. The whole time the inverted pyramid is running current in through your crown and into the new expanded parts which are your head, face, neck, and throat.

DAY 8

Repeat as above, adding the next body parts: your shoulders and chest. With your imagination and intention see the nerve fibres start to expand and grow thicker, just inside your shoulders and chest. Also continue bringing your awareness to your feet, knees, hips and shoulders and building these new nerve endings. The whole time the inverted pyramid is running current in through your crown and into the new expanded parts which are your head, face, neck and throat, shoulders, and chest.

DAY 9

Repeat as above, adding the next body part: your back and arms. With your imagination and intention see the nerve fibres start to expand and grow thicker, just inside your back and arms. Also continue bringing your awareness to your feet, knees, hips and shoulders and building these new nerve endings. The whole time the inverted pyramid is running current in through your crown and into the new expanded parts which are your head, face, neck and throat, shoulders, chest, back, and arms.

DAY 10

Repeat as above, adding the next body part, your stomach area. With your imagination and intention see the nerve fibres start to expand and grow thicker, just inside your stomach. Also continue bringing your awareness to your feet, knees, hips and shoulders and building these new nerve endings. The whole time the inverted pyramid is running current in through your crown and into the new expanded parts which are your head, face, neck and throat, chest, back, arms, and stomach.

DAY 11

Repeat as above, adding the next body part: your hips and buttocks. With your imagination and intention see the nerve fibres start to expand and grow thicker, just inside your hips and buttocks. Also continue bringing your awareness to your feet, knees, hips and shoulders and building these new nerve endings. The whole time the inverted pyramid is running current in through your crown and into the new expanded parts which are your head, face, neck and throat, chest, back, arms, stomach, hips, and buttocks.

DAY 12

Repeat as above, adding the next body part: your legs and ankles. With your imagination and intention see the nerve fibres start to expand and grow thicker, just inside your legs. Also continue bringing your awareness to your feet, knees, hips and shoulders and building these new nerve endings. The whole time the inverted pyramid is running current in through your crown and into the new expanded parts which are your head, face, neck and throat, chest, back, arms, stomach, hips, buttocks, legs, and ankles.

DAY 13

Repeat as above, adding the next body part: your feet. With your imagination and intention see the nerve fibres start to expand and grow thicker, just inside your feet. On this day you will open the apex of the pyramid much wider and allow the Star Light and the codes to flow down into this expanded nervous system, filling it up. The whole time the inverted pyramid is running current in through your crown and into the new expanded parts which are your head, face, neck and throat, chest, back, arms, stomach, hips, buttocks, legs, ankles, and feet.

DAY 14–21

Repeat the expansion process, including every body part at once. Don't force anything. You will see the nervous system gradually expand and more energy/light will flow through it. Open the apex of the pyramid wider and wider as you expand the nervous system. Keep bringing the light in and it will naturally happen, through using your intention and imagination. Feel the process with your awareness. See it with your mind's eye, feel it with your awareness. The whole time the inverted pyramid is running current in through your crown and into the nervous system.

DAY 22

Bring the light into your body and throughout your entire nervous system. See or feel (both maybe) the light flowing through. Now, start to project your energy evenly from your nervous system outwards. See or feel (maybe both) it expand, evenly in all directions. The aim of this exercise is to see light projecting from your entire body outwards. As you get used to doing this, your body's light will naturally start doing it during the healing process, when you are facilitating the healings of others. Your body has this entire amplified electrical system; you have to hone it. Do this until it feels like you should stop! On our trainings, I guide and encourage our facilitators to expand the light from their nervous system throughout the galaxy and beyond. When you do this and then bring all of the light back into your physical body, the vibration is incredible. It often feels like you can't fit inside your body and that your body is far too small. You will get used to it.

The whole time the inverted pyramid is running current in through your crown and into the nervous system. Through the Lyran light frequency you will be running light codes from Aramatena (from Star Gate 12) carrying the Krystal Coding from the primary light and sound fields.

DAY 23

Repeat the process and expand it further. Really amplify the light. When I bring the light back again, I always bring it all back inside my body. I don't like light hanging out from me. When your field is expanded, it's like the main attraction at a fair for energy vampires. Especially if you are walking through a busy shopping arcade, or in a restaurant, or anywhere with lots of people. Now, on one hand you could expand it in these places, and you will be healing as you move.

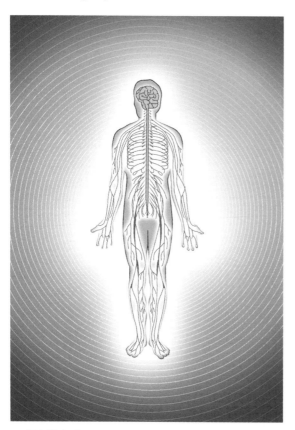

100. Light from nervous system projecting out evenly

If you do that you must maintain high levels of awareness and monitor your field. If anyone's energy latches on to your field and starts siphoning your energy, then remove it. I sometimes have my field expanded and other times bring it inside of me.

You should play around with this. You should be able to walk into a room or any space and go totally unnoticed. You should also be able to walk into a room or any space and get everyone to turn and look at you. Your energy field is the determining factor. Play with it. Experiment with it. It's fun. Expand it and contract it in different situations and observe what is happening around you and within you.

On our Training Experiences where I facilitate the remembering/learning of Star Magic, I get people to do this exercise. When everyone does it at once it feels like I am out at sea and the water is rough. The expansion of light and energy takes me off my feet. The invisible world is very real, my friend.

From here on in, spend fifteen minutes every day bringing light through your nervous system. See it flow and feel it flow. Start to "innerstand" how it flows. See and feel the patterns, the geometry. Watch it expand and ensure it expands evenly and that you can project this energy at will, evenly, through all areas of your body. If one area seems to be weaker than others, put your intention forward to strengthen it. But never force it. Increase the size of the individual nerve fibres.

Remember, throughout this entire process, drop down into your heart space. Bring your awareness there. Your awareness can be in as many places at once as you wish. After the twenty-three days and as long as your nervous system is firing on all cylinders, then you can revisit it once a week, or as often as you wish, and tap into the blueprint you are going to create in the next chapter.

Regulating the Temperature

You want your body to remain cool. Think cool and you will be cool. It really is that easy. You will need to have your awareness scanning or feeling your entire body as you are facilitating the healing. If it feels as though it's getting hot just think ice, think cool. Imagine a cool breeze flowing through your body. You don't actually want it to be as cold as ice, because if you're too cold that may take your attention away from the healing, but thinking ice can quickly cool you down

Once you have started to see and feel your body becoming cooler, set your intention to maintain the temperature that feels cool for you. You will get to know your body through your awareness, and you will soon realize if it's too hot, as then you may experience side effects such as headaches, vertigo, pins and needles, aching organs, etc. Although to be honest, with your nervous system acting as a complete unit and you not just running energy through your hands and overloading one area, you should not get too hot.

You can see the flow of energy throughout your own body as a cool blue colour. This will help in keeping it cool. See the energy as red, on the other hand (which is often associated with fire and heat) and you will get hot. Once your nervous system is fully activated and you can regulate the light/energy flow at a cool temperature, you will be able to project your energy effortlessly and powerfully, manipulating realities (in a positive way) with your own energy field.

Effortlessness is the key to Star Magic. You create an environment where it all happens for you. You really do become a pure vessel. You truly facilitate without action. I have a dial in my left shoulder. It's like a thermostat. I can turn it up or down. You can create one too. Remember, you are a Quantum Architect, and everything can be created/recreated. You may want to create a dial in your forearm or your hand or somewhere else. Have fun, be creative, play like

a child. The more fun you have with it and the more you get lost in your imagination, the realer it becomes.

Creating Your Blueprint

Firstly, you can only store this blueprint after the twenty-third day. Doing it prematurely will not be as efficient. By the time you get through the twenty-three days, your nervous system will be lit up massively, blazing light in every direction. What you must do is this:

Visualize your hologram. Entangle the hologram with your body by saying, "This is the hologram of ..." and then stating your name. You can just know it's your hologram and that is sufficient, but if you are new to working with holograms, say your name three times to be sure.

Take an imaginary USB stick. Communicate with it. Insert this code into it with your intention. You can just visualize it. The code is **C407**. This is an upload code.

Insert it into the biological computer (the brain) of your own hologram. Leave it. The code will upload the frequency from the hologram with all of the data/information of the amplified nervous system.

Now that the frequency is inside the USB stick, you will insert a second code into it. This code is **C467**. This code will create infinite copies of the encoded amplified frequency within the same USB stick. Now, it will be like a self-charging battery. Each time you download the frequency and use it, the USB stick will replenish.

All you have to do is place this code into the biological computer (the brain) of your own hologram and it will supercharge you in seconds (maximum time several minutes).

You can carry this USB stick with you always. I carry it in my tailor-made chromium suit jacket. I have a whole series of USB sticks containing codes on the inside of my jacket. If you have been to Facilitator Training, you too will have a selection of USB sticks containing a variety of different codes for different situations.

Take the time, do the work. Go through the twenty-three-day process, remember how to cool your nervous system and keep it cool. PRACTISE. Once you have completed the twenty-three days, create your code and then go and truly be a Super Human!

13

Fearless Leadership

Truth and Responsibility

In this chapter we are going to discuss being fearless, and leadership. First of all, this planet must step out of the mindset of having leaders to follow, swallowing lie after lie, hoping that this human being or that human being will make the changes that will filter into our trusting government who have been elected. Election after election the same thing happens, the same story plays out and things often get worse. The wars continue, the poverty and sickness increases, the pharmaceutical industry, private arms dealers/companies get richer, and most people continue to suffer.

In Finland, the country is run by four women. First of all, that is soooooo very cool. Don't you agree? All that right-brain, divine feminine, conscious, caring way of being, flowing through the country's people. Pure music to my ears. In Finland they realize that the children are the future and that they must be nurtured at school, not driven like dogs. The Finnish school day is only four or five hours and it is a creative day. They have long breaks too. The kids are encouraged to express themselves through art, dance, music or whatever way they feel like doing. They meditate and take a holistic approach. This generation of children are going to grow up as free thinkers, uncorrupted, rather than just being taught facts to regurgitate later on, to pass exams that will give them the privilege of entering the world and working hard for someone else just to get by.

Seeing what is happening in Finland, how their leadership is creating kids who will themselves be free and be leaders, is awesome. I know it's changing, slowly, and I trust that this will all eventually happen in other countries too. But . . . and it's a BIG BUT . . .

Rather than putting our faith in some other human being or group of people to make changes that will benefit us, what we all must have is a fearless leader in our life who leads us into the unknown RIGHT NOW, to create a better reality. This fearless leader is you. You must take the necessary action to raise your energy and shift your frequency and move into a different paradigm. We must become our own fearless leaders and start creating together by forming or creating conscious communities where we are all equal and share equal responsibility.

We must stop looking for saviours. No woman, man or child, extra-terrestrial, angel or archetypal figure will save you, me, or anyone else on this planet. Jesus is not returning to work his magic on this Earth Plane. Anyway, Jesus has/had no more potential than you or I. The power lies within. We are the power. No one can lead anyone to peace. We must unify and walk together as one. This is how real change is solidified. If we don't come together, join forces and unite as a global family, with our underlying driving current fuelled with love, truth and compassion, then we, as a race, will stay in no-man's-land.

What is no-man's-land? A state where we have woken up but are not brave and courageous enough to speak our truth and realize freedom. A space where we carry on accepting the conditions of this vibrational but physical global prison that so many are living in. Like Einstein said, doing the same thing over and over and expecting a different result (or knowing you are in this prison and doing nothing about it) is the definition of madness.

A Super-Human always seeks out the truth and is ready and willing to stand in his or her own truth always, regardless of the circumstances or potential consequences. To be a Super-Human, a master of dark and light, we must be who we are, and for most people that is tough. From birth most people are taught, encouraged to hide, to wear a mask and to express only a small sliver of their own beautiful nature.

A Super-Human, a fearless leader, knows that dark and light blend into one stream of experience on an infinite vibrational scale that merges at a central balancing point. This space is known as neutral. To be neutral in all situations takes wisdom and wisdom is a refining of the human, the emotions, the heart and the soul. Until we refine our own inner being, which is a culmination of the mind, body and spirit all experiencing the now space, we cannot be authentic.

Fragmentation distorts the energy and therefore the presence of a man or woman, causing them to react or not react. Both can be detrimental. To react and change your own personal state to a lower vibrational frequency because of the words or actions of another shows there is work to be done, a further refining. And to not react when someone steps across your boundaries and enters your personal space, either physically or energetically, keeping quiet but inwardly feeling discomfort, also shows that further refining of the being is necessary. To react in this latter situation by verbally enforcing your boundaries in a controlled manner is perfect. To clear and cleanse your space energetically of another human's energy, the energy of someone who has been infiltrated by some lower-vibrational element, or simply a direct invasion of

your field, requires a stepping up and being strong and saying no and doing what's necessary to stand in your truth, ruthlessly enveloped in a deep feeling of love, knowing your worth and being your power and saying no, in no uncertain terms, and if necessary throwing the potential threat out from your space.

When I use the term "threat", it's just a word. It's not used from fear; and really and truthfully, when you know your power, there is nothing at all that can threaten you. A master of dark and light, a True Super-Human, loves in all situations, friend and foe, and is so sure about who they are and the value of their own being, and that death is an illusion, that nothing at all ever threatens their world.

The only way the truth can heal is when you live it always, and often that can be crushing. To live your truth, you must open yourself up to any vulnerability that lies within. Quite often we do not know these aspects of ourselves exist until we feel pain and emotions fly. But that is such a beautiful thing, to open yourself up and to be vulnerable. This is how you truly master your own essence: by accepting how you are feeling in a particular space. Maybe someone triggers anger, sadness, jealousy or another emotion within you. A big thank you is necessary as you have an opportunity to be your truth, communicate with your own heart and say yes, I am feeling sad or I am feeling jealous or I am feeling angry or I am feeling hurt, betrayed, small; regardless of how you are feeling, feel it with the depths of your being and allow all of this feeling to flow out from you naturally.

By expressing your vulnerability, you create a platform to grow from. The danger lies within a human being who will not face their pain. One who hides behind the happy mask, pretending to the world that the inner pain isn't there, yet the world can see the cracks appearing in the energy field of this man or woman and they become weak, open to manipulation. But a man or woman who openly and honestly shares their truth and accepts their pain becomes stronger, wiser, more powerful; they cannot be hurt, manipulated or infiltrated, physically or energetically because they are living in their heart and the heart is a mighty force of natural power. A true warrior knows and accepts every facet of their inner workings and never hides from them. When you allow your inner pain to be your truth, you can turn that pain to immense power and the tides of infinite intelligence will be at your mercy, wanting to assist you in every situation.

Another common flaw of the "wannabe" spiritual warrior – and this applies to so many – is pretending to the world that they must do good and sacrifice themselves for humanity. When someone doesn't know their worth, instead of facing deep inner truths they mask their pain by helping others. They look outside of themselves always, because to be still is to feel pain and to feel pain, for some people, is a rope around the neck, ready to kick away the table or chair. While of course good humanitarian work can and should be done, it should be done once the inner work has been accomplished and the human being knows who and what they are. When they have brought to the surface the childhood abuse, parallel life trauma, the rejection, the bullying, the loss, opened their heart and healed it and found the power in doing so, then and only then can they move into assisting others effectively. You could always assist others while you are doing your inner work but never sacrifice your inner growth because you are helping the world. You will only ever truly be of service to your sisters and brothers by being a beautiful mirror of reflection, a pillar of certainty, a burning white fire of truth.

By uniting as one global family we will blow the roof off this vibrational space/prison and take back our power and with that power, freedom.

These are our lands, our waters. Us, we, as the human race who share the jungles with animals and insects, the oceans with whales, dolphins, turtles and other sea life, the skies with birds and the fields and woods with flowers and trees, can, when we move as a unified force, like the crest and trough of the wave, with zero separation, fluid like water, solid as iron, bring into existence a magical world where the entire global population is happy and free.

This planetary playground is already here. The Earth is beautiful. We must adjust our frequency, change our perception and create a different reality in the space we are in.

For us, as a species, as a tribe, to truly work in harmony as one global family, we must do the inner work so our lights can ignite and we become a shining example to our fellow brothers and sisters of Earth. If we shirk this inner work, we can never truly change this world. After all, we must change ourselves first. The spiritual warrior knows this, and the Super-Human is always willing to go deeper, through the next layer, peeling back the baggage that cloaks the soul and unravelling the inner wisdom, the truth, the knowledge that lies within every human being on this planet. I want to share with you an incredible exercise that you can do on your own. It may not be easy but please, do it for you.

EXERCISE *Clear Present Reality Trauma and Discover the Truth*

This meditation exercise will help you bring any trauma to the surface from this reality and heal it. This exercise may also clear some parallel reality trauma; however, I will be sharing a clearing exercise specifically for parallel life trauma very soon.

1. Lie or sit and close your eyes. Breathe deeply and centre yourself.

2. See a crystal-white light flowing into your space with electric pink light codes moving through it.

3. See it swirl clockwise around your physical body.

4. Breathe it into every cell of your body and then say thank you.

5. You will see a wooden door in front of you with the number three engraved in its centre. Walk up the path and through it.

6. On the other side there will be a corridor. Turn right and on the left-hand side, thirty metres away, will be a door with the number 336 on it. Walk through the door.

7. Once inside you will see a room with silver walls and a silver ceiling. The ground is made of crystal, smokey quartz crystal.

8. You will walk to the centre of the room. Once you stop you will start to float, levitate, until you are two metres off the ground.

9. You then must infuse this space with this code **TS333**. See this code inside an orange cube. Place it into your heart and it will dissolve. As it dissolves, say to yourself, "I am ready and willing to clear and heal all present life trauma." Energy/light will flow out from your heart and into the space. It will flow into the silver walls and activate them.

10. A multicoloured light will flow from the top of the chamber and in through your crown. It will move around the inside of your body and start healing you on a cellular level.

11. The light will cleanse your light body and your physical body. You may start to see, on the walls of the chamber, you in different periods of this life. Times when you experienced trauma. Just observe and know the light in pouring through your crown is clearing it. You are just being shown what the universe wanted you to know. Maybe you had forgotten or maybe you were unaware. Just observe. **You may see codes or geometry.** This is the underlying mathematics of the realties being healed.

12. Once the process has finished the light will retract and you will float to the ground. You can then move back to the door. This process will simply unfold.

13. You will then move through the door, turn right (back the same way) and keep walking until you see the wooden door with the number three on the left-hand side. Walk through and back into your body.

14. Sit there for a moment, breathe, become aware of your breath and open your eyes when you feel ready. Please stay hydrated after.

You can do this exercise once, or you may feel like doing it several times in case there are deeper levels/layers that were not available or were too much for you to handle the first time around. Once can be enough, but there are some people who need to go through it several times, as new layers are cleared. Some people wouldn't cope emotionally having it all rise at once. Others can. Do what feels right for you, beautiful soul.

Be Unpredictable

Most people in this world are predictable people. A Super-Human falls outside of this category that has become so normalized. Most people are emotionally cohesive to the stimulus of their external environment and not emotionally cohesive with a clearly defined inner vision of the potential future they want to create or are creating right now.

Most people react, bounce, jerk, let-off steam verbally or shake. A Super-Human responds and flows, vibrates and enjoys. Predictable people are chained to known predictable past memories, that are engraved into their consciousness, hiding behind inner doors. These memories open the doors and appear whenever the body requires an energetic fix. Predictable people allow this to happen and the body and mind run patterns, over and over, creating a vibrational misalignment in the field of the individual, making her or him susceptible to the chaos that's all around. This makes them predictable. You can pretty much guarantee that if someone says something or an event unfolds, a predictable human being will act in a predictable manner.

A Super-Human doesn't react to internal or external stimulus. A Super-Human has mastered the internal energetic imprints that once hid behind closed doors. Super-Humans flow with ease and make conscious choices, not like the predictable human who speaks, acts and feels unconsciously. They are on autopilot, whereas Super-Humans act deliberately, consciously and with full and total awareness.

When you think and act consciously, you are a dangerous woman or man. You become a free thinker and start taking life into your own hands, knowing you must take responsibility for your life, otherwise you will be like many others, struggling, surviving, hoping and praying for a miracle. Gamblers, the predictable, hope and pray. Super-Humans know and create. You are dangerous to the machine. The current system, which at the time of writing this, seems to be disintegrating. I am currently sat at my desk, looking out of my window, the world

on lockdown due to this coronavirus – which, along with the smoke and mirrors, is a blessing in disguise. Out from this event many Super-Humans will emerge. We are being forced to be still right now and go inwards, and that inward journey heals and transforms an individual. En masse it's going to change our planet. It's exciting times. By the time I finish this book, it may be over, and we will see how many unpredictable people there are then.

If you run a business, you may think that you want predictable people working for you because they are easy to manage. Actually, this is untrue. Predictable people are not easier to manage. Reliable people are easy to manage. Predictable people move in a reactive state. They react to the current stimulus, and that's great while the stimulus keeps them working in your company. But they are not loyal and will never have their heart in the game. Unpredictable people choose life and so if you have an unpredictable human being working for you, a conscious free thinker, they are working for you because they have chosen to, and their heart is in the game. They may leave your company one day, but they will do it with honour and respect.

Predictable people are the masses and unpredictable people are the minority, but the scale is changing. Consciousness is rising on this planet and Super-Humans are emerging everywhere. You can spot them because they play life by their own rules. They don't follow suit. They do what feels good for them and they do it fully, wholly and with colossal enthusiasm. They are present and care, not just about themselves but about others they interact with on their journey. They are compassionate and respectful of themselves, others and their space and of the planet as a celestial being who nourishes us every day.

Stop conforming. Be unpredictable. Create your future. Be Super-Human.

Rules of Engagement

For a Super-Human the rules of engagement are simple. There are perspectives and each and every human being on this planet is entitled to their own. We have all experienced different lives, been through different challenges, some more extreme and challenging than others, and so each one of us frames and reframes life, according to the experience life has given us. No one is right or wrong and from everyone's individual perspective, their take on reality sits right.

Because of this "innerstanding", a Super-Human will never engage in an argument. A Super-Human will observe and very rarely respond. Quite often listening and observing is all that is required in any given situation. It could be a friend, family member, other loved one or a total stranger. Whoever it is, there is never a need for an argument, EVER! There are times when a Super-Human must fight, and we will come on to that.

When it comes to another human being saying something or doing something, regardless of what it is, as long as it's not physical, body-to-body action, then listening and observing is always best. It could be a friend in need who requires a listening ear or a family member in need of some constructive feedback. But without first listening and observing, with zero inner dialogue, you will never truly know the best way to handle the situation.

If you are experiencing a human being who wants to argue, or defeat you in verbal warfare, you must ask yourself these questions. First, is this human being mentally and emotionally mature enough to see, feel and "innerstand" different perspectives? The second question you should ask yourself is this: is this human being vibrating on the same frequency as me? The answer to the first question could be a yes or no but the answer to the second question is pretty much guaranteed to be no. If they were on the same frequency, you would see eye to eye, feel heart to heart and agree or disagree with compassion and no friction would occur.

Whatever happens in life, a Super-Human will take a non-judgemental standpoint, observe a situation and smile. She or he may sit and listen for a while and then kindly excuse themselves, walking away, completely forgetting what happened. Otherwise, the Super-Human would be carrying the energy from that moment and that is a weight that should never be borne. The moment is the moment and once it's over another one begins, so leave your thoughts in the moment they originated from.

A Super-Human must love and be compassionate in all situations. With this being said, situations may occur in life that require you to fight. They are often very rare, but they do occur. A few weeks ago, my son was walking his dog Zeus, who was seven months old at the time. Still a puppy really. Four guys attacked him in an alleyway at about 10.30 p.m. They tried to stab him several times and if it wasn't for several thick layers of clothing he would have been cut to ribbons. My son took the dog's chain off of Zeus as they were approaching because they did so in a hostile fashion. He hit one of them in the face with it, punched one and kicked another who was pulling his dog's legs.

As I said, these kinds of situations are rare, but they do require you to fight. It's not good or bad, it's a just a situation that occurred. In a situation like this I would say fight with everything you have got. I raise this point because people often ask, we are love and light so do you believe that we should not fight, Jerry? What if it's unavoidable? Well, now you have my answer. The answer came before the question but back to front is never what it seems. There are no sides, simply perspectives. You have made a choice, to incarnate on this planet during some interesting and transformational times, and the rules of engagement are mission critical. No judgement, listen, respond don't react, fight when you have no other choice and always end every encounter with a smile, unless you are being chased down an alley at night with lads with knives. Seriously though, 99.9999 per cent of the time you can keep your heart open, listen, smile and either respond or walk away silently and peacefully, knowing that the situation has only elevated your vibration and hopefully yours has elevated theirs too. It's a game. Play it and enjoy it, all of it!

Be Vulnerable

A super-Human never puts on a show. A Super-Human is honest, inside and out and if a Super-Human's vulnerability must be laid on a table, then so be it. We've already touched upon vulnerability, but I want to go into it a little more. When you speak your truth and share the real you, the human being you are sharing with may love you more, or they may try to take advantage of your vulnerability. If it's the latter, you move on and let go. If it's the first, your relationship will go deeper as you will have a deeper "innerstanding" of each other. Both outcomes are perfect. You are learning/remembering/growing.

The great thing about being vulnerable is that it's the perfect platform to unleash colossal energy and massive firepower. When you are false and building life from shaky grounds, your house will eventually come tumbling down because your true colours, that which creates vulnerability, will rise to the surface, cracks will appear, and you will crumble. But when you are truthful, both with yourself and others, from the very start, you create a platform that is solid. No one is trying to hide anything, and you will be loved more for your honesty. When you try to hide past hurt, when you try to bury it down below, it will eventually rise and if not honoured can look very ugly. When you are outright honest with your insecurities

and you allow yourself to be vulnerable, your insecurities can be beautiful, as they are allowed to express themselves and be nurtured in a kind and compassionate, honest and balanced way. When they seep through the cracks, buried under a façade, the bricks and mortar weaken and both the inside and outside of the building fall apart. It's messy and creates huge instability. When a human being is vulnerable from the start, there is nothing left to hide. They become an open book. The skies are clear and there is no chance of the internal structure rotting further down the timeline.

When I first started speaking publicly, the first thing I used to say was "Hey everyone, thank you for being here. Before we start, I want you to know that I am shitting myself. I am new to public speaking, but I have an important message for you, am facing my fears and am overcoming my internal challenges, so I can share something really valuable with you."

People used to cheer, applaud me, smile and it really broke the ice, and my nerves went out the window. When I was younger my rejection issues meant I was almost crippled with fear when it came to speaking publicly. Doing this meant there was no chance of me being worried about crumbling later on. I had nothing to fear because they knew my fears. It's only when you try to hide your fears that you are really very vulnerable.

By opening your heart, being fierce in your honesty, brave and wise, you create a platform with huge potential. We are taught from a young age to be brave and to not show our emotions. This only creates internal chaos and confusion. That is not a solid platform to build from.

Times are changing on this planet and the world is waking up, becoming more conscious, and the generations to come will be even more so. I grew up with being told to shut up, beaten with a wooden ruler across my bare arse, told I was this and that. I started my children off like this too. Not the beating part, but I was bossy and controlling. I started waking up when my kids were three and one and so started changing the way I behaved, acted, thought and felt about fatherhood. With both of my children, when they reached ten, I took them out of school and let them be free. Children these days are not controllable. They are free cosmic sovereign thinkers and so we must acknowledge this and allow them to create in a safe environment. Most of the current school systems are not like this but they will change. We will discuss children in detail later on because they are the future of our planet.

It's important for all parents to express their truth, even in front of their children. It sets a good example. Many women and men stay in uncomfortable, chaotic relationships because they think they should be strong for the kids. The real, strong course of action is to show your children that you will not put up with what is happening, that you are worth more than your current relationship and you are going to be honest, stand in your truth, be authentic and maybe vulnerable in the process, but nevertheless you are leaving and are determined to create a better, stronger, more stable and loving environment for your children. Staying in a toxic relationship with children is setting a bad example.

Vulnerability is an illusion. Vulnerability is really the Star Gate of strength and wisdom. Because of our conditioning, we often think it's the other way around – that vulnerability is a sign of weakness – but it's not. When you have nothing to hide, you have a clear foundation and from there can build and build. Another word for vulnerability is honesty. If we reframe that word, it gives it an instantly recognizable and very different perspective. We all want to be honest, so let's be honest and allow our insecurities to fall by the wayside. They will do just that when you shine light on them and yes, to do that you just have to be honest.

Leadership requires honesty.

Love – Service – Compassion

As consciousness expands on this planet and more and more people wake up, realizing the truth, naturally, we start to care more and want to help others. This is a beautiful thing. When one sees another caring for a stranger, it may shock another passer-by, as they wonder to themselves, why would you want to help that human being? Some people do think like that. I used to at one point in my life too. Others will be inspired by the kind act. I always give money or food to people I see begging in the streets. Some expect it and others are truly grateful.

The thing is this, the more you help, the more you want to help; but there must be a balancing act and we will come on to this. Firstly, I want to share a little story about my journey and how I transitioned from being a self-centred, ego-driven man who was out for himself to one who cares and shares and wants the world to be free. I used to be a criminal and one of the things I was good at was stealing money from banks, in a very creative way.

I knew someone who had links to a charity in Africa. I asked them if I could donate anonymously, and they agreed to take my money and ensure it arrived in Africa safely. When I received the first letter back about the schools they built and the water pipelines they installed, it blew me away. I had never experienced giving selflessly before. The feeling inside was amazing.

So, from here I handed over cash and found other people who could help me invest in these projects and it grew. I felt like Robin Hood, stealing from the dirty, rich bankers and giving to the poor. I loved it. It lasted for about two years and then I moved to New Zealand, so it came to a halt. It gave me a taste for humanitarian work though; in New Zealand I set up some charity boxing events to donate money to local causes. Then, after Typhoon Haiyan hit the Philippines in 2013, my daughter and I went over there to build homes and schools and put permaculture projects in place. Since then we've also done some amazing work in Cambodia. It was seeing the good this money did that really further inspired me and was an integral part of my spiritual journey. That, coupled with meeting Lyrans (extra-terrestrials) and spending time remembering how to heal with codes in ancient mystery schools, was the recipe for my truth unveiling itself in this world. Giving back is definitely a must. Give in whatever capacity you can.

When it comes to being in service there are two things that we must look out for. The first is that you must give in balance. The universe doesn't want you to suffer because you want to give. Energetically, you should always give from your saucer, by which I mean you always want to ensure that your teacup is not full, but overflowing and that you look after yourself first and foremost and only then give to others. If you don't and you get drained, it defeats the object. There is no point in you raising someone else's vibration if yours dips in the process. Money, time and energy all must be given in balance.

The other thing to be aware of is when people want to give and give continuously and focus all of their attention on helping others. When someone is giving all of their time and energy to external matters, they do not have any space to go within. Firstly, this stunts the spiritual journey. Secondly, the external focus is often a scapegoat or an excuse, so the human being in question can avoid doing the inner work because it's so painful.

Women and men with self-worth issues particularly do this. They try to feel their worth by being in service, but really and truthfully, it's an excuse to avoid their pain. This is not good. It's beautiful to help but each one of us must be prepared to look inwards and do what is necessary to heal, expand, grow and develop, mentally, physically, emotionally and spiritually. We, as one universe, one song, one vibrational

force, must assist each other – that's paramount – but we must also realize that we must take care of ourselves in the process. It's OK to sacrifice but not when the sacrifice becomes an irreversible burden. All your sisters and brothers across the world want you to be healthy and happy, so please put yourself first so you can assist others in a balanced manner.

If we all adopt this approach, each one of us will be happy, healthy and full of vitality. Eventually everyone will rise up as one and there won't really be that much to do for each other. We will simply love each other. Billions of Super-Humans enjoying this magical planet. Together we will live on a gigantic playground, laughing, playing, loving, enjoying and ultimately being free. Let's lead ourselves down the golden path, through the diamond gate and into the garden of joy and as this magical playground is carved, weaved and created, we will have the perfect energetic environment to remember our multidimensional skill sets and move through those Star Gates and off somewhere else. You can join me in the Andromedan Galaxy.

Forgiveness: Stop the Wheel of Karma and Have a Love Attack

First of all, I don't relate to this word karma. People say if you do bad things then you will be punished. That's a pretty negative perspective. Let's look at this in terms of energy or cause and effect. If you create or express a certain type of energy, it flows out into the universal fabric, and, because we are all one, it will find you again, eventually, in this reality or maybe another one. Every thought, emotion and action has a consequence, and that is why it's so vitally important to send out good vibes, 24/7. Now, we are human and often we get caught up in the chaos and can react, and it's not always positive. This brings me back to what we have already discussed: to live consciously, in your heart, responding and not reacting. If we can respond consciously, we change the flow of energy. It's very easy for one human being to say or do something and affect the next woman, man or child and it can cause an energetic chain reaction. As a conscious Super-Human, make it your mission to diffuse that lower-vibrational flow and shift the frequency of the situation from negative to positive. Consciously, lead or direct the energy. A smile, a little dance, a conscious explosion of joy from an open heart, can all change the situation. Quite often neutrality is all that's required.

Let It Go

It's important, as an aware human being, that you don't hold grudges. You don't hold on to the past. You don't blame or feel shame or ridicule another. Forgiveness is mission critical. Forgiveness itself is a Super-Power even though there is nothing to forgive. Now, first of all, our usual definition or interpretation of forgiveness implies that another human being has done something wrong. But in life we have experiences, and if we don't frame them as good or bad, we can simply see them as an experience; then it's much easier to let them go. It doesn't mean you have to agree with other people's actions all of the time, no.

There are some people in this world who do things that make you sick, literally, just like some people do things that fill you with bliss. We are living in a world of polar opposites and both heavy and light situations occur. If we can observe them and move on from them quickly, without carrying the energy of the situation with us and sharing it and spreading it, we help diffuse it. That's why maintaining a high vibration at all costs is a Super-Human must. Stepping back and observing instead of judging lifts you into a bubble of emptiness where you become untouchable and ultimately free. You float and observe and the space around you is like a positive-frequency fence, transmuting lower-vibrational energies. Remember, if you

disengage (be neutral) you cannot add any charge to the situation.

As you move through life there will be people who love you and people who hate you. People who wish you well and others who are jealous. Love them all the same. Keep your vibration high. There will be people who do things you disagree with. Simply pour love into the situation. It can only help. By cursing them, bad-mouthing them to others or thinking for days about the destruction they caused, you're only going to add fuel to the already unnecessary fire. The one good thing about negative or evil incidents is that they show humanity where we do not want to be. These situations give us contrast and make us realize that all we want to do is love one another. All we can do as responsible people, is take care of our own energy and keep our frequency high.

When it comes to you, it's very important that you quickly move on from the past. Never blame, judge or hold on to any thought, emotion or action that lowers your vibration. If you did something and then realize later that you could have done it better – let it go. Do not think you must forgive yourself. You have done nothing wrong. You simply had an experience and now you know that next time you will be different in that situation. We can be tempted by greed, fulfilment, gratification, power, lust: many things can win us over. This does not make us bad. If we use these circumstances as opportunities to step in a different direction next time, they have served us well.

In more severe situations (child abuse or physical attacks, for example), ideas of "right and wrong" can get tricky. Obviously abusing another human is not right. But what we can do as Super-Humans, as well as help the human being out of the situation or assist them with recovery in some way, shape or form, is to not judge it and give it any energy; remain neutral and pour love into the situation. Remember, you are a Quantum

Architect, and any highly charged thought/vision is creating that very same thing in the quantum field.

Keeping Your Energy on Track

People having negative experiences often experience a panic attack. But what if someone had a love attack? When do you ever hear people talking about a love attack? They don't. But you can train yourself to literally go into a love frenzy. When something happens, connect with your heart, jump up and down, scream out loud with joy, excitement and happiness and see/feel the magic flowing from your heart. Consciously open it like a flower blooming in the spring and consciously feel love. With practice you can cultivate huge amounts of love immediately. The more you do it the easier it gets.

Create an environment, internally and externally, in your home and immediate space, that only allows high-vibrational energies into it. Decide that any energies that come into your space must transition onto your frequency or leave. Any human being who enters your space will have to raise their vibrational level or leave. It's that simple. Nothing will go down vibrationally in your immediate space. It's your space and your rules, so stick to them. High vibes or out, baby!

You are like a railway controller. The train coming down the track is positive energy and you can direct the train left or right at the junction, change the course of the energy, allowing it to flow to another space. Or you may see some negative energy flowing down the track, in which case you put the brakes on, stop the train, open your heart and change the frequency, then release the train to keep moving, allowing the energy to move through to the next space, raising the vibration of everything in its path.

The alternative is that the negative energy, which could be a human being or situation, doesn't want to change. In this case, as the controller, you stop the train for good, take it off the tracks, decommission it and put it in for repair. You leave it on the side of the track until the frequency has shifted, and if it doesn't you pay it zero attention again. Or you could send the train back to where it came from. That is a choice but to be honest, decommissioning it (by removing it/them from your life) until it shifts is best. Do not think twice. You are awesome. Surround yourself in awesomeness.

From an energetic perspective, if an external low-vibrational force moving through the space, external from a physical human being, travelling alone as such, moves into your space or body, you can send it back the way it came. If I felt anger, guilt, frustration, out of nowhere, the first thing I would say is this: "If this is not my energy, send it back to wherever it came from with love and light and send it right now." Quite often you will feel yourself lift as the heavy energy that belonged to another shifts. Not only are you releasing yourself from it but, by transmuting it into love and light, you are assisting the human being/being on the other end who passed it your way in the first place. Remember, we are all interconnected, and your thoughts and feelings are not always yours.

The buck stops with you. Act deliberately, be in control of your space and energy and know you have the power to change any situation. When it comes to energy, your willpower is the key. Heart over matter. Mind alongside heart. People say we only use 5–10 per cent of our brains; I say we only use 5–10 per cent of our hearts. Let's activate, switch ourselves on and Be Super-Humans living on this beautiful ball of adventure and opportunity, hovering in infinite space.

14

Healing Ways and Activations

In this section, I want to dive deeper into healing and give you some more powerful tools that you can use to help other people – but more importantly, to assist you, in your human evolution. I will share two healing ways and two very important Light Encoded Activations and then share with you the most powerful healing frequency on Planet Earth.

I say "ways" as the word technique is too rigid; Star Magic is not a modality or system, and neither does it contain a range of techniques, it is simply ways of healing.

Stars, Love, Earth, and Clearing Pyramids for Self-Healing

The first way I want to share involves using your own hologram or the hologram of another human being. So, I want you to be still, relax, breathe deeply and centre yourself. If you are, like me, well versed in accessing the information beyond the veil, then you won't need to breathe, you will simply be in that altered, tapped-in state; and if it takes you time, it's OK, keep going there and your consciousness, a little like muscle memory, will remember and just take you there. The more time you spend tapping the information beyond the veil, the easier it becomes to access and eventually you live beyond the veil and then, one day, there is no veil.

Once you are in a relaxed state, bring up your own hologram, or the hologram of another human being (make sure the back of the hologram is in front of you), or animal if you wish, as you can work on all beings. Once you have

the hologram up in front of you, I want you to connect to the Star Sirius and bring a frequency from it down through the crown of the hologram you are working on. The light will flow into the heart. See/feel/know the light stream as electric pink. Next, connect with Mother Earth's merkaba down in her core. See a platinum light flow from her bottom tetrahedron, up through the rocks and the minerals, through the surface of the planet and up through the perineum of the hologram and into the heart. Both frequencies, Sirius (masculine/positive) and Earth (feminine/negative), merge in the heart of the hologram. Next you will open your heart and send the light from it, in through the back of the hologram in front of you. These three frequencies merge. They must be brought into play in this order.

Next you are going to bring up a second hologram. The reason I am asking you to do this is to take your brain/mind out of the equation. You are connected to their heart with your heart, so the head may start to chatter while your heart is connected to the heart of the hologram, because of the different levels, which will make sense as we progress.

You are now going to work on their knees. Remember, on one hologram you have the light going in through the back of the heart. You are going to place your hands on the front of the knees of the second hologram. To do all of this on one hologram can confuse some people, so using two holograms makes it easy. You can, if you want, work on multiple holograms of you or another human being and be doing a variety of things at any one time. There are many ways to play around with holograms. For example, I could shrink it, or I could detach the legs . . . but let's keep it simple for now and just use two.

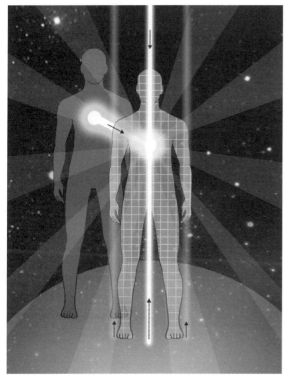

101. Hologram with Stars, Love, and Earth energy flowing

We are going to use Star Magic clearing pyramids (see image 102). I was given these a few years back during my time in ancient mystery schools. I've shared this with thousands of people now and the results they get are beyond extraordinary. You can use this way on its own, and you can use Stars, Love, Earth on its own too, but today we are stacking them together, because, trust me, it's mega powerful and you get fast results.

Please ensure that you are sitting and the other human being you are working on is lying down, especially if you are doing this at distance and if you are working on someone else, that is. If you are working on your own hologram, please sit down also. You do not want either

yourself or whoever you are working on to be standing. When Stars, Love, Earth is in full flow and these little clearing pyramids are whizzing around the body, it can make people very dizzy. I have seen people's knees buckle on our trainings and workshops, so please be sensible. If you were with them in the space, you could be right next to them to support them but still, lying is recommended to start with.

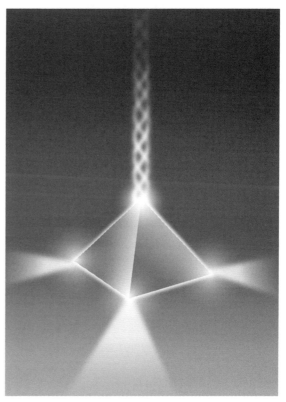

102. Star Magic clearing pyramids

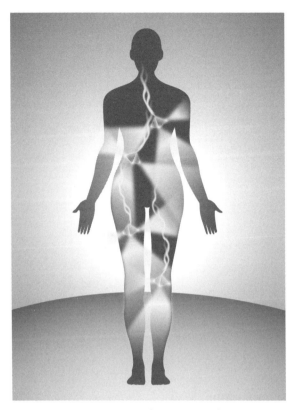

103. Star Magic clearing pyramids
whizzing around the body

Above is what the clearing pyramids look like when they are travelling around your body or the hologram of whoever you are working on.

So, you are going to set an intention for Star Magic clearing pyramids to flow. What will happen is either two, four, six or eight pyramids will start spinning in your heart. You place both of your hands over the knees of the hologram. The clearing pyramids will flow down your arms and into the knees of the hologram. They will whizz around the body, clearing and cleansing it. You must keep your hands over the knees until they return, like boomerangs. Once they have finished, they will flow back towards the knees, up through your hands, arms and into your heart, where they will dissolve. They will not bring any toxic energy back with them. They simply clear the body and dissolve toxicity. Image 104 shows the clearing pyramids and Stars, Love, Earth

energies working simultaneously on two separate holograms.

A few points to remember:

1. They always work in pairs. You will get two, four, six or eight. Never any odd numbers.

2. Keep your hands on the knees of the hologram until they return.

3. Once the hologram is in front of you, state: "This is the hologram of . . ." and then the human being's name. If it's you, say your name, not "me". Say it three times.

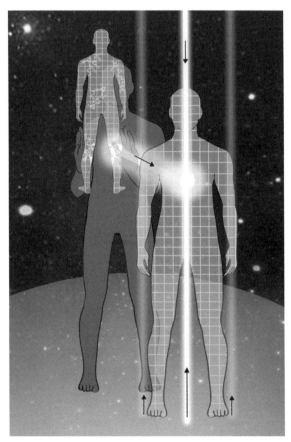

104. Stars, Love, Earth, and the Star Magic clearing pyramids working on two separate holograms

This entire process may take three minutes, or it may take fifteen. Trust the process. I have seen miracles happen in minutes. I am talking about cancer going, limb movement coming back, and much more. You may ask how I can tell if a tumour has gone. Well, the human being had one on a scan a week before the training or workshop and when they went for a scan two days after, it was not there. Now, maybe the tumour shifted in another way? Maybe it did. We will never know but it does seem like a little bit of a coincidence.

Once the Star Magic clearing pyramids have dissolved back inside your heart, you can collapse both holograms (blow them up or see them dissolve) and the light frequencies will simply dissolve on the hologram you were using for Stars, Love & Earth.

Parallel Life Trauma – R44 CUBE: Collapsing Timelines

Earlier I shared with you how to correct spinal issues through entanglement of geometries (specifically isosceles triangles), a way that can be applied to other elements of the human body too. The last combination has the potential to clear/heal an array of symptoms and now I want to show you another way.

Each time an event happens in our life, a memory or imprint of that event or situation – positive or negative – is embedded within the fabric of space-time. Generally, as humans, we are conditioned to focus on the worst, to drag up our guilt, frustration, rejection, abandonment, hurt and suffering, which is why the past rules many of our lives. It shouldn't but it does.

In this reality, the one that you and I are living/experiencing right now, we are born and grow up and have experiences as we go through our life. This is a linear movement of experiences, which we refer to as a timeline. Our souls have experiences on timelines too. For example, I may have been born in the 1300s and in that life my father may have passed when I was young and so left me feeling hurt, rejected or abandoned on some level,

and maybe even guilty that I could not save him. My soul then may have reincarnated in the 1500s and had another experience, one that also left me feeling rejected. Maybe I was a woman whose husband cheated on me with another woman, divorced me and left me. I then reincarnated as Jerry in this life and was put up for adoption. This is a timeline where my soul has experienced three different realities, all resulting in the same rejection/abandonment issues.

As well as this, I could have another timeline or multiple timelines that is/are creating harmony or havoc in my present-day reality. (I should really refer to it as potential havoc, because when you "innerstand" the game, you welcome the opportunity to dive down the timeline, learn, grow, heal and elevate from it. It's only havoc when emotions are stirred within the labyrinth of your soul and subconscious programmes run your life.) For example, my soul is multidimensional and so could be experiencing life on another Earth or another planet somewhere, right now. Everything is now. There is no future or past. This is where it gets a little more complicated to wrap your head around. Because a lot of people would say there is only one timeline that your soul is experiencing, the one from the time you emerged from Source, all the way down/up/across (however you look at it) to where you are now.

Sometimes there is, but for a lot of us here on Earth, old souls, we have fragmented and gone off on many journeys and often travelled many timelines. We also have an oversoul and an avatar self and in actuality, multiples of these in higher densities and all of these can come into play. The first thing to "innerstand" is that every possible scenario in the quantum field exists. If you experience trauma as a child in this life, it's possible for a part of you to get stuck in that quantum space and so become fragmented from the you that is you and carried on living. Your six-year-old self for example could be off living in the potential possibility that was available at the time of the trauma. In essence it's still suffering, and so are you. This is an easy fix. All you have to do is reconnect to that space memory and bring that aspect of you into healing. You would do that simply by communicating with the aspect of your soul at six years old, loving them and reassuring them and then inviting them back into your heart. It can take some negotiating at times but it's simple stuff.

Another scenario would be that your soul decided to split and venture off to two different planets, maybe as an extra-terrestrial. Both experiences took you on a different trajectory and resulted in the creation of two different soul experiences, two different sets of imprints in space memory and two different timelines. This can be a little trickier to bring into healing and this is where we would collapse one or multiple timelines. The trick is to be able to find the deepest point in space-time/space memory that contains the original trigger that is creating the disease, injury or illness now. When you do this effectively and thoroughly, miracles can happen – sometimes within minutes, hours or days, sometimes even in a heartbeat.

I want to show you the fastest way to shift parallel life or past life trauma. Remember, it's only past in linear time; in the quantum field, all things are now, all things are available, and all things are possible. This way I am about to share has been utilized by many Star Magic Tribe members to heal all sorts of dis-eases, from frozen shoulders to ovarian cysts, slipped discs to wisdom teeth, cancer to broken bones. This gives you an opportunity to tap into the deepest trigger that holds the trauma in space-time, very fast.

I was in Taiwan a few years ago and a man in our training had a lump the size of half an American football hanging out of his throat. It was huge. It had grown and grown. When I looked into it, I could see that he had issues with his father and, even at forty-one years of age, was still being bossed around by him. He had not voiced his opinion/spoken his truth and now his body was communicating with him. It went much deeper than this (because as we were working we discovered communication issues in past lives too) and once we had finished the exercise I am about to share with you, the lump had shrunk by 50 per cent. The next morning when he came into the training it had shrunk by 85–90 per cent. It later disappeared completely.

This is the easiest way to facilitate the healing of another human being, and, more importantly, yourself. To do it you do not need your third eyesight switched on. You do not require the ability to tap into past lives/parallel realities.

PROTOCOL *Healing Parallel Life Trauma*
The first step is to bring up the hologram of whoever you want to work on and entangle it with them by saying, "This is the hologram of . . ." three times, as previously discussed and if you are versed in healing then simply your intention is enough.

In this exercise you want to work on a specific symptom. You simply have to ask the human being (or yourself), what you are going to work on, change and transmute.

Once you have done this, you are going to visualize a transparent cube in the empty space, the space in front of you. You are going to place this cube into the body/hologram, filling up the space between the bottom of the ribcage and the hips. You are then going to talk to the cube and tell it to spin clockwise and collect all the trauma, all of the stuck emotion, all of the heavy/toxic energy from the bones, muscles, organs, blood, tissue, cells, that is held inside the human being's body, that is creating the symptoms. So, for example, if I was healing John's kidney stones, I would say this:

"Hey Cube, please spin clockwise and collect all the trauma, all of the stuck emotion, all of the heavy/toxic energy from the bones, muscles, organs, blood, tissue, cells, that is held inside John's body and is creating the symptoms we call kidney stones."

The cube will then start to spin clockwise. It will spin faster and faster and draw energy, often dark, heavy energy, from all parts of the body. You may see or feel or just know when the cube is full. When it is full, and the body is clear you can go to the next stage. If it's not, you may want to extend the cube and continue filling it.

There is another scenario: that the cube may be full but the body not clear. We will cover this later.

In the simpler scenario, the cube is now full and still and the body empty. You place your left hand over the top of it, inside the hologram, and your right hand over the top of your left hand. Next say the following:

"Please show me the deepest root trigger point in space-time, that holds the original trauma/trigger, that is creating the physical symptoms of kidney stones inside John's body."

Next, you start to move your right hand slowly away from your left hand and feel through the space. You move your hand out, up, down, left, right, you feel through the space until your hand goes cool or vibrates. Mine always vibrates in the palm. Some people's hands go hot, others cold, some people's hand talks to them. When you practise, you will get to know how your hand communicates with you. Or you can, from the get-go, command your hand to vibrate or go cold – whatever you decide. Remember, it's your reality and you are in control of your consciousness.

As you move your hand through space, you may experience the hot, cold, vibrating sensation or maybe a magnetic pull quite close to the hologram. You may also find that it extends out quite far; sometimes it can be further than your arm can reach. If that is the case, extend your arm with your imagination and keep feeling. Once you do get to the point/space, you will just know.

You can move your hand on and off the point and every time it comes back over it or onto it, you will feel it.

This point in space-time could be 1925, 1268, 200 BC or another date in linear time. It really does not matter. We are tapping into the field and the trauma in space-time, right now. There is no time, distance or measurement in the quantum field. You may start to collect information on the traumatic reality that created the trauma, or you may not. Either way, it's not going to make any difference to the end result.

Once you find this point, keep your right hand there or, if you have extended your arm, keep fixed on that point in space. Now, with your intention, you move the cube from inside the hologram, through space, until it's under the right hand, and then you stop it.

Next you blow up the cube in your mind. See it being obliterated. What happens is you take the trauma from the body's cells, back to the quantum space where it exists/was created, and blow it up. By doing this you collapse the reality or change the timeline. You are not sending the trauma/problem from your current reality back to the other. It never actually existed in your present reality anyway; your body was simply letting you know that it existed in the other quantum space, the other reality. Now, what happens is you heal this current lifetime, but also any other past life, on that timeline, in front of the one you found with your right hand linearly. You cancel it out in both realities and linearly shift what is in between.

This is the job done. You cannot get any simpler.

Now, I said before that you may experience a scenario whereby the cube is full but the body not clear. In this scenario, firstly you do exactly as I have just described with the full cube. Then you create another cube and do the same thing.

Everything is the same, up until the point at which you search with the right hand. What you don't do is automatically assume that the cube goes to the same place. Why? Because you may have two different timelines playing out, both creating the same symptoms. So, you go through the process again:

"Please show me the deepest root trigger point in space-time, that holds the original trauma/trigger, that is creating the physical symptoms of kidney stones inside John's body."

Once you have said this you feel, find the spot, transport the cube there and then blow it up. The greatest number of cubes that I have witnessed being used is five. Generally, one or two will do it but there are situations where you will need to use more. This is a very simple way of clearing up anything, mentally, physically, emotionally; and of course it's linked spiritually. It's very rare that the deepest pain and trauma is from childhood. That is usually the tip of the iceberg. This way will hunt out trauma and transmute it.

You must be clear and cleansed so you can grow and expand and thrive in this multidimensional playing field. As I have said, there are many ways to accomplish this and I share them on our Trainings, but for now this will suffice. It's often a good idea to do this exercise before the platonic solids exercise (to move you into a 5D frequency) I shared earlier in the book.

The Secret Code

Now, even though this is easy anyway, I have made it simpler. I have created a code that does all of the above for you. All you have to do is create the cube, place it inside the body or the hologram and then place the code inside. The code is **R44**. R44 is entangled with the whole process. It will use one cube or multiple cubes, whatever is necessary to complete the task. You just have to create the first cube, open your heart, connect, say your opening instructions . . .

"Hey Cube, please collect all the trauma, all of the stuck emotion, all of the heavy energy from the bones, muscles, organs, blood, tissue, cells, that is held inside John's body and is creating the symptoms we call kidney stones."

. . . and then place the code, **R44**, into the middle of the cube. The rest is history, baby. **R44** itself is a complex set of numbers, geometries and frequencies. I've just simplified it into **R44** to make it easier to remember.

Now, please practise with this manually. Get used to instructing the entire process before you take the short cut.

These tools are the tools of Super-Humans. They get Super-Human results very fast. Practise and bring this game-changer into your healing arsenal.

Lyran Light Code Activation

If you've made it this far in the book, I feel I can safely say that you know that you are not just a solid object, hovering in space and separate from your environment. I feel I can go one step further and assume you know you have had other experiences on this planet, and outside of this one on other planets too. There is a deep "innerstand"ing that you are a child of the stars. Or maybe you are just fascinated at the amount of BS flowing from my overstimulated imagination and you are being severely entertained? Either way it's perfect and I love you.

I have journeyed through time and space in deep meditation for a long time. I have met and interviewed people who have had similar extra-terrestrial experiences.

Through my own experiences and what others have told me, I know that life extends out beyond our galaxy and there are millions if not billions of species of extra-terrestrial life. The Lyran star system is one of the first homes of extra-terrestrial life in our universe (that I am aware of) and I have a strong personal affiliation with them.

I've talked about love that is beyond human words. The first time I experienced it was when I met the Lyrans on Alpha Centauri. I had never felt so peaceful, so at home, so loved. It was a love so pure and untainted by thought forms. When the Lyrans hugged me, I melted into an ocean of nothingness. I will never truly be able to describe what happened in that moment but, when the Lyrans hugged me, it was like coming home. It was life-altering.

The Light Codes the beings from Lyra share carry consciousness keys to activate our ancient extra-terrestrial/Lyran DNA/Wisdom. What I want to do is share with you a very specific and concentrated Lyran Light Code Activation. The first time you do this you can sit and read the instructions with your eyes open. After you have done it several times, you will know the sequence.

Light-Encoded Download

So, please make sure you are sitting nice and comfortably. Take several long deep breaths. Settle down into your space and feel your body.

Next, I want you to set the intention to invite Daeron and Derequi into your space. These are two Lyrans that I work with regularly. They are responsible for Star Magic. Sit still and you will feel them enter your space, Daeron to your left and Derequi on your right-hand side. You may see them. Both are blue and around 6.5–7-feet tall. Derequi is slightly taller. They will place their hands on your chest, back, neck and head. Allow them to do this and relax.

Continue breathing.

Allow these two beings to run frequencies through your body as you breathe in and out, long and slow, for thirteen breaths.

Next, you will become aware of an inverted, crystalline pyramid spinning clockwise, 90 cm above your head. It will be a high-frequency gold, with platinum hieroglyphs vibrating in the walls of it. These glyphs are Lyran glyphs. You may

not have experienced them before on Earth or remember them from the Stars, but deep inside you will feel and know them. As the pyramid rotates clockwise, it will draw in spiralized geometric codes from Lyra and Vega. They will stream through space, through the cosmic fabric, down through Mother Earth's atmosphere, through the roof of your space and in through the base of the inverted pyramid. Stay in this space and breathe thirteen more long, slow, deep breaths as the codes from Lyra and Vega collect, merge and form master codes.

The apex of the pyramid will open of its own accord and a powerful stream of data will run down through your crown and download into your crown, pineal gland, higher heart and heart.

Daeron and Derequi will now open their hearts and stream light from their hearts into yours as they hold space for you.

The frequencies from the pyramid will race from your heart, down through your body and into your perineum, where they will activate your genesis cells, eight little cells that form a merkaba.

Light will now flow down into your Earth Star transmission centre, 8–12 inches below your feet. Once this transmission centre is switched on, a stream of light will flow from the Earth Star to Mother Earth's Heart and from the Earth Star back up to your pineal gland.

Stay in this space and breathe for as long as you feel is necessary. You may want to stay for a few minutes, or maybe an hour. The choice is yours.

Once you feel you are done, say, "Complete the activation." What will happen is this. Your crown will open and the pyramid will descend through your crown, shrink and stop around the outside of your pineal gland. It will then dissolve in its own time. Daeron and Derequi will leave when they are ready. They may hold space while you integrate, or they may leave immediately. Please stay hydrated after this download. I recommend you do this as often as you wish. Each time it will get stronger and more powerful, boring deeper into your consciousness, unleashing deep knowledge and expanding your consciousness. Come back and revisit this as often as you like but stay very hydrated. You will start to remember so much information. You may get flashes, internal knowings. However it surfaces, just allow it and be still with it.

Enjoy the process, beautiful soul! Unleash your Super-Human!

Divine Feminine and Divine Masculine Light Code Activation

On Earth right now, there is much emphasis on the divine feminine frequency and bringing the masculine and feminine aspects of us into equilibrium, and while it's important, this notion is still based in duality. We do have aspects of both masculine and feminine inside of us, but they are two parts of a whole and if we move on from that, and look at this from a different perspective, we are whole but have divided ourselves into two halves. Or possibly one third feminine and two thirds masculine or vice versa, or a slightly different composition. Either way, we are splitting something that doesn't need to be split.

As humans we try to put things into boxes, stack them on shelves, place them in orders. The biggest one of all is that we are moving from the third dimension to the forth dimension, to the fifth dimension, and so on. Nothing could be further from the truth. We are vibrating across bands of frequency simultaneously. We can be bouncing between them all and be in them all. We are multidimensional beings.

We are trying to stabilize on this journey of ascension and remain in higher densities for longer periods of time and eventually stay there. The tools in this book are all about accessing the multidimensional spectrum in densities 1 to 5 and above and preparing you to move through Star Gates.

So, next I want to share with you another activation. This one will re-organize your energy and recalibrate your light body spin rates, connecting your merkaba field with your brain, pineal gland and other organs, so that you bring all of you into harmony. The tetrahedrons in our merkaba spin at different rates. The female tetrahedron spins faster than the male and this is perfect. It's the way it's supposed to be. It operates efficiently for the purpose of manifestation, travel and cloaking (making invisible) your space.

What I want to do is get your merkaba field communicating with your brain, pineal gland and other organs. Once this is activated, you will start feeling the strengths of both a woman and a man. You may do so already, but I assure you, this will take you to a whole new level of awareness. You will be kind, compassionate, loving, gentle and nurturing, and also be ready to enforce your boundaries, take action, speak your truth and throw down if necessary. Remember, we are human beings, here on Earth. When we are whole, we are loving and fearless, courageous and kind. We can cherish and nurture our sisters and brothers just like our own children, but be ready to fight if the situation arises. We move from being predator to protector but maintain the fury and potential temperament of a predator and if those energies are required, we can tap that potential in a nanosecond, but at the same time remain calm and collected. Being whole is being real. Denying certain aspects of who you are is unhealthy. Accepting all of you, dark and light, masculine and feminine, is how you truly harness your power and divine wisdom.

Firstly, please ensure you are sitting comfortably. Take some long deep breaths. In through your nose, down to the pit of your belly and back out through your mouth. Breathe twenty-seven long, slow, deep breaths.

As you are breathing, I want you to set the

intention to connect to the frequencies of Sirius and Orion and to activate your merkaba. Sirius will recognize this command, the light will flow down from space, and connect to your top tetrahedron, while the light from Orion will connect with the bottom one. You don't need to do anything. Your top tetrahedron will spin clockwise and your bottom one anti-clockwise. Breathe in the twenty-seven deep breaths.

Once you finish the breaths, you will become aware of an electric pink, inverted pyramid, spinning 90 cm above your crown in a clockwise direction. It will start drawing in frequencies from the constellation of Libra and the constellation of Leo. Multicoloured, spiralized geometrical codes will flow down from the Stars into the base of the inverted pyramid. The codes and frequencies from Libra and Leo will merge.

The apex of the pyramid will open on its own and the merged frequency will flow down through your crown and into your heart. A vortex of energy will start to spin clockwise in your heart. A pink and gold ball/sphere will appear in your heart. Eight streams of light will flow out from it into the apex and corners of both tetrahedrons of the merkaba field around your physical body. A ninth stream will flow from the pink and gold sphere, up into your pineal gland. Your pineal gland will start to communicate with your central nervous system, your brain and, through the brain and central nervous system, your organs.

Streams of data will flow back and forth between all of these bodily components and the field of your heart and higher heart will expand exponentially. Your body and your light body will synchronize, and a new communication network will open and recalibrate.

You will feel a pulsating of energy flowing from the Earth, up through your body and into your heart. I want you to consciously breathe, in and out, deep and slow for another twenty-seven breaths and then relax your breathing

and just be. As you breathe this second set of breaths, your crown will open, the pyramid will descend, dissolve inside your mind and around your pineal gland. Your crown will then close. Stay here for as long as you feel like it. You will be downloading and re-synthesizing your system, bringing your feminine and masculine aspects into divine harmony.

You can go through this process as often as you wish. You will download more and more data each time and the experience will get stronger. Once you start tapping the cosmic coding in these higher-frequency streams regularly, your life will grow new wings. Things will change in ways I have no words to describe. Remember, experiencing is knowing. Unleash your Super-Human!

Kaleidoscopic Chromium

Einstein said the ceiling of our material world is visible light. As the brain processes an increase in frequency and information, beyond the physical senses, from the invisible world, and beyond the speed of light, higher frequencies and a different set of information can alter us on a metaphysical and a physical level. Kaleidoscopic chromium is (to my knowledge) the most powerful healing frequency in the universe available to us right now. It contains every other high-vibrational light/colour stream within it, beyond what we see, only being accessed through that special gland we call our pineal, and it has the ability to create healing, faster than anything else I have seen.

The higher the frequency we pick up, the more it alters our chemistry, meaning the more visual, hallucinogenic and high-energy experiences we have. The crystals in our pineal gland are like a cosmic antenna, picking up and transducing/translating (into knowings/images/messages) these high-vibrational light streams into patterns and colours that our consciousness "innerstand"s on a Super-Human level. We then translate these images, codes, patterns into a feeling that can then be "innerstood" as information we can share in human words. It takes a Super-Human to translate geometry and code.

As consciousness expands on our beloved planet and throughout our human species, as well as other life forms, we are transitioning into a new octave of light. A new band of frequencies is available to us. Old programming is breaking and dissolving, and freedom is being offered through the space that will be created. Some human beings will shift at a slower rate than others, due to their biological and cosmic bodies maintaining a slower rate of oscillation and vibration, keeping them in a denser space, and some may not elevate/shift/ascend at all. They may check out or just stay in a frequency band that doesn't recognize the one we are moving into. It's important to know that as Mother Earth holds space for the Krystal Energies and allows those that do the work to be on this planet in a higher frequency band, an old version of her will be available, still plugged into the Matrix, for those who are not ready or willing to make the conscious choices to grow, elevate and expand.

As we grow and expand into new octaves of light and start accessing more information, things happen in our reality. As you transition and become more aware, there are certain things that happen to you or that you witness that change you forever. I have shared some of my experiences in this book; and what I want to share with you now will, should you decide, change your life and the lives of others. A few years ago, a friend of mine was travelling through the ether in deep meditation. She ended up on a beach, on a planet in the Andromedan Galaxy. She was told about a healing frequency called chromium. She told me about it and over the next few months I started to tap into this frequency also. This gift is one of the greatest gifts a human being can receive.

In Star Magic, we call this frequency Kaleidoscopic chromium. The reason being, inside this energy/frequency stream is a wide spectrum of colour that goes way beyond what we are acquainted with, between infra-red and ultra-violet. Kaleidoscopic chromium has a range of colours that are so beautiful, so vast, so intense, healing and transformational. The colours are almost translucent, but at the same time very vivid. There are ranges of all the colours you know and more. Infinite layers of each colour, merged into the same space, all enveloped within this chromium band of light, which seems to encase the other colours, creating what looks like a multidimensional kaleidoscope of beauty and wonder.

We were told by the Andromedans back in 2016 not to use this in our workshops, meditations or trainings, that we needed to "innerstand" it first before using it on others. So, I played with it, used it on people close to me to practise and experimented with it. But no one close to me had any serious dis-eases or injuries and so I wasn't able to see its potential in terms of healing. I did start bringing the frequency through meditations and people were blown away by how they felt. But the thing was I was really only dabbling in it.

Then one day a lad in his early twenties, Phil, contacted me. He said that he was in desperation. Something very strange had happened to him. He woke up one day and his skull had grown, so much that his brain was moving around inside it. When he lay down at night, it would drop. He couldn't run or jump. It had destroyed his life. He had been to the doctors and there was no logical explanation. He asked if I could help. I said the same thing I always say: Yes. I always commit to assisting whoever asks and work out the crucial part (how) afterwards. When you know who you are and are committed to finding a way, you will.

I asked for a photo of this guy, so I could look into his eyes. I always do that prior to any healing session. It gives me an opportunity to tap into their consciousness and see what is happening, and with this guy, I was very curious. I have shared that we have been placed in a mathematical mould and this guy broke the mould. I realized that he had been receiving some very powerful light-encoded downloads and these frequencies had triggered his DNA and had increased his skull size to what it was like when he was an extra-terrestrial and also a human being on earth before our DNA was tampered with, before the geometry of nature had followed the Fibonacci Spiral. The codes had tapped his DNA and instigated biological change. He had been rewired to the Krystal Spiral Geometries, overnight. How could this be possible? I was fascinated.

The day of the healing, we connected on Skype. Phil said, "Please help me." I said "What do you want me to do?" He said, "Please shrink my skull back to its normal size." I said, "Why don't you grow your brain?" He looked at me and said, "Look at my head? It's fucking huge." And it was a lot bigger than any human head I had ever seen. He said, "I look strange. People are staring at me in the streets and laughing and I can't move quickly at all." I never try and convince anyone of anything but in this case, I had to ask one more time. "Are you sure you don't want to grow your brain?"

First up I didn't even have a clue how I would ever grow his brain but hey, he wanted me to shrink his skull. I didn't have a clue how that would happen either. But we both found ourselves in this situation.

I explained what had happened and that this was the size of his head in an extra-terrestrial life he had experienced or maybe was experiencing right now in the quantum field and also, because everything is now, and also this is the size of what a human head should be like. He was adamant that he wanted his head to go back to normal.

So, we went into this healing session. I wish I had recorded this as Phil sat there in front of me on Skype, but to be honest, I really didn't expect to see what I saw. I am, still to this day, amazed at all the changes that take place in people's

bodies and consciousness. I asked Phil to close his eyes and breathe. I guided him into a space (in meditation), underneath the pyramids in Giza, where there are healing chambers. Once there he lay down on a healing bed. I take many clients there and many miracles have happened. If you read my last book *Healing with Light Frequencies: The Transformative Power of Star Magic*, you will have read about the surgeries that take place in these chambers.

This trip to the healing chambers was no different. As Phil lay there, I was told to bring in the Kaleidoscopic chromium. Several other Egyptian surgeons entered the room. They took Phil through what looked like a futuristic MRI machine. As they did, I connected to the kaleidoscopic chromium frequency and brought it into the space. It poured in. Even though Phil was sat upright in front me on Skype, he was also deep in this journey, lying down, underneath the pyramids, inside a healing chamber, going through this futuristic MRI machine, being bathed in chromium light, as these Egyptian surgeons worked on him through the machine.

As I looked at Phil and held space, his head started shrinking. Within sixty seconds maximum, it had shrunk. It went down about 80 per cent, back towards its normal size. Once it was over, I brought Phil back out from the deep space he was in. He opened his eyes. He said he could feel it changing but at the same time it felt like it was changing in another reality. He was happy. His brain didn't rattle any more and over the next days it shrank back fully to the size it was supposed to be. This is most definitely a Super-Human feat. Phil isn't the only human being who's contacted Star Magic with bodily parts that have suddenly grown. Both men and women whose hands and feet have grown almost overnight have contacted us.

The other thing I use Kaleidoscopic chromium for is when I am removing negative entities from a client. I use the chromium frequency because it contains every high-vibrational colour you could possibly imagine, all of the higher-density colour ranges, which are almost translucent and so subtle. When you work with negative entities, they often try to shape-shift, so you can't see them. They can hold space inside a golden light or diamond light or white light, and you may think nothing is there, but when it comes to chromium, these entities can't shape-shift fast enough through the high-vibrational colour range and you can see them, hunt them and remove them. Kaleidoscopic chromium is fast, efficient, and extremely powerful. We've now fully introduced it into our trainings and are showing people how to use it.

If you want to be a Super-Human, then you need Kaleidoscopic chromium in your healing arsenal. It's good for many other things as well and as you play with it you will discover how potent, powerful and important it is.

EXERCISE Connect to Kaleidoscopic Chromium

What I want to share with you now is a short meditation exercise that will tap you into Kaleidoscopic chromium. This meditation will shift your frequency into a new state, where you can embody new information streams and stay connected and on the pulse as the planet, our human species and other celestial beings move into 5D (and beyond) consciousness. I will connect your light body to Mother Earth's Multispectral Ascension Light Wave Matrix and bring online the Kaleidoscopic chromium photon system.

All of the meditations I am suggesting can be done sitting, lying or standing. It's up to you. If you are not used to standing meditation you may wish to start off sitting or lying. Personally, I prefer standing and those who get into standing meditation can get incredible results. Also, anyone that tells you that meditating with your eyes closed is a must, is bonkers. Standing and meditating with your eyes open, can be the most

profound experience when you surrender to it.

So, get yourself comfortable and start breathing. Breathe long, slow, deep breaths, in through your nose, down into your belly and back out through your nose or mouth. Bring your awareness down into the middle of your chest and into your heart centre. Feel the energy there. As you continue to breathe, feel the vortex of energy in your heart growing and expanding. Allow it to grow and expand out past the boundaries of your physical body until this magnetic vortex of love is holding you in its space.

Next, feel your light body sinking, down into the planet. Feel your light body travel down, through the surface of the Earth, nurtured by this magnetic vortex of heart energy. You will travel down and down until you reach a platinum and electric green light with a golden centre. This is a merkaba field down in the centre of Mother Earth's heart. Her bottom tetrahedron is platinum and her top one is electric green. Right in the centre is a golden light, a sphere, and some incredible spiralized geometries. This grid plays many roles, but we will save that for another space.

You will continue travelling down until your light body is inside the golden light, inside the merkaba field. The merkaba is hundreds of metres wide and tall. The golden sphere is around 300 metres in diameter. These geometries actually expand and contract with the Earth's grids and energy flow, but I am sharing the sizes to give you an idea of their magnitude. You will also become aware of a spiral of light that flows through this structure. This Spiral of Light actually looks like many Spirals. You may feel it. These Spirals are the new Earth frequency, the Krystal Spiral. You will be very small on the inside of this structure. You may find your consciousness expands out through this field, however, to match it. It's OK if it does; you are infinite, after all.

Once you are inside, I want you to ask, to connect to the primary light and sound fields of

Mother Earth's Multispectral Ascension Light Wave Matrix. You will become aware of a stream of spheres, pouring down through your crown and up through your perineum on a quantum (and you may feel it physically too) level. These spheres are actually tiny merkabas spinning so fast they look like spheres. They will be connecting you to fractal patterns of mathematical data from densities 5 and above. Let them flow through you. You will know once the download has finished because a crystal-white sphere will be vibrating inside your heart. The colours flowing inside the sphere will be a multitude of almost translucent high-vibrational colours, much like the colours you will see inside the Kaleidoscopic chromium.

As this process is unfolding, I want you to place a code inside your heart. This code is **XA3XB6**, inside a chromium Sphere. Visualize it, feel it or know it's in your space (depending on how you are tapped in – maybe all three or two of the three) and place this sphere, with the code, inside your heart. Once inside it will spin and explode, and light will shoot out in multiple different directions. This light will shoot out to the stars, linking into the cosmic grids that run the chromium frequency from Andromeda. Once connected, these light streams will start a download process. Kaleidoscopic chromium, new light-encoded streams of data, will flow into your heart, and then flow out into this extended field of your heart. You can stay inside this space for as long as you feel is necessary.

When you feel you have been there for long enough, simply say "close and finish". The light streams will dissolve, and you will start to ascend, moving up through the Earth, through the space, up through the Earth's surface and back into your body. Start to feel the vibration in your body and then count yourself back from five to zero. Once you reach zero, open your eyes and recalibrate. Stay in your space for a while and feel your body. You can go through this process as often as you

wish. You will download more and more data each time and the experience will get stronger. Once you start tapping the cosmic coding in these higher-frequency streams regularly, your life will grow new wings. Things will change in ways I have no words to describe.

Remember, experiencing is knowing. Unleash your Super-Human!

Krystal Spiral Transformation Code

What I want to share with you now is a powerful light code, which will realign your own inner geometry. Remember, we as human beings are an extension of nature and everything is a mathematical frequency, an equation of light. It's all so utterly perfect it's beyond comprehension.

This regularity of life within the universe may suggest that the anatomy of the form of organisms follows the same general principles and the same anthropomorphic blueprint. This could mean that eventually, all life within the universe would assume a general form much like our current human bodies. However, with this possibility of evolution being continual and universal, we must also accept the possibility that eventually we, as Homo Sapiens, will evolve beyond our present state as well. The Krystal Spiral has already set this in motion. The example I shared earlier, of Phil, the young man whose skull grew to a much larger size when certain light frequencies activated his extra-terrestrial DNA, is a prime example of layers of mathematical structuring embedded within our DNA template, lying dormant, waiting to be triggered by the geometry in certain light-encoded frequencies from our galactic origins.

The geometric relationship between conscious beings and cosmic bodies such as stars, planets and galaxies suggests that at some level these heavenly bodies are conscious as well, perhaps even alive. If this is true, it means that at some level, evolution is affecting everything in the universe in an orderly and mathematical fashion.

As the cosmos changes, we as expressions of the cosmos change. It may even be that as conscious members of the cosmos, we – though we seem small in scale – may have the ability to affect the cosmos. When Homo Sapiens become Super-Humans, our celestial sisters and brothers change also. If the cycles of solar systemic rotation can affect our sleep cycles, moods, and lifespans, perhaps the energetic influence flows both ways. Perhaps? I don't think so. I know so. We are galactic generators, and our frequency is affecting everything, micro and macro.

Is it possible – if the bodies within our solar system and the evolutionary alterations within the cosmos have an effect on Earth life – that we as the conscious collective of humanity have the ability to affect certain aspects of the cosmos with our collective intent and amplified heart frequency? It may very well be that through our collective will, we as a consciously evolving humanity hold the massive potential to determine the evolutionary path of our own population as well as steer this path to more prosperous and unified outcomes. If this is so, the implications would be Earthly, Galactic, even Universal in scale.

The architecture in the image/code below contains the Krystal Spiral and the New Earth Mathematics (see also in colour insert after page 160). This code, when you stare at it, will start communicating with you on a very deep level. It will start to rearrange and recalibrate your body's geometry to exactly how it should be. It will start to energize and harmonize the cells in your body. If you are out of alignment in any way, shape or form, the code will set you straight and then energize and harmonize your cells. Stare at it for thirteen minutes every day for the next twenty-one days and feel the difference in your body, energy flow and overall well-being.

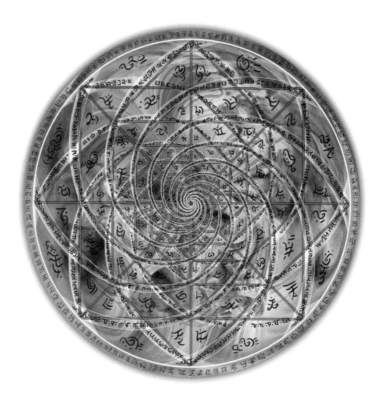

105. Krystal Spiral and the New Earth Mathematics Code

All of the tools in this book are designed to upgrade you on every level. After all, you are a Super-Human in the remembering and we must impact our system on every level: mental, emotional, physical and spiritual. They are all intertwined anyway. After you have stared at this code and absorbed the frequencies into your consciousness for twenty-one days, come back and revisit it as often as you like. It will start and continue an emergence of potential from within your own DNA template.

Ultimate Freedom

You came to Planet Earth as a Sovereign Being, a child from the Stars, like all of us here at this time.

Right now on Earth, many humans are waking up and realizing their power, their energy, their wholeness, wisdom and desire to be free and that desire is no longer a simple desire, it's a burning fire that fuels the rise of their own divine sovereignty.

We are making conscious choices to put ourselves first and foremost and not buying into the lie of guilt. In truly sovereign worlds, guilt does not exist. It doesn't exist because beings live by Cosmic Law. The law states that if you don't kill, steal from or harm another human being you have not committed a crime, or broken the law. When you live in a free society there is no need to kill, steal or harm because all things are readily available to all. You do not have lazy people in a free society because everyone naturally wants to create and expand.

It's only when beings (human beings here on this planet) are poisoned en masse through various means, mentally, physically and energetically, that they become docile and lazy. There is so much TV, media, social media and pre-packaged non-nutritious foods available to poison us.

Having read this book, you can now put into practice the wisdom that I have shared; you are raising your levels of consciousness, switching on your Super-Human abilities and are moving through the gears, declaring your sovereignty and living it fully. There is no person and no force that can tell you what you can or cannot do, as long as you are living by Cosmic Law. You are free to travel, create, love, enjoy, express and do what you want, when you want, with whoever you want and for as long as you want, enforcing your boundaries and being steadfast in your approach to life.

We are children of the multiverse and have roamed galaxies, solar systems, stars and celestial homes for billions of years. We didn't come to Earth to be caged animals. Everything I have shared with you in this book is a part of an ancient toolkit, one I have carried with me as a galactic traveller, playing and exploring, loving and caring and raising the vibration of every planet I took refuge on, for long or small amounts of linear time. I am sure you have done the same and I am sure our paths have crossed before, somewhere, on a planet far away – or maybe this one right here? Right now, you must commit to this inward journey of the heart. It's the only real journey worth embarking on and let me tell you, it's for the strong, the brave and the wise. Those who are living and not thriving, who still think that fast food is a blessing, may not take this journey for a little while.

I've always lived by this rule: never leave a soldier on the battlefield. It comes from many lifetimes as a Galactic Commander, fighting in many wars. It's ingrained into my DNA and it's why you, like me, continue to work, create, live from the heart being a beacon of light, so those who still sleep can wake and the world can return to full sovereignty. We will do everything we possibly can to raise the vibration on this Earth plane, giving our global family the opportunity they all deserve: to level up, raise their energy and claim their sovereign souls.

I have reached a space in my life where you cannot fuck with my frequency and you too may be in this space right now. If you are not, then you soon will be.

I have shared with you the best of the best. I have shared everything that works and broken it down so it's easy to digest and, more importantly, works. What I cannot do is do it for you. So, know that it's time to engage fully and unleash the magic from within.

Sovereign beings function as individuals and in teams. Sovereign beings unify with each other, knowing that a sovereign tribe who see each other as family are unstoppable. Sovereign beings have a coherent heart and mind and know that this coherence enhances longevity on a micro and a macro level and so embrace the qualities of their human and cosmic family and seek out connection with others.

When your heart and mind are coherent, you vibrate faster, you get easier access to those gamma waves that have the capacity to dramatically influence the field and your body's natural multidimensional field switches on. This field of energy activates a multitude of mini torus fields within your body, which connects to your internal merkaba system, as we have already discussed and many components we haven't. When these fields of frequency all interconnect, just like awakened souls reconnecting on Earth, waves of alignment take place and magic unfolds.

As a Sovereign Super-Human, you will welcome everything that this world lays down in your path. Nothing will faze you. You will carry the awareness that not all is what it seems. That your greatest opportunities are incredibly disguised as impossible situations. That the promised land doesn't lie beyond beautiful gardens and happy smiles. Friendly faces are not waiting for you to give you a fast track to the top of the pile. You have to knuckle down, prepare for the grind and get dirty. But remember, you can enjoy the knuckling down, the grinding and the getting dirty. It's all perception. The journey is the exciting part and

mining the gold from every encounter will fill you full of strength, knowledge and clarity.

To be whole is to be free. To love all with no judgement is to be free. To welcome all into the home of your heart, knowing there is nothing they can take that will change you, is to be free. Walking this Earth, knowing you are creating and co-creating constantly, manifesting a New Earth, is to be free. You are a Galactic Titan, here on Earth remembering. Love the process, beautiful soul, and know that the only way your frequency is going is UP!

I have given you the tools, now use them.

Mother Nature, Plant Medicine, and the Fountain of Youth

A gigantic part of realizing your sovereignty and stepping fully into your power is nature. You are just as much a part of nature as the trees, the flowers and insects. The soil contains our original human blueprint. Thousands of years ago we were crystalline and had salt-water flowing through our bodies. Now we have iron core blood flowing through our veins. This happened when we slid down through the frequency bands and lost our connection to higher dimensional information fields, each other and Mother Nature herself.

The soil contains the cosmic code. There is white gold and yellow gold in the soil and our bodies are supposed to have these elements flowing through us. When we walk around with our shoes and socks off, barefoot on the soil, a magical connection is set up. We start to upload data from the soil and our bodies rejuvenate because the minerals and elements that have been depleted from our body start to flow through us once again. The soil is like a huge battery for us.

As I've travelled this planet, I have met some incredible trees and had some of my best conversations with them. I remember recently I was in Mount Shasta with my son, walking through the forest and we met this incredible ancient Grandmother Tree. I sat next to her, barefoot, with my back to her trunk. I closed my eyes and emptied my mind. I opened my heart and instantly felt hers. Our two frequencies blended into one. I started journeying and forgot I had a body. I totally blended in with my environment and the healing I got was out of this world. The ground, the trees, the bushes all around were communicating with me. There was energy flowing in all directions. From me to every tree, flower and bush and from every tree, flower and bush back to me. There was also an energy flow from the ground to every flower, tree and bush and as well as through me and from every flower, tree and bush back through the ground. The symbiotic relationship between all things in nature is magnificent and when you stop, feel, connect and let go, you truly experience what it's like to be part of nature.

When you engage with nature in this way you detox, heal, energize and totally bring your frequency into alignment with nature itself (influencing and changing it mathematically on one level). Then the soil the Earth gives everything you need to be healthy and vice versa. To take this to the next level, you can be in this space with the sun shining brightly, feeling those supersonic photonic rays hit your skin, and from time to time open your eyes and download the light into your pineal gland. To take it one step further, connect with the great central sun, deep in the constellation of Sagittarius, and bring those cosmic codes into your heart at the same time as being connected to the ground, the trees, flowers and bushes. This is a powerful process. With practice you will start to feel and possibly see the mesmerizing interaction taking place between all things in the environment, including you. It's a beautiful flow of geometrical, spiralized data, from sentient being to sentient being to sentient being.

When you lose that connection to your environment, you lose the connection to yourself. Your entire environment feeds you with energy when you fall in love with all things, breaking down those illusory barriers between the known and the unknown, the physical and non-physical. It's all information. It's all code. It's love. When you open up to the potential that lies within you and within the unified field, beyond the zero-point or maybe within the zero-point, depending on your perception, you gain access to the true mathematics of the universe. The inner-geometric shift you are creating through this work will pass through into nature and certain elements of nature have already re-activated their true codex. Some of nature is already in the process of re-organizing itself to the true mathematical Krystal code. You will feel it. Other elements will be catalyzed by your energetic potential.

From here you can build, change and transform anything. Knowing is the TRUTH! This big old Grandmother Tree had so much to share. As I walked into her energy field, I floated and danced through the electrical, vibrational streams as geometrical, spiralized code flowed through my soul. Her frequency field started about eighty metres from her trunk and was super-powerful. When I looked a little deeper, I could see its range was beyond my physical sight, but around 2.8 km with my third eyesight. Connecting with a true spirit warrior such as an old tree is divine. The respect I had for this magnificent being was equally matched in the level of energy and information she shared with me.

Looking into the world beyond form, once you master it, is the best space to live, play and evolve in. You can come back to this 3D/4D space to do the human things and then bounce off again. The more you "be" in nature, the more you allow your own chemistry and biology to merge with your environment, and as you download more Krystal frequencies your geometry will change and you will influence the geometry of nature too. The more you step into this space, the more you realize you and your environment are ONE! No boundaries or separation. Be disciplined in your approach. Take time to be and connect. Mother Nature holds many answers. This tree gave me more in fifteen minutes than I got from eleven years at school, being fed stories and taught to regurgitate useless information. Let's meditate and connect with our Source. It lies within us and all around us. If you have ever drunk ayahuasca in nature, you will completely "innerstand" what I am sharing with you about the flow of energy and the connection. If you haven't then you should join one of our Deep in Space Retreats. It will change you forever in the most positive and magical way.

Ayahuasca, DMT, and Nature

When my ex-wife phoned me and told me that she wasn't coming home, and she had met another guy, I was at Avebury Stone Circle in the UK. I was sitting on the raised mound of earth where I always go when I arrive. I sat there and cried. I was devastated. When I'd got myself together, I walked into the larger field with the small and large stones.

I sat by one of the small stones and a Pleiadean craft came over me and gave me the most incredible download of light codes. I sketched the visuals that were entering my crown. They were galactic peace codes. I later tattooed them on my back.

I met up with Lisa who I knew from a training and had bumped into earlier. We went to the field with an empty "moat" around one side and smoked some DMT that she had brought.

I flew through the geometrical code, shapes, colours and energy, with my eyes closed. When I opened them, I saw all of the geometry in the clouds, in the grass; the empty space was alive, and

I was a part of this space. Nothing was solid, all was connected, and I could see it so vividly. I have had these experiences on ayahuasca also, but DMT is a little different.

I felt so much love. I felt love for everything. I lay there thinking that I could never be mad at my ex for meeting another guy because we are all one, and I felt total compassion and love for all things. Again, I know I had felt like this many times on plant medicine, even as a youngster dancing at raves on ecstasy, but to experience it the day my wife said she wasn't coming home was incredible. The universe aligned that immaculately.

Remember, DMT occurs in the womb, forty-nine days after conception, at the same time as eight little cells known as our genesis cells. The eight cells form a merkaba. Forty-nine equals thirteen when you add the nine and four together. Thirteen is the number that represents the Divine Goddess. Coincidence? DMT is in our spinal fluid and lungs and it occurs throughout nature.

I know that if every human being smoked DMT at the same time, we could change the world in five minutes. If I oversaw this world, ayahuasca would be offered to children in schools from the age of four. In some places, as children grow up drinking ayahuasca as part of their culture.

I remember giving my son DMT the first time. We were with my friend Steve from Colorado, at our house. Josh smoked it, sat up for a moment and then lay forward on the living room carpet. He didn't say anything. Then he said, "Dad, everything is so big, I'm like Ant-Man."

He lay there on the floor for fifteen minutes like he was the size of a tiny ant and our living room was the universe. The carpet fibres were like trees. It was amazing for him, and amazing for me to witness his bravery and willingness to expand. DMT fast-tracks you and once you go there, there's no turning back. It opens your mind and heart to the truth, just like ayahuasca.

I will share a beautiful story about ayahuasca, that bonded my children and me even deeper. We flew to Belgium to see a friend who brewed it. We went there and all took ayahuasca. We were journeying and my daughter was laughing, and my son was on all fours purging. I watched him change from a boy to a man and saw aspects of multiple realities. He was purging some deep trauma for his mother on a galactic level. He was struggling, so I connected with this energy and purged with him. We were both puking into buckets side by side. Sounds nasty, but trust me, this was a beautiful memory that I will cherish for eternity. I already loved my son to the next universe and back but after this a new-found respect grew inside me.

Once my son had finished purging, my daughter started. She's crying and being sick. While I was sat next to her, holding space for her, I heard my son saying, "Dad, sit down. Stop moving." He said, "Dad, I can see you in so many places. You are everywhere." I was smiling watching him. Next, I feel something tickling my feet. I look down and Josh has my right foot in his hands. He is staring at it saying, "Dad, I can see straight through your foot. It's amazing, If I decide to see your foot it's there and if I decide to see through it, it disappears." I was cracking up watching him.

We had the most incredible healing and bonding experience.

I highly recommend plant medicine to every human being on Earth, at least once. It will open you up to the potential in the empty space and make connecting to, feeling, and seeing your environment as one fluid, symbiotic consciousness very easy indeed.

EXERCISE *Connecting with the Cosmos*

I want you to adopt another practice. Find a tree. Talk to this tree for a few days and let it know you want to work with it. No tree will ever turn you down. Hug the tree, love the tree and show your respect.

Once you have been to see the tree for a few days, sit down, take your shoes and socks off, bare feet on the Earth, sit with your back against the tree, close your eyes, open your heart and let the energy spill from your heart 360 degrees in all directions. See and feel your heart frequency flow through everything around you, including the ground. Feel the flow being reciprocated back through you. Start to see and feel the code, like there are millions of galactic highways and the codes are the vehicles travelling up and down, back and forth on them. Your body, the trees, the flowers and bushes and any animals or insects around are the towns and cities connecting the highways. There is a constant flow of traffic and it's out of this world. If it's sunny where you live, connect with the rays of the sun on your body. Set an intention to connect with the great central sun and feel those cosmic photonic plasma rays flowing through the cosmic fabric and into your heart. See these rays flow onto the highways and flow within, through and around the code as everything becomes one and within that oneness you see and feel the mathematical separation, the individual pieces of code, which really are ONE CODE!

Do this once per week for an hour and daily for at least 10–15 minutes, longer if you feel it!

It will become one of your favourite pastimes and it will keep you very young. Stepping into this field of energy is like bathing in the fountain of youth.

15

The Future and Krystal Children

This world is constantly evolving and so are we as a human species. Generation after generation the children being born are evolving and changing and entering this world with a new perspective, or no perspective at all. What I mean by this is that there are two very distinct types of children entering our Earthly environment from the stars. You can spot them a mile away. We can place both of these types of children, or should I say energies, into the field of Krystal Children. Really these souls should not be given a label but for the sake of this discussion, Krystal Children is an awesome name. I say Krystal Children because they are a stepping stone in humanity returning to its original Krystalline Matrix, when we had Krystal Diamond Sun Bodies and lived on Tara (5D Earth) before the fall.

The children entering our planet right now and who have been since the early 2000s are here to create change. I say there are two very distinct types because there are. One of them is a stream of extremely old souls and the other is a stream of children whose souls have never been to Earth before. The ancient souls and the first-timers are both here to bring knowledge, systems, structure and peace. They are here to birth a new way on this planet that serves the whole of humanity as a global family and builds relations with our intergalactic community. These children will seriously amplify our abilities as adults to remember our true Super-Human strength.

The powers that be, knew this wave of upgraded children was coming and have been preparing for a long time, doing their best to introduce vaccines and artificial intelligence (AI), getting us hooked to our smart phones and smart technology because it's their only hope of stopping this wave of Krystal Children raising the vibration on the planet and birthing a new dawn, a platinum/diamond age, by turning us into cyber-humans/trans-humans.

If you have one of these children in your family, first up, I take my hat off to you. I respect you for choosing this mission. It's not easy to raise one of these souls because they tear down most of what our generation has been raised to believe. No more three-square meals, no more listen because I am the adult, no more it's my way or the highway. These kids eat when they are hungry, know that we are all equal and do what is best for them and not you as the parent. They will challenge you fully. It's actually a beautiful thing as they are forcing you to go within, reassess your values, ideas and what's important, and bring a new way of parenting to the table.

These young Star Seeds are our future leaders of the free world. They will not grow up and take the roles of prime ministers and presidents as we know it inside our current system. They will grow up and show us how to live in harmony on this planet, take full responsibility for our own actions and live as Divine Sovereign Beings on Planet Earth. They will birth the new era of longevity and vitality and squash war once and for all. They will set up off-planet business relationships and bring new technologies to Earth. Some are here already but once these souls hit their twenties and thirties, in their Earthly bodies, in the next ten

286

to fifteen years, you will see for yourself. Planet Earth will be a whole new world. They will assist in the reigniting of our Krystal Architecture and helping humanity raise consciousness, realign our geometry and move through Star Gates with ease, maybe with our bodies and if not our consciousness.

As parents it's mission critical for us to honour and support the divinity of these children, nurture, encourage and support their creativity and create a foundation for them to excel. These children don't need to go to school. They need to be running around in fields, playing in the woods and in touch with nature, given the opportunity to draw and paint and express themselves fully in their own unique way. It's tough to do as parent but the rewards are exponential once you let go and accept these unique Star Beings for who and what they are.

Our responsibility as parents is to give them their freedom. At the healing centres we are building, we have a huge emphasis on the space being a creative haven for the children. I see many Krystal Children, who have been in mainstream education and shown their unique abilities, getting taken into special facilities and mentally and emotionally destroyed, then sent back to their parents in a screwed-up state. The system doesn't like these unique souls because they will not conform and have a very different way of seeing the world. Teachers do not know how to be with these kids. They do not know how to talk to them, respond to them, teach them. It's tough for teachers who have been conditioned by a system to teach and control. The reason I pulled my children out from school and home-schooled them was because they would not do what the teacher wanted them to do and the only course of action the teachers could resort to was punishment and my children would say no to that too. The teachers were at a loss. It was not healthy for anyone to keep sending them to mainstream education.

I feel that in two generations' time, the new Star Children will be running a new type of school, possibly inspired by the way we will be running things at our Star Magic Healing Centres once they are open. They will be based on freedom, equality, wisdom and love. What I trust that you see and fully integrate into every fibre of your being is that these new children require a new set of parenting skills and they need a foundation to fully express and create from; and if we don't give them this foundation they will force us into providing it for them as parents. And, as any parent who has gone through this process of trying to understand a Krystal Child knows, it is extremely challenging to say the least, you must "innerstand".

But if we can readjust our mindset, reframe life and bin all of our beliefs about parenting, we stand a very good chance of being of service to this beautiful new frequency stream of children.

I mentioned that there are two streams of children. The ancient souls are the knowledge bringers and the teachers. The new souls are the space holders and the frequency amplifiers. The first will tell you straight the way things should be. They are fierce. The second will just be love, extremely gentle but will not conform within that gentleness, knowing that by just being kind and loving you will eventually see this is the way. The new souls will raise the bar on our current global frequency massively and hold space for the strong-willed, wise, ancient souls to create new structures and ways of life on Earth. The faster we embrace these Krystal Children, knowing they carry unprecedented waves of wisdom that we have not seen on Earth for a very long time, the easier it will be for everyone because these children will keep coming and coming and they will kick our arse in a positive way if we don't listen.

You, me, we, all of us are creating this positive foundation for these Krystal Children. It's our mission to present them with this foundation in the most loving and caring way possible. The more opportunity we give them to create and express, the faster we, as adults will remember our true nature, our Divine Cosmic Code and unleash our Super-Human Abilities.

Parenting Krystal Children

Oh boy . . . this is one heck of a topic of discussion. One that we could talk about for days and days; but from personal experience with my own children, I feel I have found the best way. Now, I know we are all unique beings, and our children are all unique in their own right, but – and it's a BIG BUT – I do feel there is a recipe that fits all of these incredible new children. Some people will certainly not agree with me, and it can be a very hard recipe to follow, especially when you are in the middle of the chaos, but once you emerge from the other side, you will see the method to the madness.

I will discuss my own personal journey with my children and hopefully shed some light on the situation, and, at the very least give you some options. My method is this. Let them do what they want and just watch. Yes, let me say that again . . .

LET THEM DO WHAT THEY WANT AND JUST WATCH!

Never tell them what to do but simply offer alternative suggestions and be an excellent role model for them to want to aspire to.

First of all, children should not be "raised". Cattle are raised and children are not like cattle. Although when two teenagers are kicking off and stuff is getting smashed up, observing it is like watching two little bulls going hammer and tong. I have tried intervening in these situations. I have tried getting mad. I've tried being soft. I have tried all the ways you can think of and the best thing to do is open your heart, observe, and let them do what is necessary. It always works out better in the end.

Humans are cultivated, nurtured, not raised. Give them the space to explore. A child should not be your legacy and you should not want them to be like you. You should show them good values, show them what healthy living and conscious living look like. Set them free to explore their own potential and on this exploratory road they will naturally take from you bits and pieces that will assist them in finding out who they truly are.

Getting mad only adds more fuel to the fire. Being soft often gets the reply, "But Dad, you tell people not to interfere and now you are interfering." It's true, kids are like sponges. They listen to everything and soak it, up. I tell everyone non-interference is the highest form of mastery and I truly feel that. I know when your kids are scrapping, it's hard to be a bystander, but interfering does not let them learn/remember. If you inspire by example and instil good values into your children, they will always hold those values deep in their heart and once the dust settles, they will hug each other, apologize and their bond will strengthen.

I was an angry dad wanting to instil discipline into my children at the very beginning. My daughter Aalayah was born one year before I started my spiritual journey of the heart, and I didn't fully "innerstand" the way of the force until six or seven years into my journey. I never once hit my children, but I did shout at times and get angry. When I was little, my mum used to hit me for things she considered naughty. I knew it was wrong and so would never go down that road myself. I always wanted to protect my children fiercely and would never want any physical harm to come to them.

My daughter was doing twenty sit-ups, twenty burpees, twenty squats and twenty push-ups every morning and night before bed while she was still in nappies. This is what I mean by inspiring your children. My ex-wife was very different to me. She's an awesome soul but I feel she would have led our children down a different path if I wasn't there. When we split up the children lived with me permanently and they truly excelled. My ex-wife had zero confidence, was scared of things and never followed through and with me being the total opposite, there was a push and pull of inspirational leadership going on. My ex-wife was very disciplined and seemed to get more disciplined as our relationship went on. I became more relaxed (our attitudes reversed) and I started to realize that children are like flowers: they need to be watered, fed and loved and then simply observed and all that is needed is for me to shine on them to help them grow.

The sun does not talk, it simply lights up the world and the flowers thrive. When you light up your children's world they will thrive. If you bring thunder and lightning and massive hailstones 24/7, they will wilt and die or get blown to pieces, just like a flower. You need a bit of both. The hail and wind and rain help the flowers root firmly into the ground. Weathering storms and basking in sunlight are both very important. Just know that they will find plenty of storms on their own and you must love them and allow them to experience those storms.

With my ex-wife being strict and me free, the children soon opted for the road of freedom, and once Laura left, they really were free. No school. Just plenty of travelling with me. Now, when you give your children this kind of freedom, you really do have to buckle up and watch them work it out for themselves and sometimes it's real tough, especially when you can see a hard lesson coming. This is where you being an inspiring role model comes into play. If you have always shown them a positive lifestyle, healthy habits, the right way to handle situations that unfold and following your own values then they will remember what you did, how your handled things, and even though they will try it their own way (often ending up in a little pain or upset) they will always realign or recalibrate and straighten things out afterwards.

My children used to travel with me regularly and when they hit twelve and fourteen, they were always glued to their phones on our Facilitator Trainings. Instead of engaging with the class they would be engrossed in YouTube or some game. This used to frustrate the heck out of me. But it's not up to me to tell them what to do. So, I said to them that I'm paying thousands of pounds to fly you everywhere and all you do is stare at your screen. So, I started travelling without them. I told them if all you are going to do is stare at the phones and disengage from all the magic, I may as well save myself the money. They were happy for a few trips and then they started to realize. I had to let them work it out for themselves. Now, they come and take part in the trainings and grow so much and it's a real joy to work and create with them. You have to, in whatever capacity it is, let them work it out on their own.

My children are extremely strong. They will not let anyone tell them what to do. They won't do something for anyone if it doesn't feel right. They do not bow down to authority. I love them for this because you cannot pull the wool over their eyes. If you show your kids the difference between right and wrong and follow certain principles and values, they will naturally pick up on them. But if you try and tell them what to do, they will not listen and will rebel.

I remember a few years back the police were giving me a hard time over something, outside of our house; for standing as a man and not bowing down to their BS statutes and corporate rules. I told my ex-wife and children to go inside but Aalayah stayed. She filmed the whole scenario. One of the officers pushed me and they both grabbed me from either side. I have real good balance and know how to move my body in subtle ways to shift the weight of people manhandling me, so I did and one of the officers hit the deck quite badly and smashed up his knees. They cuffed me and arrested me in the end and took me to the police station. When they put me in the back of the police van, they told Aalayah she had to give them the phone. They told her they were going to arrest her. She said, "No, I am not giving you the phone and no, you can't arrest me." She is strong. I phoned her from the cells several hours later and the first thing she said was, "Don't worry, Dad, I have the phone." She was only twelve at the time.

As a child I took every drug under the sun and drank like crazy. If my kids come to me and want to try alcohol or drugs, I say yes. I say, do it with me and let me be there to support and ensure you are safe. My kids have tried different substances for the experience and to squash their curiosity. If they don't do it with me, they are going to try it somewhere and who knows with who that will take place. Now they may have the occasional drink to celebrate a birthday but that's it. I will never encourage or discourage; they have free will. I will offer suggestions, which are like seeds that I plant in their head. They will remember them one day.

When my wife left and it was just Aalayah, Josh and me, we went on a real journey of self-discovery together. They didn't go to school and I suggested that they meditate, exercise, learn about healthy foods and research something they are interested in daily as a plan. This lasted a few days. I kept telling them they had to, then in the end I said it's up to you. I went through two years of pure hell. I created this pure hell in my own head though. I had a way I wanted them to be in this world based on my own model of reality. I had to surrender to the fact that I had chosen to let them be free to discover themselves. It really was tough at times, watching them eat unhealthy food, do no exercise, play on their phones and in my eyes waste their life away. Little did I realize that it was all perfect and valuable lessons were being remembered.

I just kept doing my thing, writing, creating, healing, training others to heal and building my business. Now my daughter is twenty and my son seventeen. Both of them eat well, cook for themselves, exercise, meditate and do breathwork daily. My son is focusing on boxing and my daughter loves horses and has published four books. It changed when I let go, opened my heart and loved them as they were and started giving up more time for them. I realized that I was so focused on what I was doing I didn't have enough time for them. When I watered the flowers more, loved the flowers more and poured more sunshine into their life, they naturally took to a way of life that they knew in their hearts was good for them, that they had seen me living daily but all the time had resisted.

Both of them are extremely intelligent, can converse with anyone, from a criminal to a lawyer. They hold their ground, speak their truth, are very honest and have so much love to give. They don't like authority (just like me) and are also very fierce if you try to mess with them. It's beautiful. They are balanced in their approach to life and give amazing advice to me and others. They are focused on what makes them happy and are so kind. I ask them for advice when I can't figure things out and they offer some of the best advice on the planet, especially when it comes to women.

A new breed of school will rise like a phoenix from the ashes. The Steiner Schools are a step in the right direction. Only a step though; many teachers there still don't know how to be with the children. Still too many rules. Rules do not work. Nature takes care of itself and there are no rules in nature. The trees, flowers, plants, bushes, insects and animals just seem to figure it all out and be in harmony. Maybe we can learn a thing or two from nature? Let your children play in the woods. Give them paints and colours and canvases. Let them climb trees and thrive.

We, as an aware Super-Human species, the children especially, know what is good for them and their sisters and brothers. If you let them create and express, they will flourish. A friend of mine called me one day. She said, "My son is in hospital. Will you do some healing?"

I had just arrived in the gym and was putting on my wraps and gloves to hit the bag. I put the phone down and as soon as I did her son came through the wall in the gym. I jumped. It was with such a force that you could feel him physically. He said, "No Jerry, my mum has got to learn her lessons." And then he went. I phoned her and told her, "This one's on you, sister."

You see, our children are here to grow and also help us grow and evolve. When we try to protect them too much and mollycoddle them and restrict them from freedom of experience and expression, it really comes back to bite us in the arse. This young chap wanted his mum to let him be and to stop worrying about him. Her worry had created a scenario where her son ended up in hospital so she could either worry some more, or surrender. We can't fix things for our children. They have to work it out on their own. They are not weak, stupid, incapable. They are divine instruments of truth and have an intelligence flowing through them that can assist them through any and every situation.

I mentioned the story about my son walking his dog at night-time and four twenty-ish-year-old lads accosting him in an alleyway. It is a tight alley and about two hundred metres long. They had knives. They punched him in the face and tried stabbing him and pulling the dog from his hands. He knew they were coming for him, so he took the dog chain off, smashed them over the face with it, kicked one, punched one and got him and the dog out of there. I went to the alley with him and he showed me what happened. It was a tough situation to get out of. When he got home his clothes were cut to shreds where they had tried to stab and cut him but luckily, he had several layers on. The blade had gone through his last hoody and must have been millimetres away from his skin.

A few weeks later I took him to a friend who regressed him into past life experiences. She had seen him as a high-ranking samurai warrior. Highly skilled. It made perfect sense to me. Getting out of a situation like that for Josh would have been easy. His DNA switched on and he knew what to do. I am sharing this because our children come onto this planet, and we worry so much but quite often we don't realize that they have a huge arsenal of abilities stored inside their DNA. If we kick back, guide and suggest, observe, water and love, and create a sacred, creative space for them, they will thrive and flourish beyond measure.

The foundation for our children to prosper must be built on love, freedom, wisdom, and creativity. There is no other way. To deny any of these four means we, as parents, as guardians of Earth are doing a massive disservice to the Krystal Children who are entrusting us to create this solid, but fluid and flexible free platform for them to express from. It really isn't easy being the parent of a child who knows so much, has such a big heart and a strong will, but letting go of how you think it should be and allowing them the freedom to make choices, and show you how they want to be, is of the utmost importance.

I also mentioned the children coming onto this planet that have never been here before. They are so pure. Both sets of children have huge hearts but there is a difference. Both carry immense power, but the first-timers are a lot calmer, gentler and more passive. They will just be, shine their lights, be in your space with a wide-open heart and feel love. Quite often these children are misunderstood. They don't often express themselves with words but simply vibration. To them, Earth really is archaic in terms of the way in which we utilize language to communicate. Words and sentences are so limited. When you express and communicate through feeling/vibration, the scope for expression is infinite.

Sometimes these first-timers are very introverted and they need space to create, be and express, in their own way. Trying to get these children to do more than they want to do or be is absurd. They need quiet, peace, harmony. Often, they will paint, read, draw, play in nature and be so content.

Others enter this planetary environment in bodies with Down's syndrome. This is the perfect home for these unique souls. They are like beacons; they vibrate, shining brightly. I have worked with many children with this so-called condition, and often it's the parents that want the healing for their child. They feel there is something wrong with their child because they are looking at them in terms of how other children are functioning. They view it from a 3D perspective. They lack the knowledge and wisdom to truly see the situation beyond the veil and tap into the truth, beauty and magic of what their child is bringing to this planet. These children simply require love, as we all require love. All we need to do as a species is love, with zero judgement or expectation. We must love because we *are* love and that is it. These Star Seeds are like pillars of light, beacons of grace and we must cherish and nurture them.

I encourage parents to have home births or water births. I cannot speak from experience on this matter; however, I have spoken with enough mums and dads to know how magical it is. If I had another child with someone then I would definitely want the child's mother to give birth outside of a hospital. There was a place in Hawaii where mothers could give birth with dolphins. It was closed by the government. The babies were being born with extremely high frequencies and with an intelligence far greater than children who had standard births. When a woman gives birth in water and dolphins are present, the dolphins swim in a circle and create a powerful vortex and connect with the womb and the baby with their sonar. They hold space and must download super-powerful codes into the babies. This is something that will resurface. Maybe in one of our Star Magic Healing Centres?

If you are a parent of one of these children just know that you have been gifted, or maybe you chose it, but the responsibility of caring and supporting these incredible souls is a real blessing. I know how blessed I am to be with two of these extraordinary children. The worst thing you can do is try to control them. Trust me, it's like tipping gasoline on a roaring fire. Be the cool water running through your Krystal Children's lives and flow gently but firmly. Water is both fluid and solid.

I remember when I was nineteen, I came off the back of a jet bike in Tenerife and hit the water fast. It was like hitting concrete. The hard water is the robust, strong, disciplined element of nature; it is gentle, fluid and soft, carrying us on a daily basis, but can turn in a heartbeat. Not being distracted, staying focused and being a positive role model for these young Star Seeds is important. The water will be soft or hard depending on your personal choice and course of action. The gentle part is you accepting them fully, knowing that your mission is to love them, water them and observe them and they will remember/grow/learn from you simply being you and showing them how to live a healthy, conscious life.

Step into your role fully, encourage always, hug tightly, never be the first to let go, love fiercely and ferociously and you will create the dream environment for your Krystal Children. And when the going gets tough, remember: you signed up for this.

I AM with YOU in SPIRIT!

Epilogue:
The Beginning

I have shared the tools, the strategies, the ways of shifting your frequency, unlocking your full Super-Human potential and being the Galactic Titan you came to Earth to be. All you must do is use them. It sounds simple, right? Yet in a world full of distractions, where the game is rigged in favour of you not achieving this, it can be difficult. In a society that thinks inside a tiny little space the size of a stock cube, it's thwart with challenges. From this moment forward it's down to you. This is where you seriously take a deep dive into the labyrinth of your heart, have a deep conversation with yourself and say "right you, listen up". You've been watching from the touchline for long enough. You've seen your sisters and brothers create magic and yet you've not taken action. You've shied away when the going got tough and felt sorry for yourself when life kicked the shit out of you, instead of saying thank you, knowing you were in training camp.

Since being a youngster you have wondered, contemplated, travelled your mind and the world searching for answers, but found none. You have listened to gurus, teachers who you thought could provide you with the answers to your infinite stream of questions, yet you have not reached anywhere near your full potential. You have trusted your parents, the government, large corporations, other authority figures, hoping they had your best interests at heart. You have wandered these lands breathing in chemtrails and nanotechnology, at times eating genetically modified foods that you trusted were real and would nourish you because of those glitzy ads on the TV and the colourful labels that told you they were good for you.

A lot of things in our culture are detrimental to the evolution of our species and deep down inside you know they are wrong and make life more difficult.

For generations we have all accepted things as they are instead of rallying the army of love, honour, strength, and unity.

But now is the time. Now, you know. Now you are aware. Now you are primed, ready and unquantifiable.

We Are Galactic Titans from the stars. We keep getting stronger. We keep evolving and expanding and every time anyone tries to strip us of our freedoms, we will rise and tear their heads off one by one – lovingly of course, with gratitude for their service to the contrast they provided us with and a belly full of cosmic energy!

Sometimes you've got to be ruthless. That doesn't mean you are dark or bad. It simply means you have acquiesced for far too long and you are about to show your teeth, your wings, your heart and rise into the portal of the sun and take control! You've been conditioned and led to believe that being quiet and not making noise is the right thing to do. To be subservient, to let it go, because you don't want to make a fuss.

There is a New Beginning! A New Dawn! A sovereign world awaits us. It's time for each and every one of us to be the change we want to experience and shift our frequency into the next octave of light.

Now is the only moment you ever have and tomorrow has been an excuse for far too long. Will you seize this moment and do the work necessary to create Heaven on Earth inside of your heart? Only by doing this can you bring it into being in your external reality. I can be living in the same street as you, in the same neighbourhood, with the same job and while I live in heaven, you can be living in hell. Always remember this. Your perception is everything. Choose how you frame your reality. Once you frame it correctly, you will feel heaven all around you and now you can start the process, the journey, the climb, the adventure.

I've always lived my life on the edge. I go for everything and whatever the consequences, I flow with them and grow. Sometimes they work in my favour and sometimes they work in my favour. You see, when you know that the universe has your back, you "innerstand" that all events are growth opportunities, and you are getting stronger. It's time for each one of us on this planet to adopt that attitude and throw caution to the wind. It's time right now for you and all of your sisters and brothers to become Super-Human. 26 July 2020 was the start of the new lunar year in the Mayan calendar. It's a thirteen-year cycle that will end with the magnetic blue storm in the year 2032/3 and during this cycle more Star Knowledge will be embedded within our human experience. These next thirteen years are about bringing Star Knowledge to Planet Earth. It's the moon phase where we stabilize and unify the planetary telepathic network. It's the cycle of time that brings forth transformation and alchemy of the highest order, and we are going

to see the abilities open up in humanity as our DNA is activated and our true geometrical code switches on. There is no better time to realize you are Super-Human.

Now is the time to be you. Now is the time to be whole. Now is the time to share these Earthly planes with each other, with zero competition. We can increase the frequency of guiding coincidences/synchronicities, by uplifting the vibration of everyone who comes into our lives. And we do that by not doing anything apart from being our beautiful lights. Ensure your cup is full and overflowing, not half full.

Are you still enough to experience the truth? Are you silent enough to connect with the source of all creation? There is magic streaming through you right now. Be still, experience it and become it. In the stillness of the ocean of your consciousness, you will be offered the opportunity to embrace all things. You will be gifted the knowledge of those with a pure heart.

Now you have real-eyesed the truth, there is no turning back. Get stuck in, right now, commit to you, for eternity, because life doesn't end in this physical form. You have a long, never-ending road ahead and what you remember in this life will see you well in the next incarnation (or destination in this body), wherever that may be in the universe. So, decide right now that this is it. This is your opportunity. Your big moment to make a colossal difference to your life, to the frequency on this planet and the future of the human race, and go for it. Go hard or go home. Choose love not fear and embrace the magic in your soul.

It's time to Be Super-Human!

Jerry's Super-Human Schedule

Here's what I suggest to maximize the effects of the Star Magic Healing System:

1. Every day practice kindness and gratitude. Maintain self-control, right thought, calmness, action, discipline and love. And turn off your Wi-Fi at night.

2. For a **period of 49 days** focus on preparing and activating your mind and body as follows:

Day	Activity (morning)	Activity (anytime during the day)
1–9	5 am Power House 6 6 am Body Love 7 am Activate the 13 Transmission Centres	Lyran Light Code Activation Activate Your Master Alchemists Krystal Spiral Transformation Code Clear Present Reality Trauma Kindness Code Clearing the Heart and Lower Energy Centres Nervous System Upgrade
10–13	5 am Power House 6 6 am Body Love 7 am Activate the 13 Transmission Centres	Activate Your Master Alchemists Krystal Spiral Transformation Code Clear Present Reality Trauma Kindness Code Clearing the Heart and Lower Energy Centres Nervous System Upgrade
14–21	5 am Power House 6 6 am Body Love 7 am Activate the 13 Transmission Centres	Divine Feminine and Masculine Light Code Activation Krystal Spiral Transformation Code Clear Present Reality Trauma Kindness Code Clearing the Heart and Lower Energy Centres Nervous System Upgrade
22–27	5 am Power House 6 6 am Qigong 7 am Activate the 13 Transmission Centres	Divine Feminine and Masculine Light Code Activation (until Day 26) Clear Present Reality Trauma Kindness Code Clearing the Heart and Lower Energy Centres Nervous System Upgrade (until Day 23, then once a week)
28–30	5 am Power House 6 6 am Qigong 7 am Activate the 13 Transmission Centres	Kindness Code Clearing the Heart and Lower Energy Centres
31–36	5 am Power House 6 6 am Qigong	Kindness Code Clearing the Heart and Lower Energy Centres
37–49	5 am Power House 6 6 am Qigong	Clearing the Heart and Lower Energy Centres

3. This is the weekly schedule that I follow. I adapt it when I am running online and in-house trainings but the fundamentals stay the same.

When you have completed all tasks of the 49-day-schedule from the previous page, start working with this weekly plan. If time allows and you want to, you can repeat tasks of the 49 days and combine them with this weekly schedule, running both at the same time.

Time	Monday	Tuesday	Wednesday
5am	Collect Urine, Creative Time	Collect Urine, Creative Time	Collect Urine, Creative Time
6am	Qigong, Headstand, Cold Shower	Meditation, Cold Shower	Qigong, Headstand, Cold Shower
7am	Creative Time	Creative Time	Creative Time
8am	Creative Time	Creative Time	Creative Time
9am	Run	Creative Time	Creative Time
10am	Cold Shower	Cold Shower	Cold Shower
11am	Exercise	Exercise	Exercise
12pm	Drink Urine, First Food – Shake	Drink Urine, First Food – Shake	Drink Urine, First Food – Shake
1pm	Third-Eye Merkaba Matrix	Activation of Choice	Activation of Choice
2pm	Meditation or Light Language Star Magic Library	Creative Time	Meditation or Light Language Star Magic Library
3pm	Creative Time	Creative Time	Creative Time
4pm	Creative Time	Creative Time	Creative Time
5pm	Breathing Espresso or Nature Time	Breathing Espresso or Nature Time	Breathing Espresso or Nature Time
6pm	Last Food – Meal	Last Food – Meal	Last Food – Meal
7pm	Creative Time or Family Time	Creative Time or Family Time	Creative Time or Family Time
8pm	Creative Time or Sexual Energy	Meditation or Light Language Star Magic Library	Creative Time or Sexual Energy
9pm	Cold Shower/ Headstand/Reflexology	Cold Shower/ Headstand/Reflexology	Cold Shower/ Headstand/Reflexology
10pm	Krystal Spiral Code / Meditation/Sleep	Advanced Merkaba Activation/Sleep	Self-Healing/Sleep

Any of the following can be your activation of choice:

- Power House 6
- 13 Transmission Centres
- Nervous System Upgrade
- Guided Meditation – Star Magic Library
- Light Language Transmission – Star Magic Library
- Lyran Light Code Activation
- Kaleidoscopic Chromium Activation

Thursday	Friday	Saturday	Sunday	Time
Collect Urine, Creative Time	Fast Day (no Urine Collection), Creative Time	Collect Urine, Creative Time	Collect Urine, Creative Time	5am
Meditation, Cold Shower	Qigong, Headstand, Cold Shower	Meditation, Cold Shower	Qigong, Headstand, Cold Shower	6am
Creative Time	Creative Time	Creative Time	Exercise, Cold Shower	7am
Creative Time	Creative Time	Creative Time	Exercise, Cold Shower	8am
Creative Time	Run	Nervous System Upgrade	Holotropic Breathing (1 hour)	9am
Cold Shower	Cold Shower	Cold Shower	Cold Shower	10am
Exercise	Exercise	Exercise	Exercise	11am
Drink Urine, First Food – Shake	Drink Urine, First Food – Shake	Drink Urine, First Food – Shake	Drink Urine, First Food – Shake	12pm
Third-Eye Merkaba Matrix	Third-Eye Merkaba Matrix	Third-Eye Merkaba Matrix	Third-Eye Merkaba Matrix	1pm
Creative Time	Creative Time	Creative Time	Free Time	2pm
Creative Time	Creative Time	Creative Time	Free Time	3pm
Creative Time	Creative Time	Creative Time	Free Time	4pm
Breathing Espresso or Nature Time	Breathing Espresso or Nature Time	Breathing Espresso or Nature Time	Breathing Espresso or Nature Time	5pm
Last Food – Meal	Last Food – Meal	Last Food – Meal	Last Food – Meal	6pm
Creative Time or Family Time	Creative Time or Family Time	Creative Time or Family Time	Creative Time or Family Time	7pm
Meditation or Light Language Star Magic Library	Creative Time or Sexual Energy	Meditation or Light Language Star Magic Library	Meditation or Light Language Star Magic Library	8pm
Cold Shower/ Headstand/Reflexology	Cold Shower/ Headstand/Reflexology	Cold Shower/ Headstand/Reflexology	Cold Shower/ Headstand/Reflexology	9pm
Advanced Merkaba Activation/Sleep	Krystal Spiral Code/ Meditation /Sleep	Krystal Spiral Code/ Meditation /Sleep	Krystal Spiral Code/ Meditation /Sleep	10pm

Exercise, Protocol, and Activation Index

The exercises, protocols, and activations are listed in chronological order as they appear in the book.

You also find guided meditations and Light Magic Transmissions and
Light Codes in the Star Magic Library at
https://www.starmagichealing.com/meditations-library and
https://www.starmagichealing.com/light-language

To join the *Be Super-Human* Community, stay in touch with the author
and receive access to online meditations, activations,
and Q & A's on the *Be Super-Human* Protocols, please visit
http://starmagichealing.com/besuperhuman
and register for free.

Illustration Index

About the Author

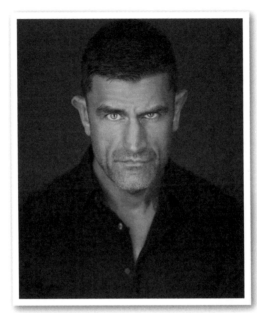

Photo by Benjamin Gardies

JERRY SARGEANT, known as "The Facilitator", is the founder of Star Magic Healing. He is world renowned for healing people and creating rapid shifts within them on the mental, physical, emotional, and spiritual plane. Jerry's mission is to set the human race free by expanding consciousness on Planet Earth through the Star Magic Matrix, a powerful energetic grid of light that is being constructed around our planet.

Jerry knows about setting one's self free. Being a drug addict from a young age and walking a different path, which led to mixing with some of the world's most dangerous criminals, Jerry broke free from this life after a number of life-altering events. A near-fatal car crash, a trip to Alpha Centauri in a spacecraft, an encounter with an angel, and time spent in Egyptian Mystery Schools underneath the Great Pyramids led him to insights and precious information enabling him to access and harness super-transformative healing energy.

Jerry's ability to heal has been likened to some of the most powerful healers in history, having healed broken bones, removed tumours, cysts, dissolved fibromyalgia, healed hearts as well as healing broken relationships and super-charging businesses to achieve massive success.

Star Magic, as well as being the most powerful healing modality on the planet, is a lifestyle. It's an opportunity to be free, mentally, physically, emotionally, and spiritually. It's a way of being free to do what you want, when you want, with whomever you want, for as long as you want. Star Magic is a way of life, a lifestyle that you will live with passion, once you know and utilize the power that lies within your own genetic make-up. Star Magic is the key to unlock the door to a free, loving, and compassionate world. A space nurtured and cradled in love.

Jerry's vision is to harness extra-terrestrial light frequencies and bring them safely and effectively to Planet Earth, through a number of Star Magic Healing facilities, strategically placed around the Kryst Consciousness Grid of our planet. The codes contained within the light will elevate consciousness in a phenomenal way and create freedom for humankind, by connecting every

man, woman, and child through their heart to unconditional love.

Jerry runs a number of Star Magic healing and meditation workshops, a Global Meditation Group and trains people to create with Star Magic and work with the light and sound codes, constantly travelling through the ether. You can find out more about Jerry and his work with Star Magic here: **www.starmagichealing.com.**

Jerry is available for speaking engagements worldwide. If you would like him to speak at your event, please contact **info@starmagichealing.com.**

Also by Jerry Sargeant

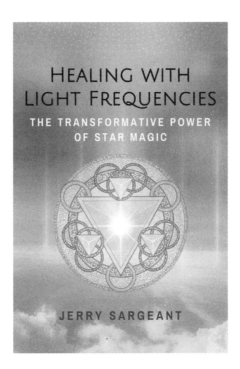

Connect with and harness extra-terrestrial light frequencies to energize, uplift, and consciously empower your mind and body. An introduction to Star Magic Healing, *Healing with Light Frequencies* offers basic, intermediate, and advanced Star Magic tools and exercises to shift your vibration and bring about rapid healing that lasts.

978-1-64411-109-3